Diagnostic Imaging: Chest, Breast, Heart and Vessels

Diagnostic Imaging: Chest, Breast, Heart and Vessels

Editor: Olivia Hunt

MURPHY & MOORE
www.murphy-moorepublishing.com

www.murphy-moorepublishing.com

MURPHY & MOORE

Cataloging-in-Publication Data

Diagnostic imaging : chest, breast, heart and vessels / edited by Olivia Hunt.
p. cm.
Includes bibliographical references and index.
ISBN 978-1-63987-159-9
1. Diagnostic imaging. 2. Chest--Imaging. 3. Breast--Imaging. 4. Heart--Imaging.
5. Blood-vessels--Imaging. I. Hunt, Olivia.
RC78.7.D53 D53 2022
616.075 4--dc23

Murphy & Moore Publishing,
1 Rockefeller Plaza,
New York City, NY 10020, USA

ISBN 978-1-63987-159-9 (Hardback)

Diagnostic Imaging: Chest, Breast, Heart and Vessels

Editor: Olivia Hunt

MURPHY & MOORE
www.murphy-moorepublishing.com

www.murphy-moorepublishing.com

MURPHY & MOORE

Cataloging-in-Publication Data

Diagnostic imaging : chest, breast, heart and vessels / edited by Olivia Hunt.
p. cm.
Includes bibliographical references and index.
ISBN 978-1-63987-159-9
1. Diagnostic imaging. 2. Chest--Imaging. 3. Breast--Imaging. 4. Heart--Imaging.
5. Blood-vessels--Imaging. I. Hunt, Olivia.
RC78.7.D53 D53 2022
616.075 4--dc23

Murphy & Moore Publishing,
1 Rockefeller Plaza,
New York City, NY 10020, USA

ISBN 978-1-63987-159-9 (Hardback)

Contents

Preface

I am honored to present to you this unique book which encompasses the most up-to-date data in the field. I was extremely pleased to get this opportunity of editing the work of experts from across the globe. I have also written papers in this field and researched the various aspects revolving around the progress of the discipline. I have tried to unify my knowledge along with that of stalwarts from every corner of the world, to produce a text which not only benefits the readers but also facilitates the growth of the field.

Diagnostic imaging is a process used to view the interior parts of the body for clinical analysis. It is also used to get a visual representation of the function of some tissues and organs. Diagnostic imaging reveals the internal structures of the body which are hidden by the skin and bones so that the diseases can be diagnosed and treated. Diagnostic imaging of the chest involves the usage of plain X-rays, magnetic resonance imaging, computed tomography, nuclear scanning and ultrasonography. The non-invasive imaging of the heart by using ultrasound, computed tomography and magnetic resonance imaging is known as cardiac imaging. This book is a compilation of chapters that discuss the most vital concepts and emerging trends in the field of diagnostic imaging. Most of the topics introduced herein cover new techniques and the applications of diagnostic imaging of chest, breast, heart and vessels. Researchers and students in this field will be assisted by this book.

Finally, I would like to thank all the contributing authors for their valuable time and contributions. This book would not have been possible without their efforts. I would also like to thank my friends and family for their constant support.

Editor

1

A Systematic Approach to Chest Radiographic Analysis

Jeffrey S. Klein and Melissa L. Rosado-de-Christenson

Learning Objectives

- List the nine components of a chest radiographic examination to be systematically analyzed.
- Identify key technical quality aspects to be assessed prior to interpretation of a chest radiograph.
- Identify the normal anatomic structures and interfaces routinely displayed on chest radiographic examinations.
- Detail the different patterns of lung disease seen radiographically.
- Describe the different appearances of pleural disease seen on chest radiography.

1.1 Introduction

The chest radiograph remains one of the most commonly performed examinations in radiology. It is typically the first radiologic examination obtained in patients presenting with chest pain, shortness of breath, or cough. In the hospital setting, chest radiographs are performed in the emergency room, critical care unit, and following the placement of monitoring and support devices. Chest radiographs are routinely obtained prior to major surgical procedures, as part of annual physical examinations, and to screen for metastatic disease in patients with malignancy or paraneoplastic syndromes.

The accurate interpretation of chest radiographs requires an understanding of the normal frontal and lateral chest radiographic appearances, as obscuration of normally visualized structures may be the only clue to the presence of an abnormality.

Radiography allows visualization and assessment of the chest wall, mediastinum, and hila including the heart and great vessels, central airways, the lungs including the pulmonary vasculature, the pleural surfaces including the fissures and the diaphragm.

The superimposition of complex structures of various radiographic density (gas, water, calcium, metal, and fat) makes radiographic interpretation challenging. An understanding of normal interfaces allows for detection of conditions that manifest with chest symptoms or as asymptomatic abnormalities.

1.2 A Systematic Assessment

We present a systematic approach to the analysis of chest radiographs (Table 1.1). This should begin with an assessment of technical aspects of the radiographic study including patient positioning, mediastinal penetration, sharpness of structures (to detect motion), lung volumes, and presence of artifacts [1] to allow for accurate detection of abnormalities. The orderly assessment of each anatomic region and structure will yield a comprehensive imaging evaluation, will allow identification of subtle abnormalities, and will minimize interpretive errors. The following must be evaluated in each chest radiograph: support and monitoring devices (if present), chest wall, heart and mediastinum, hila, lungs, airways, pleura, and diaphragm.

J. S. Klein (✉)
Department of Radiology, University of Vermont College of Medicine, Burlington, VT, USA
e-mail: jsklein@uvm.edu

M. L. Rosado-de-Christenson
Department of Radiology, Saint Luke's Hospital of Kansas City, Kansas City, MO, USA

Department of Radiology, University of Missouri-Kansas City, Kansas City, MO, USA
e-mail: mrosado@saint-lukes.org

Table 1.1 Systematic analysis of chest radiographs

Component evaluated	Assessment
Technical quality	Positioning, penetration, motion, lung volumes, artifacts
Support/ monitoring devices	ET/NG tube, vascular catheters, pacemaker
Chest wall	Absence of normal contour, swelling, mass, calcification, air, osseous abnormality
Mediastinum	Cardiomegaly, mass, widening, position, calcification, air
Hila	Height (right vs left), size, density, contour
Lungs	Atelectasis Air space opacities Interstitial lung disease Focal opacities (solitary pulmonary nodules/ masses Abnormal lucency-localized/unilateral/diffuse
Airways	Tracheal diameter, course, nodule/mass Bronchiectasis
Pleura/diaphragm	Costal/diaphragmatic/fissural pleural surfaces Diaphragmatic contour/position

1.3 Technical Quality (Table 1.2)

The initial evaluation of any chest radiograph should include a determination of the technical adequacy of the examination to confirm that it is of adequate quality for interpretation. This step is often overlooked, which can lead to both overdiagnosis (as low lung volume may simulate lung disease) and underdiagnosis (motion or rotation may limit proper evaluation of the lungs, mediastinum, and hila). There are five main factors to be assessed.

On a properly positioned frontal chest radiograph, the spinous processes should align with an imaginary vertical line drawn midway between the clavicular heads. The dorsal wrists should be placed on the waist with elbows oriented anteriorly to rotate the scapulae laterally so that they are not superimposed on the upper lungs. Radiographic penetration should allow faint visualization of the vertebral bodies and disc spaces through the mediastinum, with the lungs gray in density and the pulmonary vessels easily seen. Motion is detected by noting the sharpness of the superior cortices of the ribs, vessel margins, and diaphragmatic contours. Proper inspiration is assessed by noting the position of the top of the right hemidiaphragm with respect to the ribs; this point should correspond to the sixth anterior rib or tenth posterior rib at the mid-clavicular line. Artifacts including faulty detectors or visible grid lines can be seen in the digital radiography systems used for obtaining virtually all conventional chest radiographs in a modern radiology department [1].

Key Point

- Evaluation of proper chest radiographic technique involves analysis of patient positioning, proper mediastinal penetration, absence of motion, adequate lung volumes, and the detection of artifacts.

Table 1.2 Evaluating the technical adequacy of chest radiographs

Technical parameter	Assessment
Positioning	Rotation, kyphosis/lordosis
Penetration	Visualization of vertebral interspaces
Motion	Sharpness of hemidiaphragms, ribs, vessels
Lung volumes	Position of diaphragm relative to ribs
Artifacts	Detector drops, grid lines

1.4 Support/Monitoring Devices (Tubes/Lines/Catheters/Pacemakers) (Table 1.3) [2]

Chest radiographs, particularly those obtained in a critical care setting, can demonstrate a broad array of different tubes, vascular catheters, cardiac pacemakers/defibrillators, and other monitoring or therapeutic devices. While in the hospital setting, chest radiographs are typically obtained to confirm proper positioning and to exclude complications following placement of a tube or line; the recognition of one or more of these devices can provide important clues to underlying disease entities.

1.5 Chest Wall

The symmetry of normal chest wall structures such as the breast shadows in females and the spine, ribs, and shoulders should be analyzed to detect chest wall abnormalities. Poland syndrome is a congenital anomaly in which there is unilateral underdevelopment of the musculature of the chest wall. Nonsurgical absence of a portion of a rib or vertebral body may be instrumental in making the diagnosis of malignancy. Congenital deformities such as pectus excavatum can mimic middle lobe disease, as this chest wall deformity creates a vague opacity overlying the region of the middle lobe on frontal radiography (Fig. 1.1). Rib destruction adjacent to a peripheral lung mass is virtually diagnostic of chest wall involvement by lung cancer. Benign pressure erosion of a rib is characteristic of neurogenic neoplasms or chest wall vascular abnormalities such as dilated intercostal arteries in a patient with coarctation of the aorta. In patients with anasarca

Table 1.3 Common support/monitoring devices on chest radiography

Device	Normal appearance
Endotracheal tube	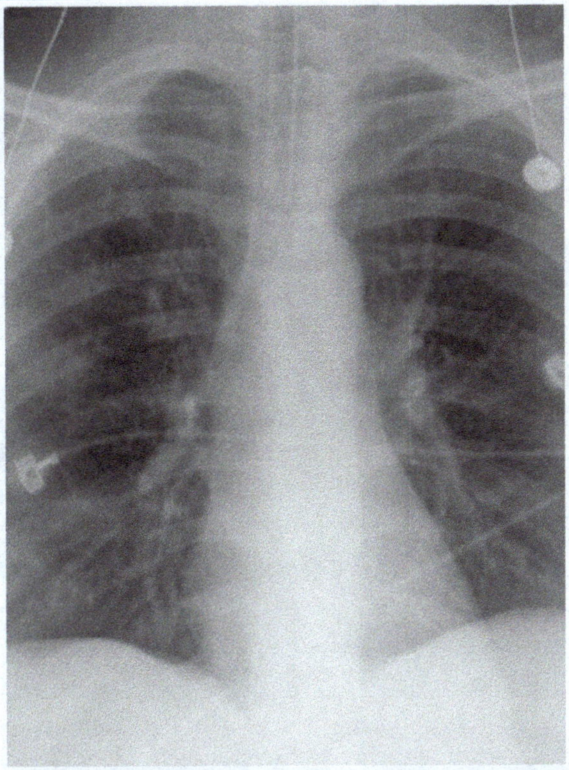
Nasogastric feeding tube	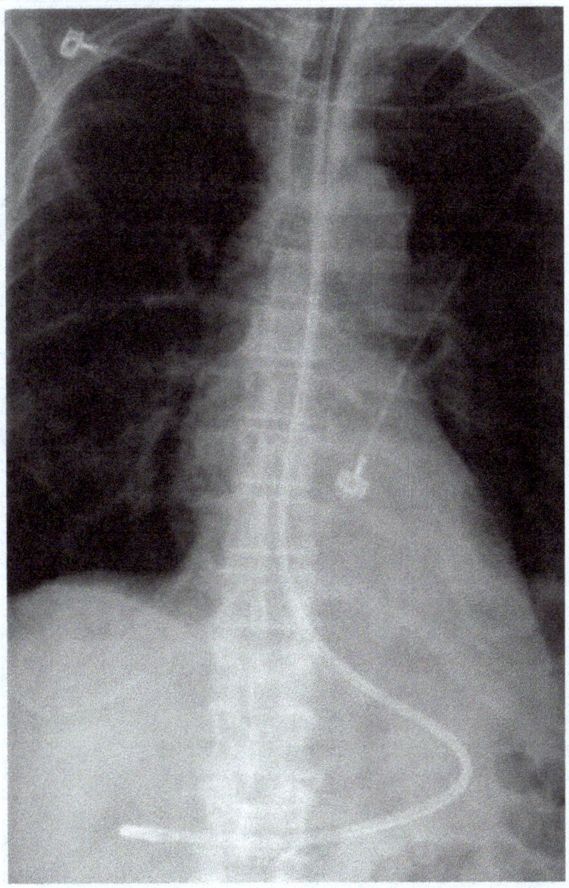

Table 1.3 (continued)

Device	Normal appearance
Central venous catheters	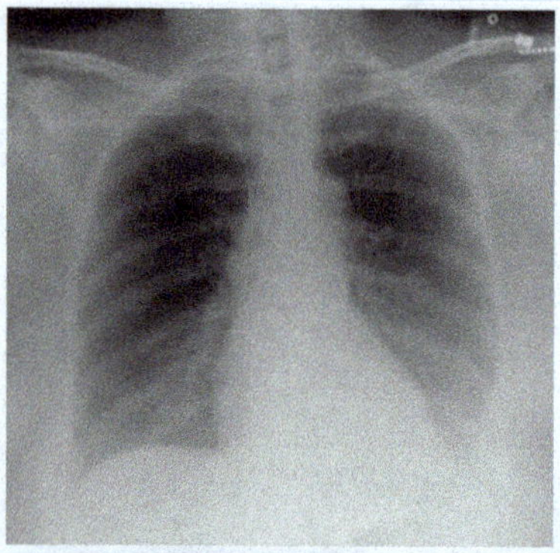
Pacemaker/defibrillator	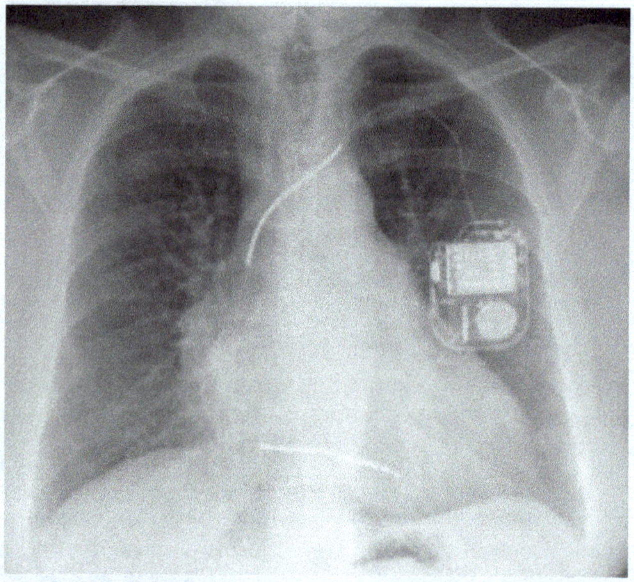
Chest tube	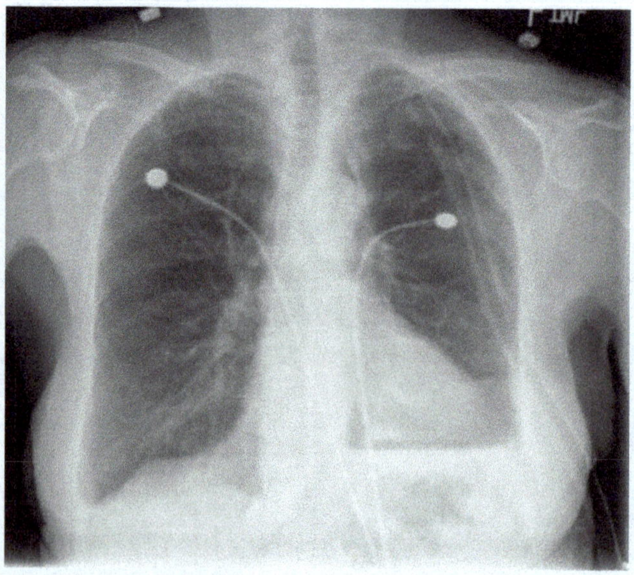

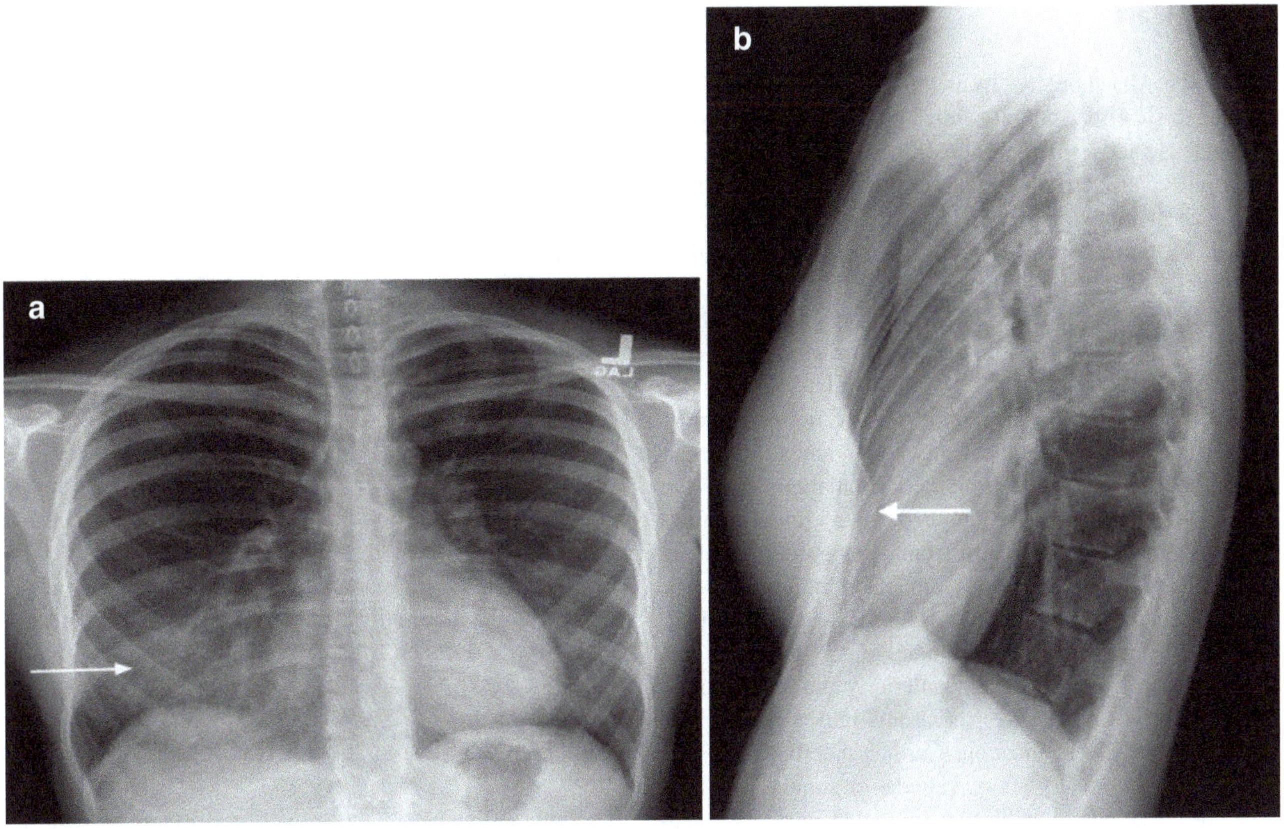

Fig. 1.1 (**a**, **b**) Pectus excavatum chest wall deformity mimicking middle lobe disease. (**a**) Frontal chest radiograph of a 25-year-old female demonstrates a vague opacity overlying the medial right lower lung (arrow). (**b**) Lateral radiography shows the characteristic posterior deformity of the lower sternum (arrow) representing pectus excavatum

Table 1.4 Chest wall abnormalities

Finding	Condition
Absence	S/P mastectomy, Poland syndrome
Shape	Pectus excavatum, carinatum
Bone destruction	Peripheral lung cancer, metastasis, infection
Swelling	Anasarca, localized edema
Mass	Breast cancer
Calcification	Dermatomyositis, sarcoma, tumoral calcinosis
Gas	Air leak from chest, S/P laparoscopy, S/P drainage of pneumothorax

due to fluid administration, there may be marked swelling of the soft tissues lateral to the ribs. Larger chest wall masses may produce an "incomplete border sign" radiographically, as the mass creates a visible interface with atmospheric air (or if intrathoracic with the adjacent lung). Soft tissue calcification may indicate prior trauma (myositis ossificans), collagen vascular disease (dermatomyositis), or the presence of a vascular lesion (hemangioma) or a bone-forming malignancy (osteosarcoma or chondrosarcoma) [3]. Gas within the chest wall could indicate an air leak in the setting of trauma, pneumomediastinum, or pneumothorax (Table 1.4).

Key Point

- Chest wall masses typically demonstrate an incomplete border sign as only a portion of the circumference of the mass is typically outlined by atmospheric air or intrapulmonary gas.

1.6 Mediastinum

The mediastinum is the space between the mediastinal pleural reflections bound anteriorly by the sternum and posteriorly by the thoracic vertebrae. It courses from the thoracic inlet superiorly to the diaphragm inferiorly. It contains the heart, pericardium, central great vessels, esophagus, trachea, carina and proximal main stem bronchi, the thoracic duct, lymph nodes, and mediastinal fat. The radiologist must be familiar with the normal mediastinal structures, their contours, and the normal mediastinal lines, stripes, and interfaces to detect mediastinal abnormalities radiographically [4].

1.6.1 Heart

The right cardiac border is formed by the right atrium. From inferior to superior, the left cardiac border is formed by the left ventricle and a small portion of the left atrial appendage. The right ventricle projects anteriorly and inferiorly on the lateral chest radiograph, with the posterior cardiac border formed by the left ventricle inferiorly and the left atrium superiorly.

The heart must be assessed for its shape, size, and location. Abnormal cardiac shift may reflect ipsilateral loss of volume (e.g., lobar atelectasis) or contralateral increased volume (e.g., a large pneumothorax). The normal pericardium is not visible radiographically. Enlargement of the cardiac silhouette may result from cardiac enlargement and/or pericardial effusion. When large, the latter may manifest with a "water bottle heart" on frontal chest radiographs or with the "epicardial fat pad sign" on lateral radiography. The "epicardial fat pad sign" results from visualization of pericardial effusion as a curvilinear band of soft tissue >2 mm thick outlined by mediastinal fat anteriorly and subepicardial fat posteriorly. Constrictive pericarditis may manifest with linear pericardial calcification. Cardiac calcifications may correspond to coronary artery, valvular or annular calcifications, or curvilinear calcification in a left ventricular aneurysm from prior myocardial infarction.

1.6.2 Systemic Arteries

The normal aortic arch is readily visible on radiography and characteristically produces an indentation on the left tracheal wall. With increasing aortic atherosclerosis and tortuosity, a larger portion of the aorta is visible and may exhibit intimal atherosclerotic calcification. The left para-aortic interface projects through the left heart and courses vertically toward the abdomen. The left subclavian artery is seen as a concave left supra-aortic mediastinal interface on frontal chest radiography. A right aortic arch is usually associated with a right descending thoracic aorta. In the absence of associated congenital heart disease, right aortic arch is usually associated with non-mirror image branching characterized by an aberrant left subclavian artery which may be seen as an indentation on the posterior trachea on lateral chest radiography.

1.6.3 Systemic Veins

The azygos arch is visible at the right tracheobronchial angle and normally measures <1 cm in the upright position. The azygos arch may be contained within an accessory azygos fissure, an anatomic variant. Enlargement of the azygos arch may occur in azygos continuation of the inferior vena cava, in which the vertical portion of the azygos vein manifests as a right-sided vertical mediastinal interface.

The right lateral margin of the superior vena cava is normally visible as it interfaces with the medial right upper lobe. The inferior vena cava may be visible as it creates a concave interface with the right lower lobe in the right cardiophrenic angle prior to its entry into the right atrium. The posterior margin of the inferior vena cava is most evident on lateral radiography as its posterior concave margin is outlined by lung.

1.6.4 Pulmonary Arteries

Enlargement of the central pulmonary arteries may represent pulmonary hypertension and is typically associated with enlargement of the pulmonary trunk. The pulmonary trunk is visible as a left mediastinal interface located above the heart and below the aorta on frontal chest radiography.

1.6.5 Lines, Stripes, and Interfaces [5]

The anterior and posterior junction lines represent the interface between the right and left upper lobes anterior to the great vessels (anterior junction line) (Fig. 1.2) and posterior to the esophagus, superior to the aortic arch, and anterior to the upper thoracic spine (posterior junction line). These lines may be thickened by fat, lymphadenopathy, or mediastinal masses. The paravertebral stripes may be thickened by lymphadenopathy fat or may be displaced laterally by a paravertebral hematoma or infection. An abnormal convex contour of the upper azygoesophageal recess may result from subcarinal lymphadenopathy or a bronchogenic cyst, while a hiatus hernia often produces convexity of the lower 1/3rd of the azygoesophageal recess. Convexity of the aortopulmonary reflection normally a flat or concave interface below the aortic arch and above the main pulmonary artery may be caused by lymphadenopathy in the aortopulmonary window, mediastinal mass, or anomalous vasculature.

1.6.6 Mediastinal Masses (Table 1.5) [6]

Mediastinal masses include primary and secondary neoplasms, mediastinal cysts, vascular lesions, glandular enlargement (thyroid and thymus), and hernias (hiatus and Morgagni). As 10% of mediastinal masses are vascular in etiology, a vascular lesion should always be considered in a patient with a mediastinal contour abnormality.

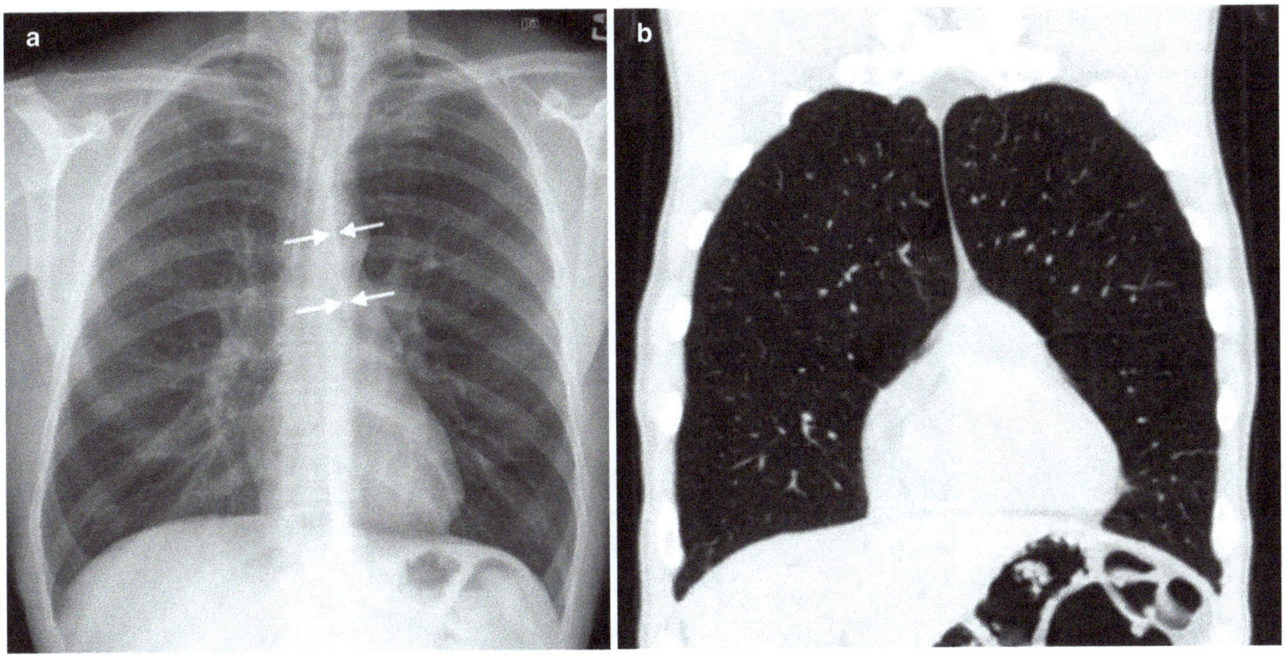

Fig. 1.2 Anterior junction line on frontal chest radiograph with CT correlation (**a**,**b**). (**a**) Frontal chest radiograph shows an obliquely oriented linear opacity (arrows) overlying the upper mediastinum. (**b**) Coronal multi-detector CT scan at lung windows through the anterior chest shows that the anterior junction line represents the right and left upper lobes (and corresponding pleural layers) that contact one another anterior to the mediastinum

Table 1.5 Differential diagnosis of mediastinal masses

Anterior	Middle	Posterior
Lymphoma	Lung cancer	Schwannoma/ neurofibroma
Thymic neoplasm	Lymph node enlargement/mass	Ganglion cell tumor
Germ cell neoplasm	Foregut/pericardial cyst	Descending aortic aneurysm
Thyroid goiter	Hiatus hernia	Paravertebral hematoma/abscess

The first step in the assessment of a mediastinal mass is determining that there is indeed a mediastinal abnormality. Focal unilateral mediastinal masses are typically primary neoplasms, enlarged lymph nodes, cysts, and vascular aneurysms or anomalous vessels. While diffuse symmetric mediastinal widening without mass effect can be seen in mediastinal lipomatosis, when lobulated or asymmetric, it should suggest lymphadenopathy in advanced lung cancer, metastatic disease, or lymphoma (Fig. 1.3) or in patients with chest trauma mediastinal hematoma associated with vascular injury. Mediastinal masses should then be localized within a mediastinal compartment based on the lateral chest radiograph. For the purposes of localizing masses and providing a concise differential diagnosis, the mediastinum is divided radiographically into the anterior, middle, and posterior compartments [6]. The middle mediastinum encompasses the heart, pericardium, aorta and great vessels, systemic and pulmonary veins, trachea, carina, and esophagus. Ancillary findings should be noted such as benign pressure erosion in patients with paravertebral masses (typical of neurogenic tumors). The cervicothoracic sign or obscuration of an abnormal mediastinal contour as it extends above the clavicle into the neck allows lesion localization in both the thorax and the neck, for which the most frequent etiology is intrathoracic goiter. Clinical factors such as age, gender, and presence or absence of symptoms allow the radiologist to provide a focused differential diagnosis prior to proceeding to cross-sectional imaging. Mediastinal widening in the setting of trauma may represent hemorrhage from traumatic vascular injury.

Key Point
- The most common anterior mediastinal masses in adults are lymphoma and thymic neoplasms.

1.6.7 Mediastinal Calcification

The most common cause of mediastinal/hilar calcifications is calcified lymph nodes from prior granulomatous disease such as tuberculosis, histoplasmosis, and sarcoidosis. Patients with treated mediastinal lymphoma may

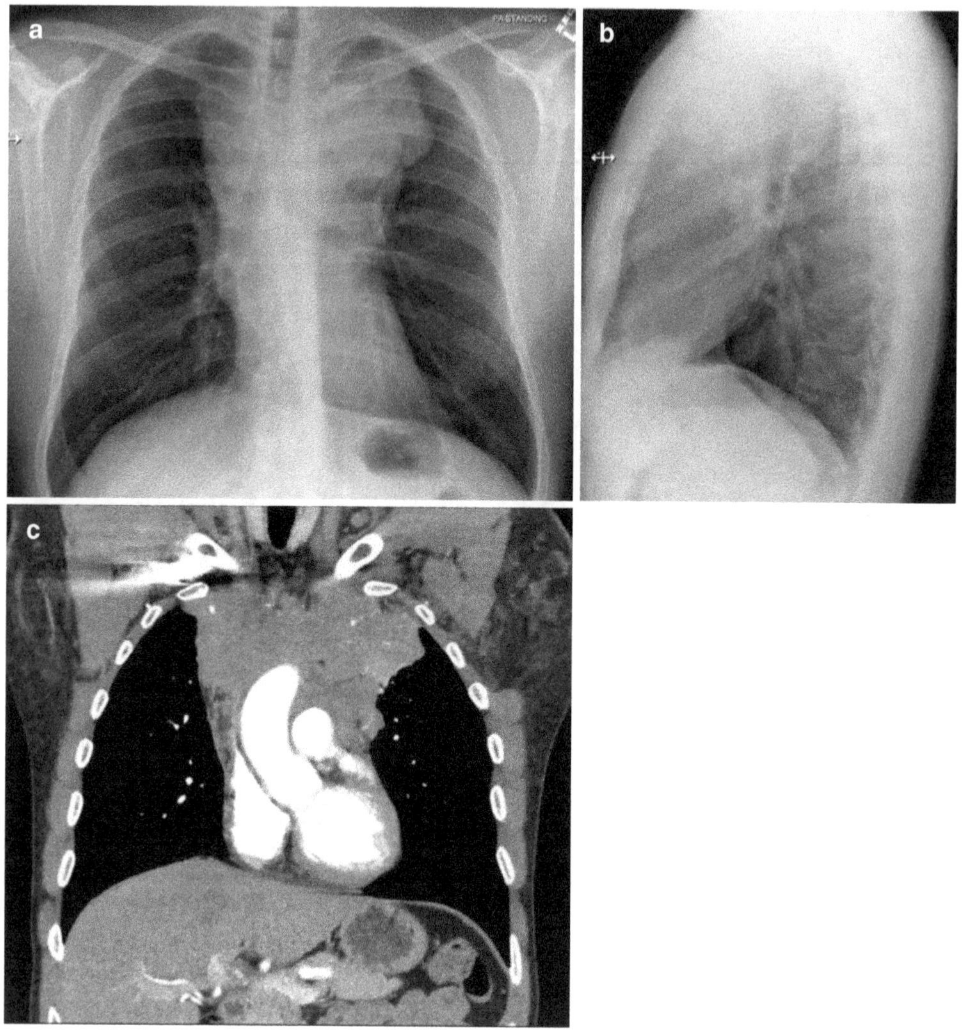

Fig. 1.3 Anterior mediastinal mass due to Hodgkin lymphoma (**a-c**). (**a,b**) Frontal (**a**) and lateral (**b**) chest radiographs of a 37-year-old man with cough and weight loss show a large lobulated mass mediastinum. (**c**) Coronal contrast-enhanced CT through the anterior chest shows a large, locally invasive soft tissue mass subsequently proven to reflect nodular sclerosing Hodgkin lymphoma

demonstrate mass-like calcification, while specific mediastinal neoplasms such as thymoma and mature teratomas may contain de novo calcification evident radiographically.

1.6.8 Pneumomediastinum

While gas may normally be evident radiographically within the trachea, central bronchi, and esophagus, mediastinal gas located outside of these structures is abnormal and usually reflects air leak from the lung or disruption of the central airways or esophagus. Pneumomediastinum is seen as linear and curvilinear lucencies outlining mediastinal structures such as the heart, trachea, and central diaphragm. The most common cause of pneumomediastinum is alveolar rupture in patients with airway obstruction due to asthma or intubated patients receiving mechanical ventilation. Blunt chest trauma can also lead to alveolar rupture and pneumomediastinum. The combination of pneumomediastinum with left lower lobe lung consolidation and a left pleural effusion or pneumothorax in a patient who has had prolonged vomiting or retching should prompt consideration of esophageal rupture or Boerhaave syndrome, which is a surgical emergency associated with high mortality.

1.7 Hila

On normal frontal chest radiographs, the right hilum is lower than the left in 97% of cases, and the hila are at the same level in 3% of cases [7]. Alterations of this relationship should suggest volume loss on the affected side due to atelectasis, scarring, or prior lung resection. The right hilum is anterior to the left on lateral chest radiography. The intermediate stem line, visible on the lateral chest radiograph, represents the posterior wall of the bronchus intermedius and should be assessed for abnormal thickening which may be seen in interstitial edema and central malignancies.

Hilar disease may manifest radiographically as increase (Table 1.6) or decrease in size, an increase in density, or abnormal convexity of the hilum or hila. Hilar enlargement most often results from a central neoplasm, lymph node enlargement (Fig. 1.4), or enlarged central pulmonary arteries as in pulmonary hypertension. The *hilar convergence sign* refers to enlarged vessels coursing toward the enlarged hilum and signifies a vascular etiology.

Table 1.6 Causes of hilar enlargement

Unilateral	Bilateral
Lung cancer	Sarcoidosis
Infection (granulomatous)	Metastatic lymph node enlargement
Metastatic lymph node enlargement	Pulmonary arterial hypertension
Lymphoma	Lymphoma
Valvular pulmonic stenosis (left)	Infection (granulomatous)

1.8 Lungs

1.8.1 Lung Volumes

Lung volume may be increased in obstructive diseases such as emphysema and is reduced in restrictive diseases such as pulmonary fibrosis and in patients with pleural fibrosis ("trapped lung"), neuromuscular disease (myasthenia gravis, amyotrophic lateral sclerosis, diaphragmatic dysfunction in systemic lupus erythematosus), or extrathoracic disorders (obesity, ascites).

Atelectasis may involve the entire lung, a lobe (Fig. 1.5), and a pulmonary segment [8] or may be subsegmental. Obstructive (resorption) atelectasis is characterized by absence of intrinsic air bronchograms. It may result from endoluminal obstruction, most often from a mucus plug as seen in asthma, bronchitis, or mechanically ventilated patients, although a centrally obstructing neoplasm such as lung cancer must be excluded.

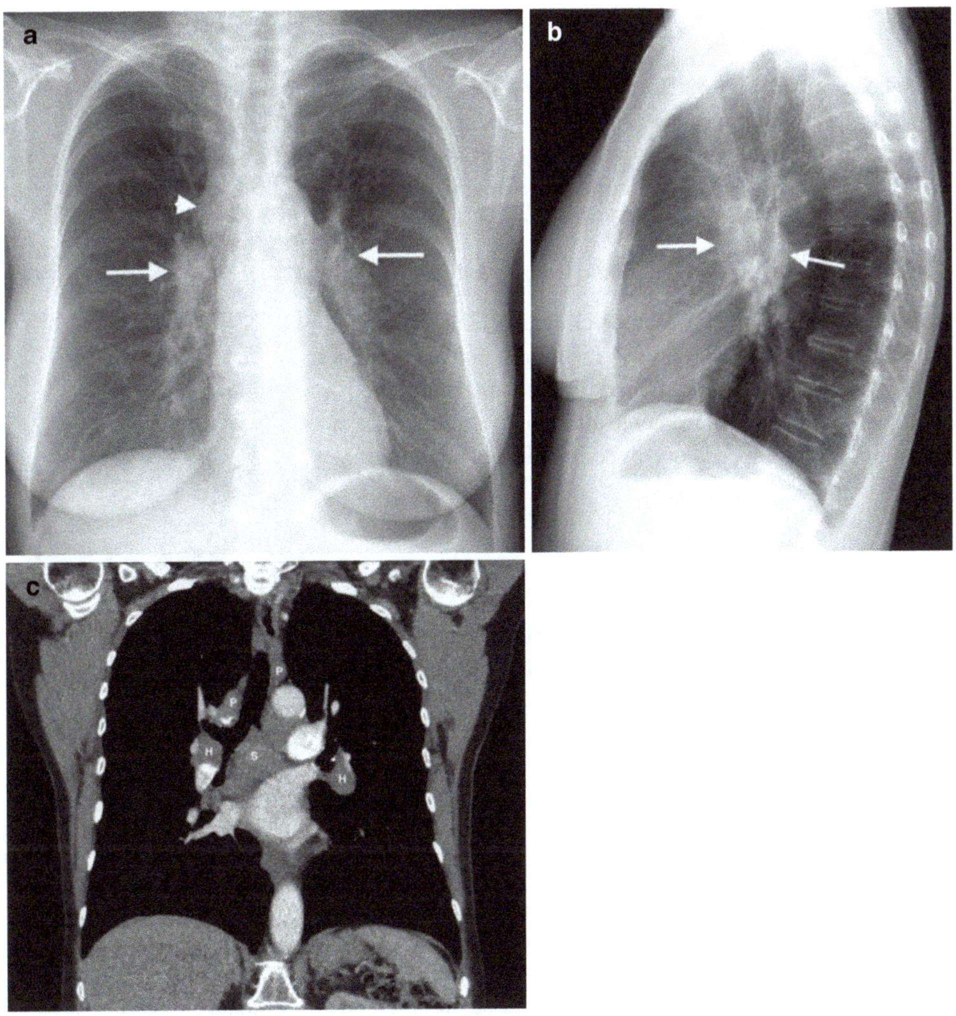

Fig. 1.4 (**a**–**c**) Sarcoidosis manifesting as bilateral hilar and mediastinal lymph node enlargement. (**a**) Frontal chest radiograph of a 71-year-old woman with nonproductive cough shows bilateral hilar (arrows) and right paratracheal (arrowheads) lymph node enlargement. (**b**) Lateral radiograph confirms enlargement and increased density of the bilateral hila as well as soft tissue in the inferior hilar window (the so-called doughnut sign) consistent with bilateral hilar and mediastinal lymphadenopathy (arrows). (**c**) Contrast-enhanced coronal MIP at mediastinal windows at the level of the carina confirms enlarged hilar (H), bilateral paratracheal (P), and subcarinal (S) lymph nodes

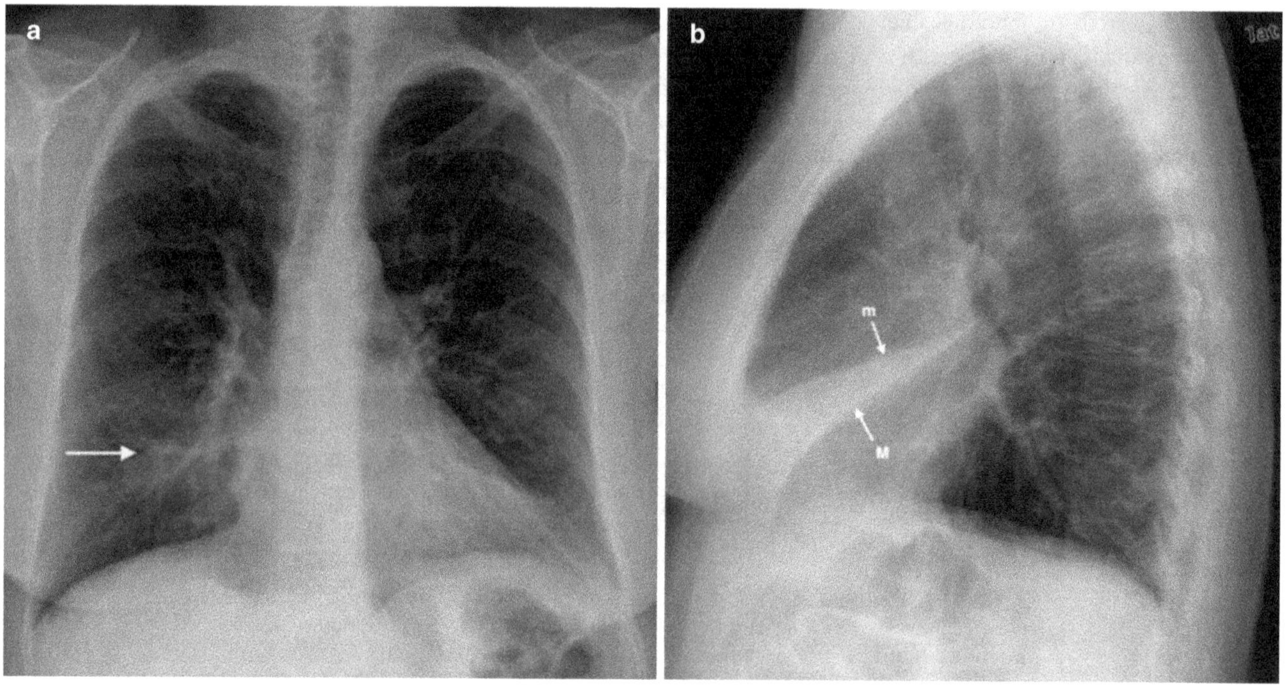

Fig. 1.5 Middle lobe atelectasis (**a**,**b**). (**a**) Frontal radiograph shows a vague opacity (arrow) overlying the lower medial right lung partly obscuring the right heart border. (**b**) The lateral radiograph shows an atelectatic middle lobe outlined by displaced minor (m) and major (M) fissures

Relaxation (passive) atelectasis often results from mass effect upon the lung, most commonly pleural effusion. Cicatricial atelectasis is due to pulmonary fibrosis. Rounded atelectasis occurs adjacent to pleural thickening in which the subpleural lung, most commonly in the lower posterior part of the chest, "folds" upon itself.

Direct signs of lobar atelectasis include fissural displacement (Fig. 1.5), bronchovascular crowding, and shift of a preexisting lung nodule or calcified granuloma. Indirect signs include increased pulmonary density, ipsilateral mediastinal shift, hilar displacement, ipsilateral hemidiaphragm elevation, and compensatory hyperinflation of the adjacent lung.

Key Point

- The most concerning cause of obstructive (resorptive) atelectasis in an adult is an endobronchial neoplasm such as lung cancer or a carcinoid tumor.

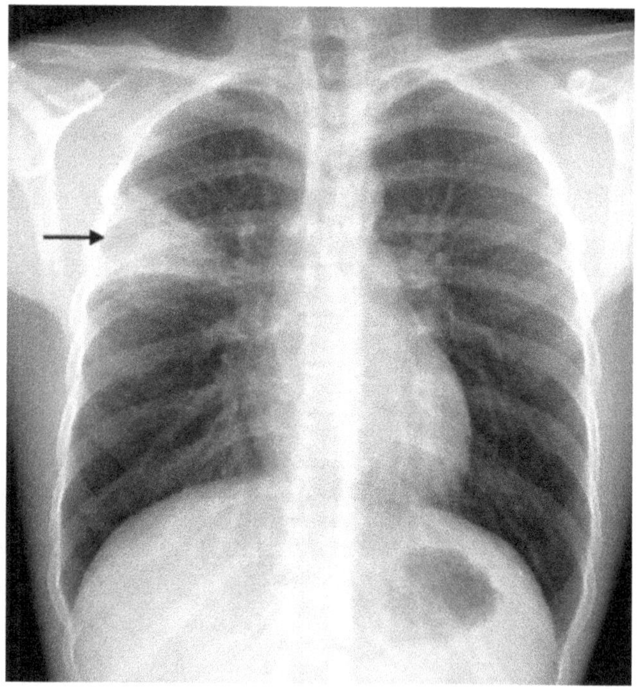

Fig. 1.6 Subsegmental right upper lobe pneumonia as air space opacification. Frontal chest radiograph of a 17-year-old with cough and fever shows a focal area of subsegmental right upper lobe air space opacification (arrow) reflecting pneumonia

1.8.2 Parenchymal Opacities

Parenchymal opacities include air space and interstitial processes. Pneumonia typically manifests with air space opacification due to alveolar filling by purulent material and may be lobar or sublobar (Fig. 1.6) or may manifest with patchy pulmonary opacities. Air space opacification often exhibits intrinsic air bronchograms and may also result from alveolar edema or hemorrhage (Table 1.7).

Interstitial opacities may manifest with reticular, linear, and/or small nodular opacities. As the normal interstitium is not visible radiographically, visualization of peripheral subpleural reticular opacities is always abnormal. A reticulonodular pattern occurs when abnormal reticular opacities are superimposed on micronodular opacities. Interstitial opacities frequently result from interstitial edema characterized by perihilar haze, peribronchial thickening, septal thickening (Kerley B lines), and subpleural edema often associated with cardiomegaly and pleural effusion. Associated radiographic findings can help limit the differential diagnosis of interstitial disease (Table 1.8).

Cells and fibrosis may also infiltrate the pulmonary interstitium, producing reticular and reticulonodular interstitial opacities in diseases such as sarcoidosis, silicosis, and lymphangitic carcinomatosis.

The idiopathic interstitial pneumonias are a distinct group of disorders often characterized by basilar predominant pulmonary fibrosis associated with volume loss [9]. The diagnosis usually requires further imaging with high-resolution chest CT (HRCT) (Fig. 1.7).

Table 1.7 Differential diagnosis of air space opacification (ASO)

Finding(s)	Disease
Focal/segmental	Pneumonia, contusion, infarct, lung cancer (adenocarcinoma)
Lobar	Pneumonia, endogenous lipoid pneumonia, adenocarcinoma
Patchy	Pneumonia, aspiration, organizing pneumonia, contusions adenocarcinoma, metastases
Diffuse	Edema, hemorrhage, pneumonia
Perihilar	Edema, hemorrhage
Peripheral	Eosinophilic pneumonia, organizing pneumonia, acute respiratory distress syndrome, contusions
Rapidly changing/ resolving	Edema, eosinophilic pneumonia, hemorrhage

Table 1.8 Ancillary findings in patients with ILD and differential considerations

Finding(s)	Disease
Hilar lymph node enlargement	Sarcoidosis, lymphangitic carcinomatosis, viral pneumonia
Clavicular/osseous erosions	Rheumatoid arthritis associated UIP
Pleural effusions	Infection, edema
Pleural plaques	Asbestosis
Hyperinflation	Langerhans cell histiocytosis, stage IV sarcoidosis, lymphangioleiomyomatosis, emphysema with UIP
Esophageal dilatation	Scleroderma associated UIP, recurrent aspiration
Conglomerate masses	Silicosis/coal worker's pneumoconiosis, sarcoidosis, talcosis
Basilar sparing	Langerhans cell histiocytosis, sarcoidosis
Basilar predominance	UIP, fibrotic NSIP, aspiration

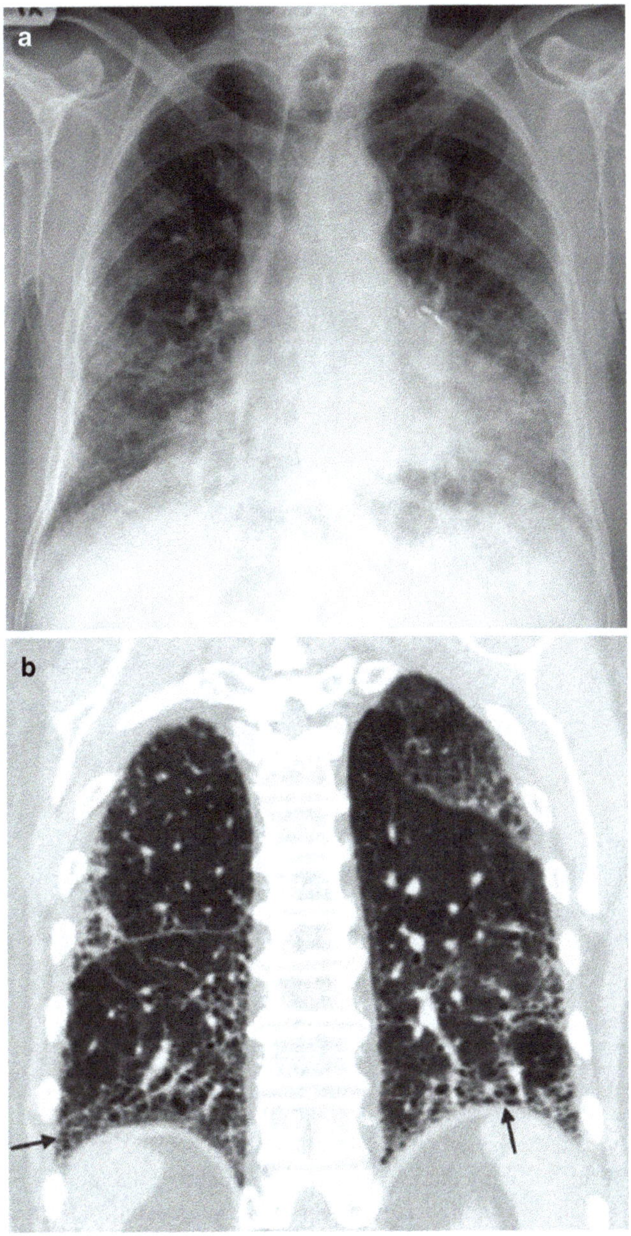

Fig. 1.7 Usual interstitial pneumonia (UIP)/idiopathic pulmonary fibrosis (IPF) as coarse basilar reticular ILD (**a**,**b**). (**a**) Frontal chest radiograph of an 84-year-old man with progressive shortness of breath demonstrates basal predominant coarse reticular opacities. (**b**) Coronal CT through the posterior chest at lung windows shows lower lobe subpleural reticulation with honeycombing (arrows) diagnostic of a UIP pattern

Key Point

- Chronic, basal predominant ILD is most often due to usual interstitial pneumonia (UIP) or fibrotic nonspecific interstitial pneumonia (NSIP). Both conditions produce basilar reticular interstitial opacities with fibrosis and can be difficult to distinguish clinically and on imaging; biopsy is often necessary for definitive diagnosis in patients lacking CT findings of UIP.

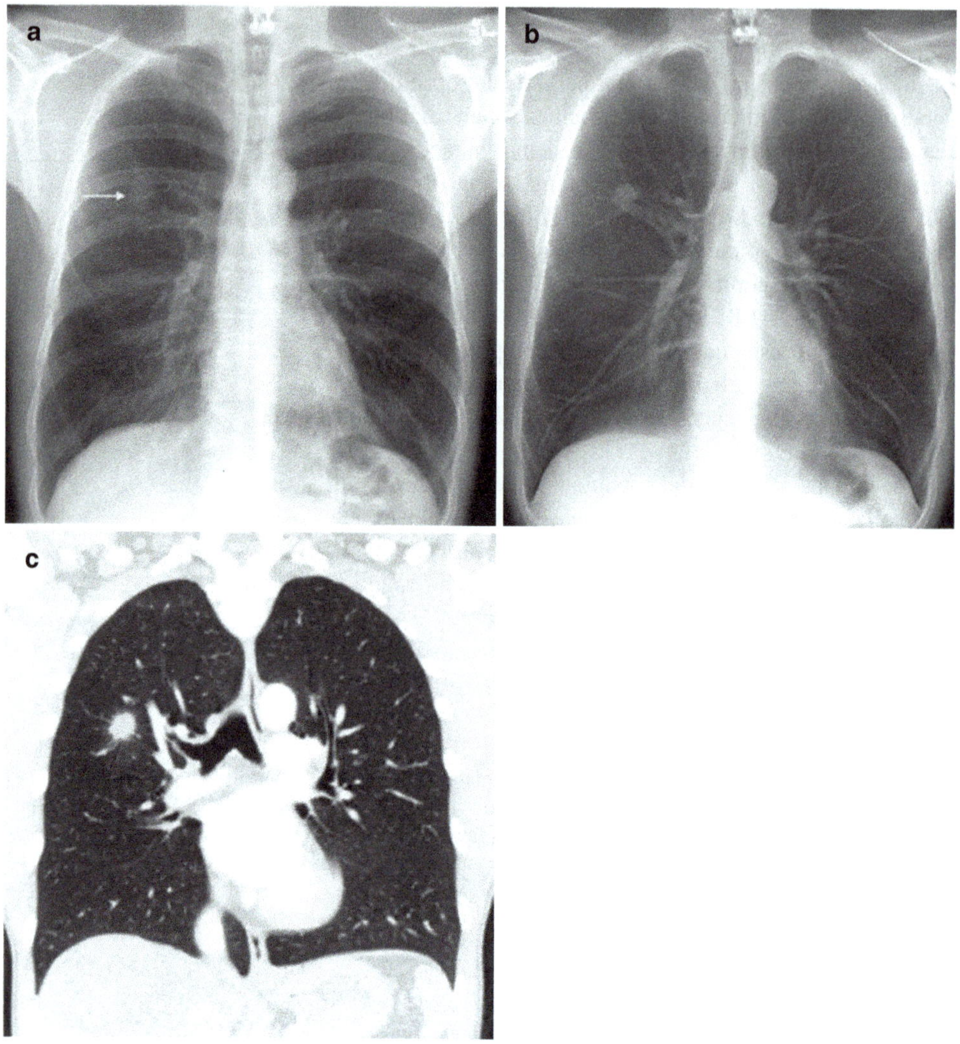

Fig. 1.8 Solitary pulmonary nodule with spiculation (**a**–**c**). (**a**) Frontal chest radiograph of a 43-year-old asymptomatic smoker shows a right upper lobe nodule (arrow) (**b**,**c**). Frontal digital tomographic image through the nodule (**b**) shows a spiculated margin, confirmed on coronal CT at lung windows through the nodule (**c**). Diagnosis was lung adenocarcinoma

A solitary pulmonary nodule (SPN) is defined as a round or ovoid opacity <3 cm in diameter. A benign pattern of intrinsic calcification in a smooth or slightly lobulated SPN reflects a granuloma or hamartoma and precludes further imaging evaluation [10].

However, the presence of calcification can be difficult to discern on standard high-kVp chest radiographs. CT provides superior contrast resolution, and thin-section scans can detect calcification that is not evident radiographically. The majority of SPNs are indeterminate on radiography and require further assessment and characterization with thin-section computed tomography (CT) to exclude malignancy (Fig. 1.8)(Table 1.9).

> **Key Point**
> - While chest radiography can detect a solitary pulmonary nodule (SPN), thin-section CT will almost invariably be needed to characterize an SPN for possible malignancy.

Table 1.9 Common causes of a solitary pulmonary nodule

Granuloma
Hamartoma
Malignancy: lung cancer, carcinoid tumor, metastasis
Focal organizing pneumonia

A pulmonary mass is a round or ovoid pulmonary opacity ≥3 cm in diameter and is highly suspicious for malignancy, typically lung cancer. The radiologist should look for pertinent ancillary findings of malignancy including other lung nodules, local invasion of adjacent structures, lymphadenopathy, and pleural effusion.

Abnormal lucency can be difficult to detect radiographically as the lungs are predominantly air filled. The most common localized lucent lesion is a bulla, seen as a focal lucency >1 cm diameter demarcated from adjacent lung by a uniform, thin (<1 mm) wall [11]. Unilateral lucency can relate to technical issues, chest wall defects, or parenchymal abnormalities as seen in the Swyer-James or unilateral hyperlucent lung syndrome, which is a post-infectious obliterative bronchiolitis that results in air trapping and decreased lung vascularity. Bilateral hyperlucency is most often seen in severe emphysema or in patients with acute asthma exacerbation.

1.9 Airways

The trachea and bronchi should be assessed for size, patency, and course. Tracheal narrowing may be focal or diffuse (Table 1.10) [12]. Focal tracheal narrowing or stenosis most often occurs secondary to mucosal or cartilaginous damage from prolonged intubation. More diffuse tracheal narrowing is most common in patients with COPD in which there is narrowing of the transverse diameter of the tracheal lumen, the so-called saber-sheath trachea. Primary or metastatic airway neoplasms may manifest as endoluminal soft tissue nodules that may be associated with volume loss. Endotracheal tumors may grow to obstruct up to 75% of the airway lumen before symptoms ensue (Fig. 1.9). Airway neoplasms may also manifest as focal or diffuse airway stenosis and must be differentiated from inflammatory conditions. Tracheal dilatation seen in the Mounier-Kuhn syndrome is a rare congenital condition characterized by tracheal and bronchial dilatation due to atrophy of the muscular and elastic tissues of the trachea and main bronchi. The trachea may deviate toward a region of upper lobe volume loss, as seen in upper lobe fibrosis, or may be displaced by a mass in the thoracic inlet such as an enlarged thyroid.

Bronchiectasis is abnormal irreversible bronchial dilatation and may result from infection, cystic fibrosis, primary ciliary dyskinesia, or allergic bronchopulmonary fungal disease. It is seen radiographically as tram tracks which represent the thickened bronchial walls in cylindrical bronchiectasis and clustered, thin-walled cystic lesions in cystic bronchiectasis.

1.10 Pleura/Diaphragm

Pleural abnormalities manifest radiographically as gas (pneumothorax) or fluid (pleural effusion) in the pleural space or as abnormalities of the pleural surfaces including thickening (pleural plaques, neoplasms) and calcification (pleural plaques, fibrothorax) [13].

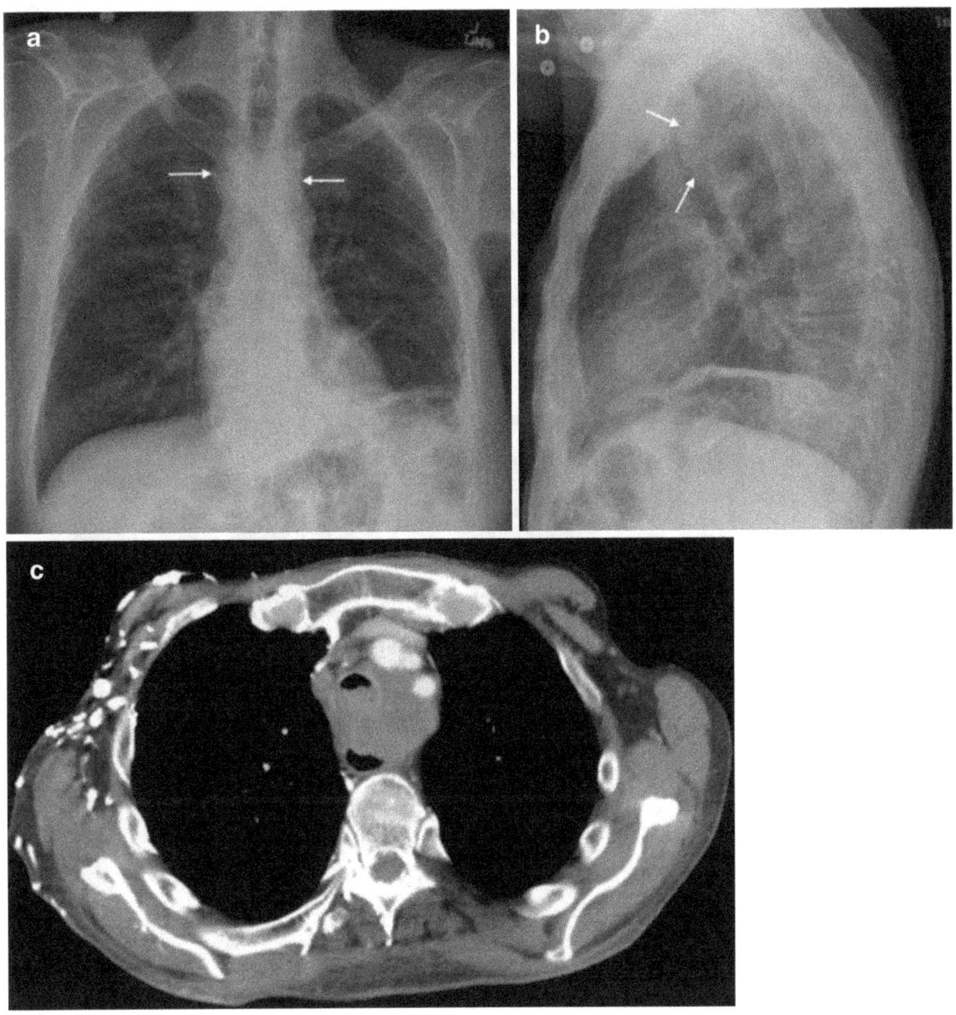

Fig. 1.9 Tracheal mass reflecting local invasion by esophageal carcinoma (**a**–**c**). (**a**) Frontal chest radiograph shows lobular contours of the upper mediastinum and thickening of the bilateral paratracheal stripes (arrows). (**b**) The lateral chest radiograph demonstrates thickening of the anterior and posterior tracheal walls and smooth stenosis of the upper trachea (arrows). (**c**) Axial contrast CT through the upper chest at mediastinal windows shows a lobulated soft tissue mass involving the anterior wall of the esophagus with invasion of the mediastinum and posterior trachea with marked narrowing of the tracheal lumen

Table 1.10 Tracheal abnormalities seen radiographically

Tracheal deviation	Ipsilateral	Upper lobe volume loss (fibrosis)
	Contralateral	Thyroid/thoracic inlet mass
Tracheal narrowing	Focal	Stenosis post intubation, tracheostomy
		TB, fungal infection
		Thyroid mass (extrinsic)
	Diffuse	Saber-sheath trachea
		Relapsing polychondritis
		Granulomatosis with polyangiitis
		Amyloidosis
		Congenital (complete tracheal rings)
Tracheal dilation	Focal	Tracheomalacia
	Diffuse	Pulmonary fibrosis
		Mounier-Kuhn syndrome (tracheobronchomegaly)
Tracheal mass		Squamous cell carcinoma
		Metastasis
		Adenoid cystic carcinoma
		Hamartoma
		Foreign body/mucus

Pneumothorax is seen on upright chest radiography as a superior lucency that parallels the chest wall and outlines the curvilinear visceral pleural line that is inwardly displaced from the chest wall. Pneumothorax may be spontaneous or traumatic. Spontaneous pneumothorax is categorized as primary (no underlying lung disease) and secondary (underlying lung disease).

The radiographic appearance of pleural effusion depends on the amount of fluid, whether the fluid is free-flowing or loculated, and the position of the patient when the radiograph is obtained. A small, free-flowing pleural effusion in an upright patient manifests radiographically as a meniscus blunting the posterior costophrenic sulcus on lateral radiography, with larger effusions blunting the lateral costophrenic sulcus on frontal radiography and effusions exceeding 500 mL in volume obscuring the hemidiaphragm. Loculated pleural effusions are typically infected (so-called parapneumonic effusions and empyemas) and produce biconvex mass-like opacities along the dependent costal pleural surfaces (Fig. 1.10). In such cases, an air fluid level in

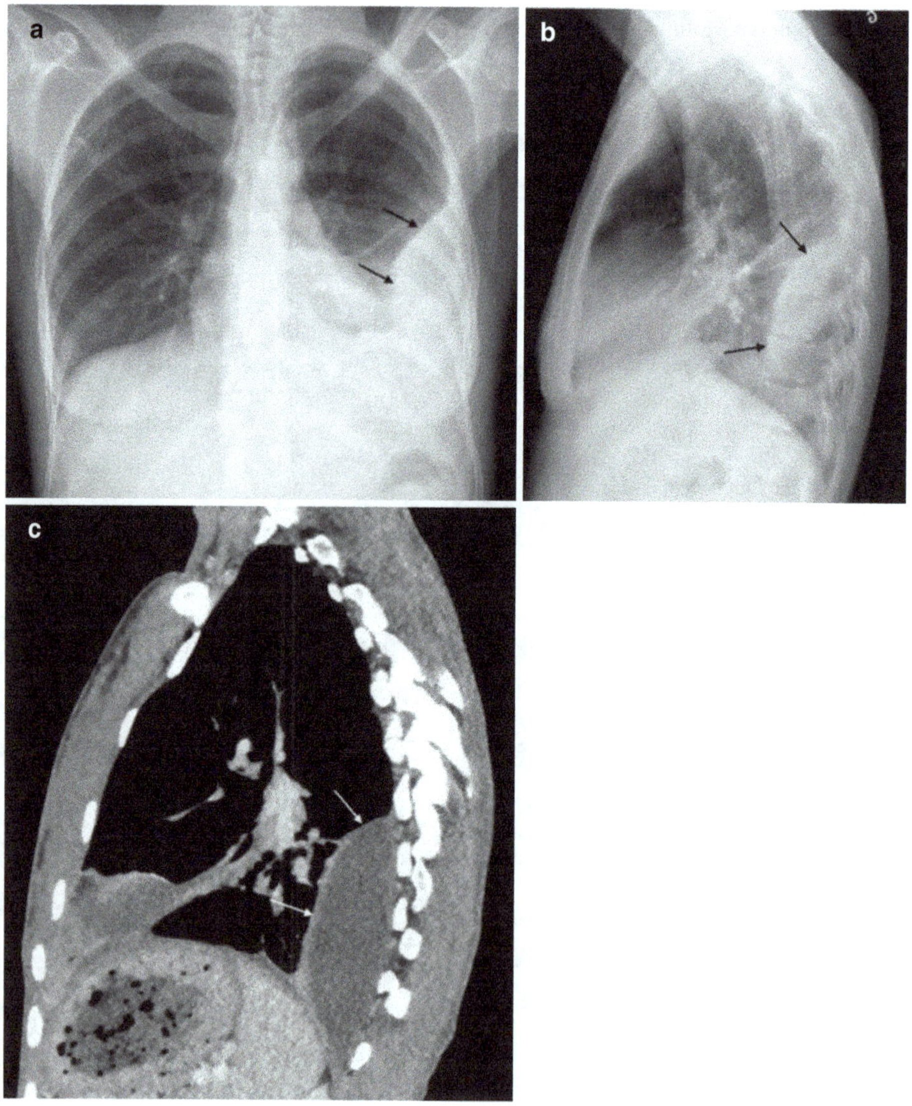

Fig. 1.10 Empyema as a loculated pleural effusion (**a–c**). (**a**,**b**) Frontal chest radiograph of a 37-year-old woman with a history of intravenous drug use who presented with fevers and chest pain shows a loculated left basilar and lateral (**a**) and posterior (**b**) pleural collection (black arrows), confirmed on contrast-enhanced sagittal CT (**c**) (white arrows)

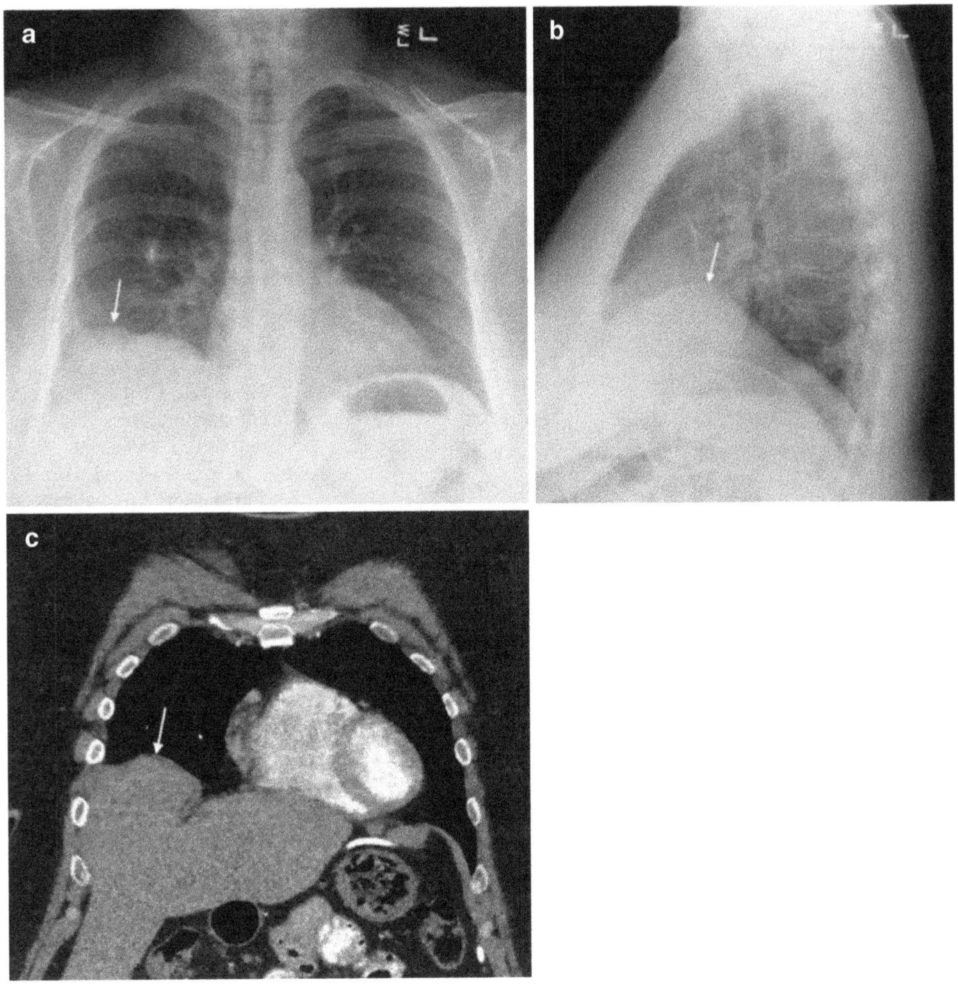

Fig. 1.11 Diaphragmatic eventration (**a-c**). (**a**) Frontal and lateral (**b**) chest radiographs show a focal bulge in the lateral (arrow in (**a**)) and anterior (arrow in (**b**)) right hemidiaphragm. (**c**) Coronal contrast-enhanced CT through the anterior chest at mediastinal windows show the liver projecting into the lower right chest due to eventration of the lateral right hemidiaphragm (arrow)

the pleural space in the absence of prior intervention is diagnostic of a bronchopleural fistula. Massive pleural effusions and pleural effusions with associated pleural nodules should suggest malignancy in the absence of trauma. Identification of circumferential nodular pleural thickening is virtually diagnostic of malignancy, with the main diagnostic considerations including metastatic disease, malignant pleural mesothelioma, and lymphoma.

The diaphragm is a domed structure, with the right slightly higher than the left owing to the position of the heart on the left. A uniformly elevated diaphragm is most often due to weakness or paralysis of the diaphragm, while focal bulges in the diaphragmatic contour are typically due to eventration (thinning) of the diaphragm (Fig. 1.11) or diaphragmatic hernia through a congenital or acquired diaphragmatic defect [14].

Key Point

- Loculated pleural effusions often manifest radiographically as vertically oriented biconvex pleural opacities and are usually associated with underlying lung infection (termed parapneumonic effusions).

1.11 Concluding Remarks

Although considered relatively "low tech" in the age of multi-detector CT, MR, and ultrasound, conventional chest radiography remains an important imaging study in the evaluation of patients with chest symptoms, in assessing hospitalized patients who have tubes or catheters placed for monitoring or treatment, and in screening the chest for asymptomatic disease. Each study should first be evaluated for technical adequacy, followed by a consistent, systematic review of the normal anatomy and structures to allow detection of abnormalities or exclude the presence of disease. Each component of the chest radiograph should be reviewed with findings reported in the same, consistent fashion, ideally in a systematic way that provides the referring clinician with a structured report that parallels the radiographic analysis. While many chest radiographic findings are nonspecific, there are important conditions evident radiographically such as pneumothorax or pneumonia that can direct specific treatment or, as in the case of a non-calcified SPN, allow the radiologist to make recommendations of appropriate imaging follow-up or management.

Take-Home Messages

- An analysis of the technical adequacy of a chest radiographic study is necessary prior to interpretation.
- In critically ill hospitalized patients, chest radiographs performed for the assessment of monitoring or support devices provide important information regarding proper device positioning and help detect complications of placement.
- The radiographic detection of mediastinal abnormalities requires a detailed knowledge of normal mediastinal imaging anatomy and interfaces.
- Lung radiographic abnormalities can be divided into air space and interstitial diseases, solitary pulmonary nodules or masses, and abnormal decreases in density that can be localized, unilateral, or diffuse.
- Diaphragmatic contour abnormalities may be localized, such as in patients with eventration or hernia, or diffuse as in diaphragmatic weakness of paralysis.

References

1. Walz-Flannigan AI, Brossoit KJ, Magnuson DJ, Schueler BA. Pictorial review of digital radiography artifacts. Radiographics. 2018;38(3):833–46.
2. Godoy MCB, Leitman BS, de Groot PM, Vlahos I, Naidich DP. Chest radiography in the ICU: part 2, evaluation of cardiovascular lines and other devices. Am J Roentgenol. 2012;198(3):572–81.
3. Nam SJ, Kim S, Lim BJ, et al. Imaging of primary chest wall tumors with radiologic-pathologic correlation. Radiographics. 2011;31(3):749–70.
4. Whitten CR, Khan S, Munneke GJ, et al. A diagnostic approach to mediastinal abnormalities. Radiographics. 2007;27:657–71.
5. Gibbs JM, Chandrasekhar CA, Ferguson EC. Lines and stripes: where did they go?—from conventional radiography to CT. Radiographics. 2007;27:33–48.
6. Carter BW, Benveniste MF, Madan R, et al. ITMIG classification of mediastinal compartments and multidisciplinary approach to mediastinal masses. Radiographics. 2017;37(2):413–36.
7. Webb WR. Chapter 3: The Pulmonary Hila. In: Webb WR, Higgins CB, editors. Thoracic imaging: pulmonary and cardiovascular radiology. 3rd ed. Philadelphia: Wolters Kluwer; 2017. p. 78–82.
8. Abbott GA. Approach to atelectasis and volume loss. In: Rosado-de-Christenson ML, editor. Diagnostic imaging—chest. Salt Lake City: Amirsys; 2012. p. 1–56.
9. Sverzellati N, Lynch DA, Hansell DM, Johkoh T, King TE, Travis WD. American thoracic society–European respiratory society classification of the idiopathic interstitial pneumonias: advances in knowledge since 2002. Radiographics. 2015;35(7):1849–71.
10. Hodnett PA, Ko JP. Evaluation and management of indeterminate pulmonary nodules. Radiol Clin N Am. 2012;50:895–914.
11. Hansell DM, Bankier AA, MacMahon H, McLoud TC, Müller NL, Remy J. Fleischner society: glossary of terms for thoracic imaging. Radiology. 2008;246(3):697–722.
12. Heidinger BH, Occhipinti M, Eisenberg RL, Bankier AA. Imaging of the large airways disorders. Am J Roentgenol. 2015;205:41–56.
13. Qureshi NR, Gleeson FV. Imaging of pleural disease. Clin Chest Med. 2006;27(2):193–213.
14. Nason LK, Walker CM, McNeeley MF, Burivong W, Fligner CL, Godwin JD. Imaging of the diaphragm: anatomy and function. Radiographics. 2012;32(2):E51–70.

2

Missed Lung Lesions: Side-by-Side Comparison of Chest Radiography with MDCT

Denis Tack and Nigel Howarth

Learning Objectives

- To be aware of the actual risks of misdiagnosis when reading chest radiographs
- To learn the best tips and tricks for reducing your error rate
- To understand the limitations of chest radiographs compared with multi-detector CT

2.1 Introduction

Missed lung lesions are one of the most frequent causes of malpractice issues [1–3]. Chest radiography plays an important role in the detection and management of patients with lung cancer, chronic airways disease, pneumonia and interstitial lung disease. Amongst all diagnostic tests, chest radiography is essential for confirming or excluding the diagnosis of most chest diseases. However, numerous lesions of a wide variety of disease processes affecting the thorax may be missed on a chest radiograph. For example, the frequency of missed lung carcinoma on chest radiographs can vary from 12 to 90%, depending on study design [4]. Despite the lack of convincing evidence that screening for lung cancer with the chest radiograph improves mortality, chest radiography is still requested for this purpose. The chest radiograph will also help narrow a differential diagnosis, help to direct additional diagnostic measures and serve during follow-up. The diagnostic usefulness of the radiograph will be maximized by the integration of the radiological findings with the clinical features of the individual patient. In this chapter, we will review the more important radiological principles regarding missed lung lesions in a variety of common chest diseases, with a special focus on how correlation with multi-detector CT (MDCT) of missed lung lesions can help improve interpretation of the plain chest radiograph.

D. Tack (✉)
Department of Radiology, Epicura, Ath, Belgium
e-mail: denis.tack@epicura.be

N. Howarth
Institut de Radiologie, Clinique des Grangettes, Genève, Switzerland
e-mail: nigel.howarth@grangettes.ch

2.2 Reasons for Missed Lung Lesions

Conditions contributing to missed lung lesions, especially carcinomas, have been extensively studied [2, 4–6]. Poor viewing conditions, hasty visual tracking, interruptions, inadequate image quality and observer inexperience are amongst the most important [5, 7, 8]. Features of lesions themselves, when faced with nodules, such as location, size, border characteristics and conspicuity, also play a role [5]. Missed lung nodules during initial reading of a chest radiograph are not uncommon. Missing a nodule which may represent malignancy will have adverse consequences on patient management, essentially through delayed diagnosis, which may carry medicolegal implications. A number of authors have explored the reasons why lesions are overlooked [9–14]. Specific studies have focussed on size [7], contrast gradient [15], conspicuity [16] and anatomic noise [17]. Importantly, other types of errors, named systemic errors, can also occur [18] and include inappropriate orders or imaging utilization, procedure phase errors (patient identification, laterality, technique) and post-procedure phase errors (lighting conditions, transcription errors, communication failures).

One interesting study [19] examined the imaging features of non-small-cell lung carcinoma overlooked at digital chest radiography and compared general and thoracic radiologists' performance for lung carcinoma detection. Frontal and lateral chest radiographs from 30 consecutive patients with lung carcinoma overlooked during initial reading and 30 normal controls were submitted to two blinded thoracic radiologists and three blinded general radiologists for retrospective review. The location, size, histopathology, borders, presence of superimposed structures and lesion opacity were recorded. Interobserver agreement was calculated, and detection performance between thoracic and general radiologists was compared. The average size of carcinomas missed by the thoracic radiologists was 18.1 mm (range 10–32 mm). The average size missed by general radiologists was 27.7 mm (range 12–60 mm). Seventy-one percent (5/7) of missed lesions were obscured by anatomical superimposition. Forty-three percent of lesions were located in the upper lobes, and 63% were adenocarcinomas. Compared with general radiologists, the lesions missed by thoracic radiologists tended to be smaller but also had significantly lower CT density measurements and more commonly had an ill-defined margin. The clinical stage of the overlooked lesions did not differ between the two groups ($p = 0.480$). The authors concluded that the lesion size, location, conspicuity and histopathology of lesions overlooked on digital chest radiography were similar to those missed on conventional film screen techniques.

The detection of carcinoma on a chest radiograph remains difficult with implications on patient management. Nowadays, it is still by far the most frequent cause of malpractice suits (42% of cases) [3]. Whereas overlooking chronic airways disease, pneumonia and interstitial lung disease may not have the same potential medicolegal implications, the consequences for patient care could be critical.

We propose to review how correlation with multi-detector computerized tomography (MDCT) of missed lung lesions can help improve interpretation of the plain chest radiograph. During the course of clinical work, when reporting chest CT, whenever available, every effort should be made to review previous chest radiographs and their reports, thereby providing one of the best learning tools for chest radiograph interpretation.

Artificial intelligence will probably replace or modify our work as chest radiologists, minimizing detection errors and helping us to reduce our error rate. Convolutional neural networks have already been reported to provide a sensitivity of 97.3% and specificity of 100% in the detection of tuberculosis on chest X-rays [20].

A CT scan can be performed in patients with a negative chest radiograph when there is a high clinical suspicion of chest disease. CT scan, especially MDCT reconstructed with high-resolution algorithm and iterative reconstruction, is more sensitive than plain films for the evaluation of interstitial disease, bilateral disease, cavitation, empyema and hilar adenopathy. CT is not generally recommended for routine use because the data for its use in chronic airways disease and pneumonia are limited, the cost is high, and there is no evidence that outcome is improved. Thus, a chest radiograph is the preferred method for initial imaging, with CT scan reserved for further characterization (e.g., evaluation of pattern and distribution, detecting of cavitation, adenopathy, mass lesions or collections).

Many methods have been suggested for correct interpretation of the chest radiograph. There is no preferred scheme or recommended system. The clinical question should always be addressed. An inquisitive approach is always helpful and being aware of the areas where mistakes are made is essential. Hidden abnormalities can thus be looked for. The difficult "hidden areas" which must be checked are the lung apex, superimposed over the heart, around each hilum and below the diaphragm. We will concentrate on difficult areas such as lesions at the lung apices or bases or lesions adjacent to or obscured by the hila or heart. For a systematic approach, we will divide the review into three sections representing specific problems: missed nodules, missed consolidation and missed interstitial lung disease. Finally, we will illustrate some of the common signs that may help to detect lesions located in difficult anatomical areas of the chest.

Key Points

- Missing lesions is frequent.
- Hidden areas are at highest risks for missing lesions.
- Missing lesions is a frequent cause of medicolegal issues.

2.3 Specific Problems

Specific problems of missed lung lesions can be divided into missed nodules, missed consolidation and missed interstitial lung disease. In cases of a missed nodule or missed consolidation, the overlooked pathology may have been detected if special attention were paid to known "difficult areas". The examples which follow will show how a side-by-side comparison of the chest radiograph and CT images improves our understanding of the overlooked lesion. There is no harm done by learning from one's mistakes!

2.4 Missed Nodules

2.4.1 Nodular Lesions: Tumours

Nodular lesions are frequently due to lung cancer, which may be primary or secondary. Lung cancer is probably one of the most common lung diseases that radiologists encounter in practice. Berbaum formulated the concept that perception is better if you know where to look and what to look for [21]. Our first example is that of a 53-year-old man who complained of pain in the right axilla for 4 months and underwent chest radiography. The postero-anterior and lateral radiographs were interpreted showing normal findings (Fig. 2.1a and b). The subsequent MDCT showed a right

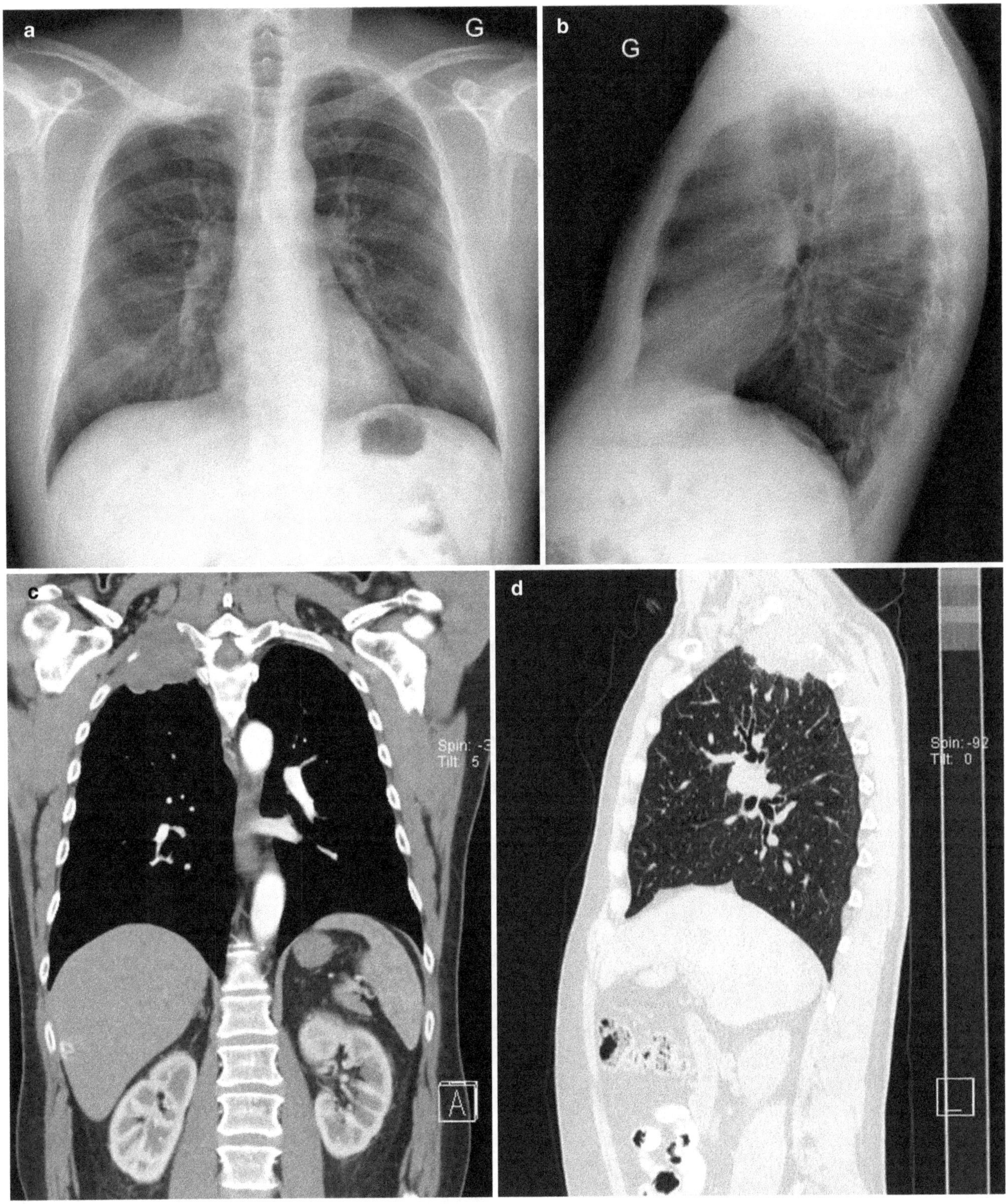

Fig. 2.1 A 53-year-old man who underwent chest radiography for pain in the right axilla. Postero-anterior (**a**) and lateral (**b**) radiographs interpreted as normal. With hindsight bias from MDCT the right apical mass is obvious. MDCT coronal and sagittal images with soft tissue (**c**) and bone (**d**) windows showing a right apical mass with bone destruction

superior sulcus mass with rib destruction (Fig. 2.1c and d). Needle biopsy established a diagnosis of bronchogenic carcinoma (adenocarcinoma). Hindsight bias [22] with the information available from the MDCT makes the initial lesion extremely obvious. Careful scrutiny of both apices is essential when reporting a frontal chest radiograph.

Radiologic errors can be divided into two types [23]: cognitive, in which an abnormality is seen but its nature is misinterpreted, and perceptual or the "miss", in which a radiologic abnormality is not seen by the radiologist on initial interpretation. The perceptual type is estimated to account for approximately 80% of radiologic errors [24].

Our second patient illustrates the complexity of the detection of a lung nodule close to the hilum. A 77-year-old man with known prostate cancer underwent chest radiography for right upper quadrant abdominal pain (Fig. 2.2a and b). The

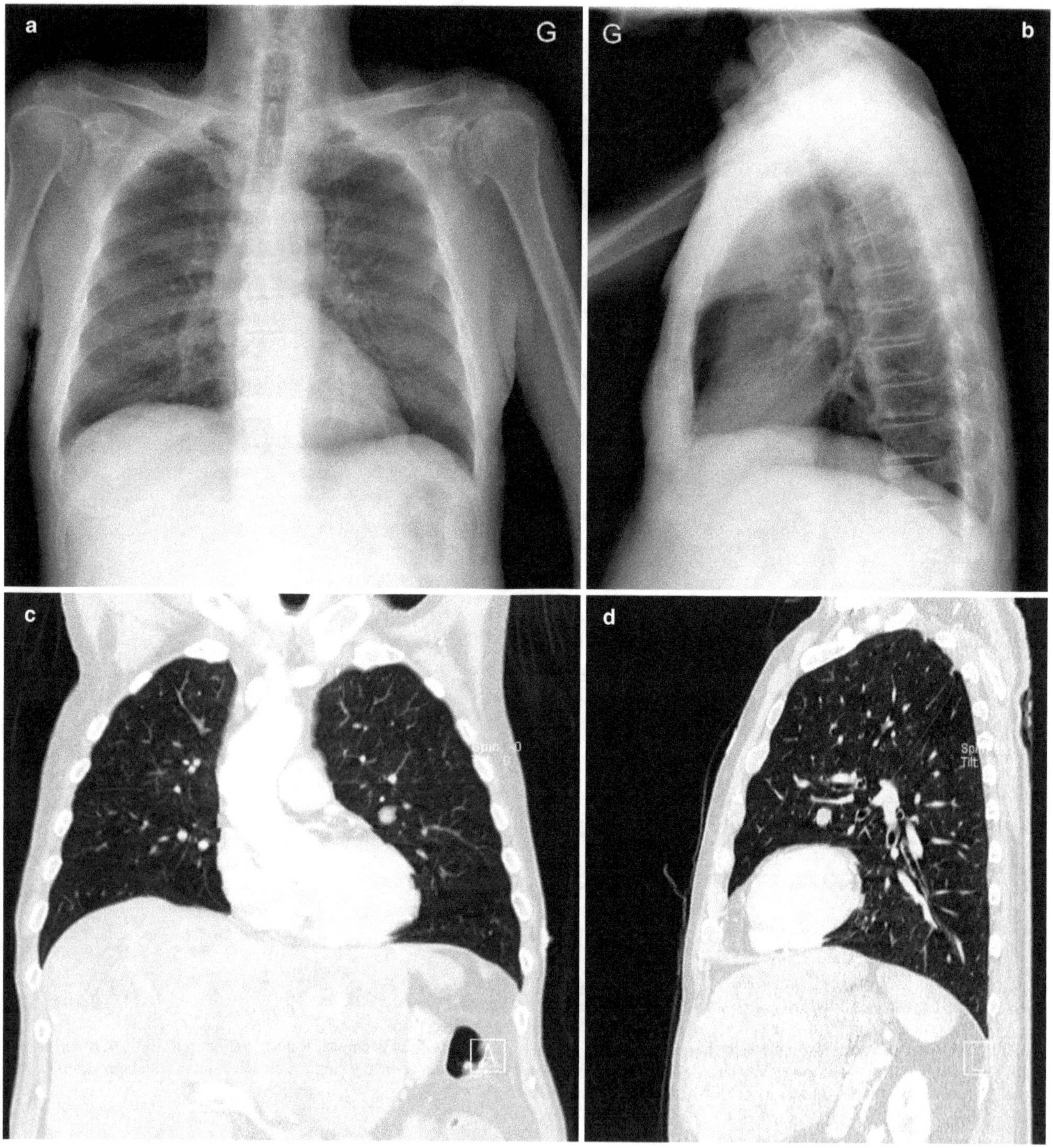

Fig. 2.2 A 77-year-old man with right upper quadrant pain. Posteroanterior (**a**) and lateral (**b**) radiographs interpreted as normal. With hindsight, the 13 mm nodule in the superior segment of the lingula can be seen. Coronal (**c**) and sagittal (**d**) reformats (lung window) show the position of the lingular nodule, close to the hilum

radiographs were reported as normal. The coronal and sagittal reformats demonstrate the position of the nodule (Fig. 2.2c and d), which can be seen clearly with hindsight on the postero-anterior and lateral chest radiographs.

2.4.2 Nodular Lesions: Infections

Nodular lesions attributed to pulmonary infections are most often seen in nosocomial pneumonias and in immunocompromised patients. They may be caused by bacteria such as *Nocardia asteroides* and *M. tuberculosis*, septic emboli and fungi. *Nocardia asteroides* causes single or nodular infiltrates with or without cavitation. Invasive pulmonary aspergillosis (IPA), *mucor* and *Cryptococcus neoformans* may present with single or multiple nodular infiltrates, which often progress to wedge-shaped areas of consolidation. Cavitation (the "crescent sign") is common later in the course of the infiltrate. In the appropriate clinical setting, CT may aid in the diagnosis of IPA by demonstrating the so-called halo sign. Figure 2.3 shows a 43-year-old woman with fever after a bone marrow transplant. The postero-anterior radiograph was interpreted as normal (Fig. 2.3a). With hindsight, a subtle infiltrate can be seen at the left apex. Conspicuity is lessened by the overlying clavicle and first rib. Axial CT image (Fig. 2.3b) shows nodular consolidation

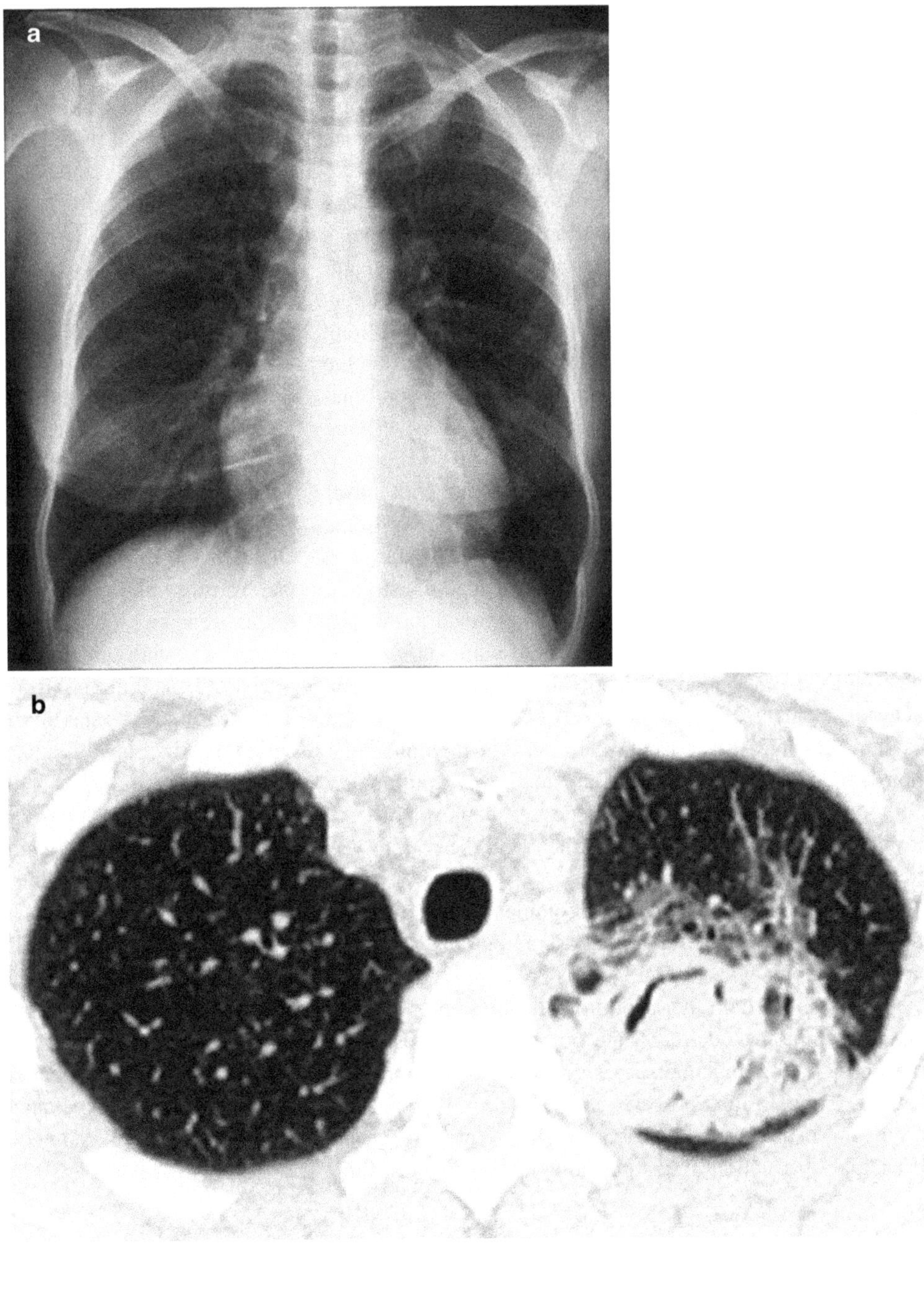

Fig. 2.3 A 43-year-old woman with fever after a bone marrow transplant. Postero-anterior radiograph interpreted as normal (**a**). With hindsight, a subtle infiltrate can be seen at the left apex. Conspicuity is lessened by the overlying clavicle and first rib. Also note the indwelling catheter from the left brachial vein to the superior vena cava. Axial CT image (lung window) shows nodular consolidation with crescentic cavitation (air-crescent sign) and surrounding ground-glass infiltrate (halo sign) (**b**)

with crescentic cavitation (the "crescent sign") and surrounding ground-glass infiltrate (the "halo sign"). These characteristic findings of IPA are best identified on CT.

> **Key Points**
> - Nodule location in hidden areas is the most frequent cause for missing nodules
> - Low nodule attenuation favours missing the lesion
> - Calcified nodules are easiest to detect but not clinically relevant

2.5 Missed Consolidation

2.5.1 Airspace Disease

Airspace disease is usually caused by bacterial infections. However, airspace disease can be seen in viral, protozoal, fungal infections and malignancy, typically brochioloalveolar carcinoma. Acute airspace pneumonia is characterized by a mostly homogeneous consolidation of lung parenchyma, well-defined borders, and does not typically respect segmental boundaries. An air bronchogram is very common. Progression to lobar consolidation may occur. As with lung nodules, whether consolidation is detected or missed on the plain chest radiograph may be determined by any combination the same factors of size, density, location and overlying structures. Location is a significant factor for missed consolidation. Consolidation in the middle lobe and both lower lobes can be difficult to diagnose, especially when only the postero-anterior view is obtained. Figure 2.4 shows a 46-year-old woman with cough and right-sided chest pain. The postero-anterior radiograph was interpreted as normal (Fig. 2.4a). Due to a clinical suspicion of pulmonary embolism, MDCT was requested, showing consolidation in the anterior segment of the right lower lobe. The coronal and sagittal reformats demonstrate the extent of the consolidation (Fig. 2.4b and c). There were no signs of pulmonary embolism on the contrast media study. A diagnosis of right lower lobe pneumonia was established, and the patient was treated successfully with antibiotics.

Chest radiography is the first recommended imaging test for the diagnosis of pneumonia. Chest radiography can diagnose pneumonia when an infiltrate is present and differentiate pneumonia from other conditions that may present with similar symptoms, such as acute bronchitis. The results of the chest radiograph may occasionally suggest a specific aetiology (e.g., a lung abscess) and identify a complication (empyema) or coexisting abnormalities (bronchiectasis, bronchial obstruction, interstitial lung disease). Chest radiography remains a valuable diagnostic tool in primary care patients with a clinical suspicion of pneumonia to substantially reduce the number of patients misdiagnosed. MDCT imaging is useful in patients with community-acquired pneumonia when there is an unresolving or complicated chest radiograph and at times in immunocompromised patients with suspected pulmonary infections. MDCT can help in differentiating infectious from non-infectious abnormalities. MDCT may detect empyema, cavitation and lymphadenopathy when the chest radiograph cannot. MDCT should be performed in immunocompromised patients with a clinical suspicion of pneumonia when the chest radiograph is normal. This is especially true when the early diagnosis of pneumonia is critical, as is the case with immunocompromised and severely ill patients.

> **Key Points**
> - Chest radiography is the first imaging test for the diagnosis of pneumonia.
> - Chest radiographs may help identify complications of pneumonia.
> - Hidden areas are the most frequent reasons for missing pneumonia.

2.6 Missed Interstitial Lung Disease

2.6.1 Diffuse (Interstitial or Mixed Alveolar-Interstitial) Lung Disease

Diffuse lung disease presenting with widely distributed patchy infiltrates or interstitial reticular or nodular abnormalities can be produced by a number of disease entities. An attempt is usually made to separate the group of idiopathic interstitial pneumonias from known causes, such as infections, associated systemic disease or drug related. The most common infectious organisms are viruses and protozoa. In general, the aetiology of an underlying pneumonia cannot be specifically diagnosed because the patterns overlap. It is beyond the aim of this chapter to discuss in detail the contribution of MDCT to the diagnosis of diffuse infiltrative lung disease. For over three decades, the development and then refinement of high-resolution computed tomography (HRCT) have resulted in markedly improved diagnostic accuracy in acute and chronic diffuse infiltrative lung disease. The chest radiograph remains the preliminary radiological investigation of patients with diffuse lung disease but is often non-specific. Pattern recognition in diffuse lung disease has been the subject of controversy for many years. Extensive disease may be required before an appreciable

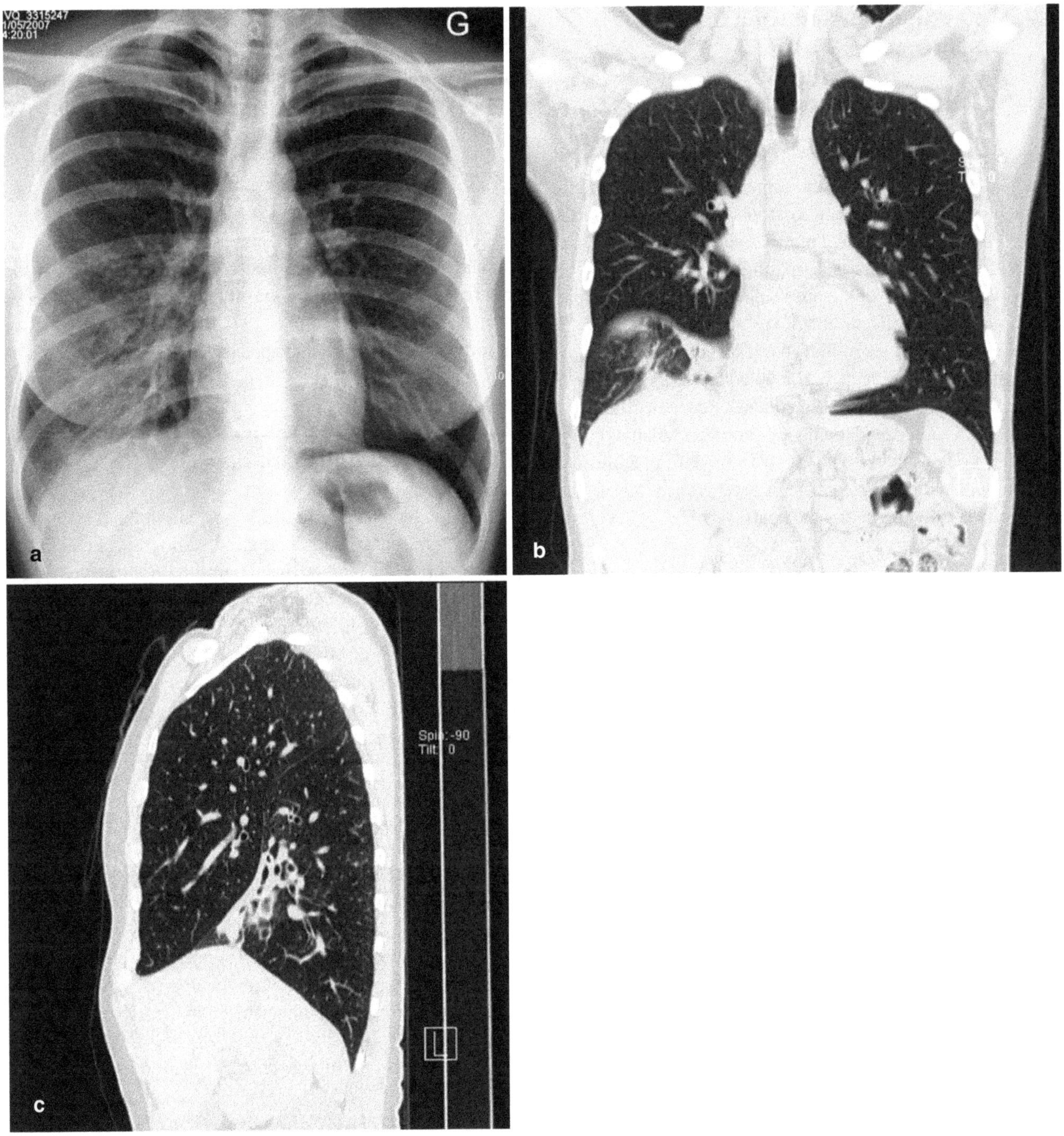

Fig. 2.4 A 46-year-old woman with cough and right-sided chest pain. Postero-anterior radiograph interpreted as normal (**a**). Coronal (**b**) and sagittal (**c**) reformats showing consolidation in the anterior segment of the right lower lobe

change in radiographic density, or an abnormal radiographic pattern can be detected on the plain chest radiograph. At least 10% of patients who are ultimately found to have biopsy-proven diffuse lung disease have an apparently normal chest radiograph. HRCT and now MDCT have become an integral component of the clinical investigation of patients with suspected or established interstitial lung disease. These techniques have had a major impact on clinical practice.

Key Points

- Chest radiography is less sensitive and less specific than MDCT.
- If the chest radiograph is normal, MDCT may be indicated.
- Chest radiographs may be helpful for the follow-up of ILD.

2.7 Key Signs for Reducing the Risk of Errors in CXRs

2.7.1 Deep Sulcus Sign

The deep sulcus sign (Fig. 2.5) is seen on chest radiographs obtained with the patient in the supine position [25]. It represents lucency of the lateral costophrenic angle extending toward the abdomen. The abnormal deepened lateral costophrenic angle may have a sharp, angular appearance. When the patient is in the supine position, air in the pleural space (pneumothorax) collects anteriorly and basally within the nondependent portions of the pleural space; when the patient is upright, the air collects in the apicolateral location. If air collects laterally rather than medially, it deepens the lateral costophrenic angle and produces the deep sulcus sign. In Fig. 2.5, a deep sulcus sign is seen on the left, in addition to a continuous diaphragmatic sign, seen when air is seen between the diaphragm and the heart.

2.7.2 Spine Sign

On the normal lateral chest radiograph, the attenuation decreases (the lucency increases) as one progresses down the thoracic vertebral bodies. If the attenuation increases, locally or diffusely, there must be a posterior located lesion (Fig. 2.6). This lesion might not be seen on the frontal view, hidden by the heart or the hila. Interestingly, the positive predictive value of the spine sign is high (up to 97%) [26].

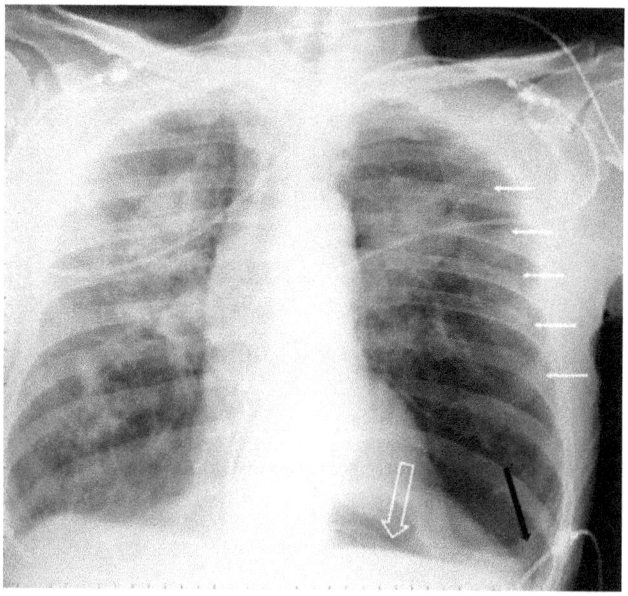

Fig. 2.5 A 78-year-old man with acute left chest pain and previous history of pneumoconiosis. Bedside chest radiograph showing a thin white line near the left chest wall (white arrows), corresponding to the left lung visceral pleura and indicating a pneumothorax. The deep lucency of the left lateral costophrenic angle extending towards the abdomen is an indirect sign of pneumothorax (black arrow). The continuous diaphragmatic sign is also seen as air separating the diaphragm from the heart (white hollow arrow)

2.7.3 Silhouette Sign

In a chest X-ray, non-visualization of the border of an anatomical structure that is normally visualized shows that the area neighbouring this margin is filled with tissue or material of the same density (Fig. 2.6) [27]. The silhouette sign is an important sign indicating the presence and the localization of a lesion.

2.8 Concluding Remarks

Despite the increasing use of CT imaging in the diagnosis of patients with chest disorders, chest radiography is still the primary imaging method in patients with suspected chest disease. The presence of an infiltrate on a chest radiograph is considered the "gold standard" for diagnosing pneumonia. Extensive knowledge of the radiographic appearance of pulmonary disorders is essential when diagnosing pulmonary disease. Chest radiography is also the imaging tool of choice in the assessment of complications and in the follow-up of patients with pulmonary diseases.

MDCT plays an increasing role in the diagnosis of chest diseases, especially in patients with unresolving symptoms. CT will aid in the differentiation of infection and non-infectious disorders. The role of CT in suspected or proven chest disease can be summarized as follows:

1. CT is valuable in the early diagnosis of chest disease, especially in patient groups in which an early diagnosis is important (immunocompromised patients, critically ill patients).
2. CT may help with the characterization of pulmonary disorders.
3. CT is an excellent tool in assessing complications of chest disease.
4. CT is required in the investigation patients with a persistent or recurrent pulmonary infiltrate.

A side-by-side comparison between the chest radiograph and MDCT when confronted with a missed lung lesion is very instructive. The radiologist should be able to understand the reasons for missing certain lesions. By adopting this inquisitive approach, both our cognitive and perceptual errors could be reduced.

Awareness of the dangers of systemic errors has become of upmost concern, as a result of the high examination volume

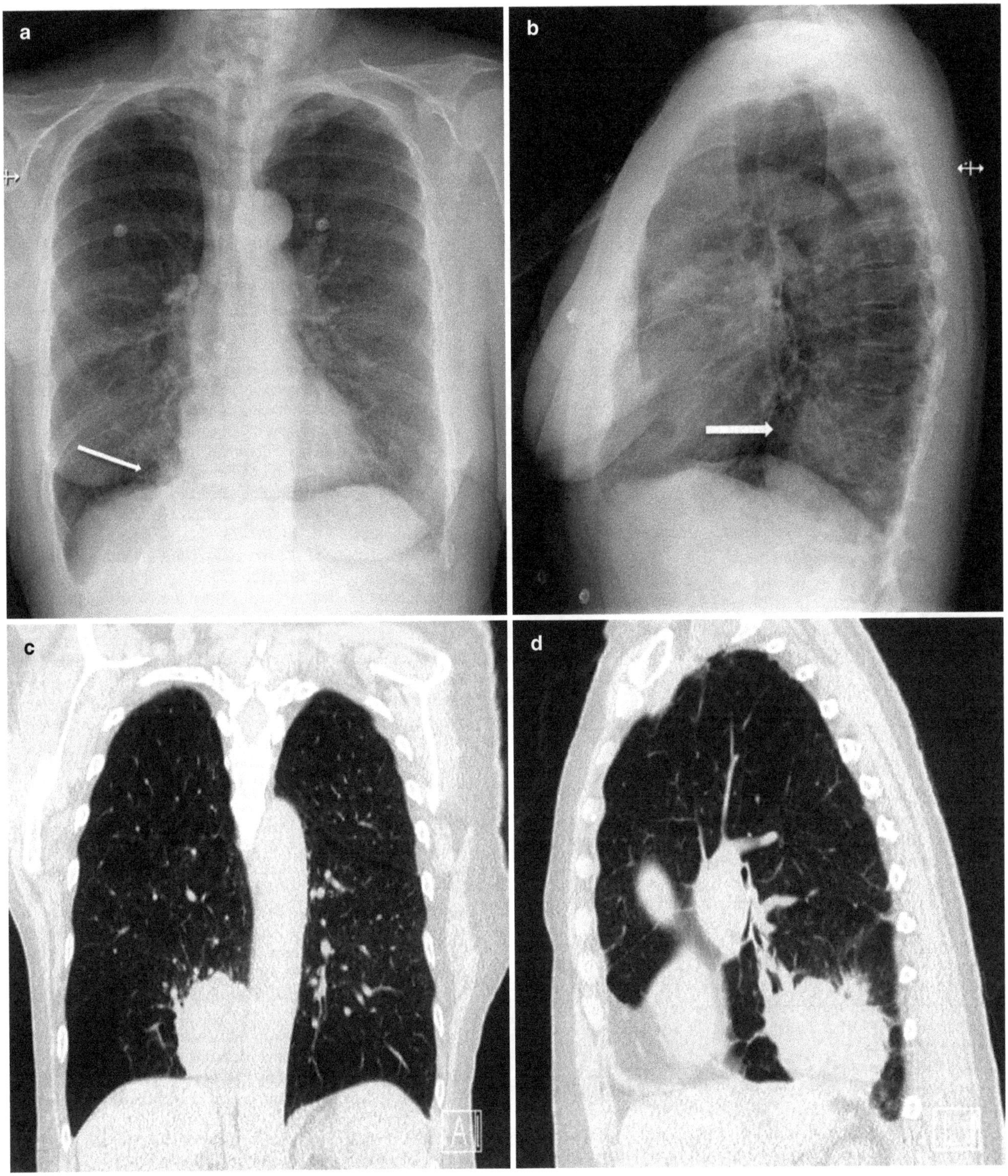

Fig. 2.6 A 69-year-old woman with COPD and haemoptysis. Posteroanterior chest radiograph (**a**) showing an opacity next to the right border of the heart (arrow) and obliterating the right side of the spine. This silhouette sign of the right posterior mediastinal border indicates that the lesion is in a posterior location in the right lower lobe. Lateral view (**b**) showing an increased density (arrow) of the lower spine compared with the upper and middle thoracic spine (spine sign). This increased density is due to a large mass in the right lower lobe. Coronal CT image (**c**) showing the right lower lobe mass obliterating the border of the mediastinum. Sagittal CT image (**d**) showing the posterior location of the mass

and long shifts experienced by radiologists [28]. Double readings and subsequent readings by subspecialists may become common practice, especially if medicine shifts toward physician payment based on quality or outcomes, rather than volume [29]. Artificial intelligence will undoubtedly offer opportunities to improve our diagnostic accuracy, as systems will be developed as adjuncts to human cognition and perception [30].

Artificial intelligence generates fear about the future role of radiologists and their employment. Let us remember that although we analyse many images, we still decide on what imaging examinations should be prescribed and how they are performed best, we confer on difficult diagnoses, we discuss treatment plans with patients and we translate the conclusions of the research literature into real-life practice. If some of the more repetitive tasks can be handled safely by a computerized helper, radiologists will be able to focus on the rewarding ones, improving patient care and safety.

Take-Home Messages
- Be aware that missing lesions is frequent.
- Always look at hidden areas.
- Beware of satisfaction of search.
- Take time to read the lateral view of the chest.
- Learn the key radiologic signs to reduce your error rate.

References

1. Garland LH. Studies on the accuracy of diagnostic procedures. Am J Roentgenol Radium Therapy, Nucl Med. 1959;82(1):25–38.
2. Potchen EJ, Bisesi MA. When is it malpractice to miss lung cancer on chest radiographs? Radiology. 1990;175:29–32.
3. Baker SR, Patel RH, Yang L, Lelkes VM, Castro A. Malpractice suits in chest radiology: an evaluation of the histories of 8265 radiologists. J Thorac Imaging. 2013;28:388–91.
4. Quekel LG, Kessels AG, Goei R, et al. Miss rate of lung cancer on the chest radiograph in clinical practice. Chest. 1999;115:720–4.
5. Austin JH, Romney BM, Goldsmisth LS. Missed bronchogenic carcinoma: radiographic findings in 27 patients with a potentially resectable lesion evident in retrospect. Radiology. 1992;182:115–22.
6. Kim YW, Mansfield LT. Fool me twice: delayed diagnoses in radiology with emphases on perpetuated errors. AJR. 2014;202:465–70.. W.
7. Krupinski EA, Berger WG, Dallas WJ, et al. Searching for nodules: what features attract attention and influence detection? Acad radiol. 2003;10:861–8.
8. Busby LP, Courtier JL, Glastonbury CM. Bias in radiology: the how and why of misses and misinterpretations. Radiographics. 2018;38(1):236–47.
9. Kundel HL, Nodine CF, Krupinski EA. Searching for lung nodules. Visual dwell indicates locations of false-positive and false-negative decisions. Invest Radiol. 1989;24:472–8.
10. Samuel S, Kundel HL, Nodine CF, et al. Mechanism of satisfaction of search: eye position recordings in the reading of chest radiographs. Radiology. 1995;194:895–902.
11. Quekel LG, Goei R, Kessels AG, et al. Detection of lung cancer on the chest radiograph: impact of previous films, clinical information, double reading, and dual reading. J Clin Epidemiol. 2001;54:1146–50.
12. Tsubamoto M, Kuriyama K, Kido S, et al. Detection of lung cancer on chest radiographs: analysis on the basis of size and extent of ground-glass opacity at thin-section CT. Radiology. 2002;224:139–44.
13. Shah PK, Austin JH, White CS, et al. Missed non-small cell lung cancer: radiographic findings of potentially resectable lesions evident only in retrospect. Radiology. 2003;226:235–41.
14. Samei E, Flynn MJ, Peterson, et al. Subtle lung nodules: influence of local anatomic variations on detection. Radiology. 2003;228:76–84.
15. Kundel HL, Revesz G, Toto L. Contrast gradient and the detection of lung nodules. Investig Radiol. 1979;14:18–22.
16. Kundel HL. Peripheral vision, structured noise and film reader error. Radiology. 1975;114:269–73.
17. Kundel HL, Revesz G. Lesion conspicuity, structured noise, and film reader error. AJR. 1976;126:233–8.
18. Waite S, Scott JM, Legasto, et al. Systemic error in radiology. AJR. 2017;209:629–39.
19. Wu M-H, Gotway MB, Lee TJ, et al. Features of non-small cell lung carcinomas overlooked at digital chest radiography. Clin Radiol. 2008;63:518–28.
20. Lakhani P, Sundaram B. Deep learning at chest radiography: automated classification of pulmonary tuberculosis by using convolutional neural networks. Radiology. 2017;284:574–82.
21. Berbaum KS. Difficulty of judging retrospectively whether a diagnosis has been “missed”. Radiology. 1995;194:582–3.
22. Berlin L. Hindsight bias. AJR. 2000;175:597–601.
23. Berlin. Defending the “missed” radiographic diagnosis. AJR. 2001;176:317–22.
24. Berlin L, Hendrix RW. Perceptual errors and negligence. AJR. 1998;170:863–7.
25. Kong A. The deep sulcus sign. Radiology. 2003;228:415–6.
26. Medjek M, Hackx M, Ghaye B, De Maertelaer V, Gevenois PA. Value of the “spine sign” on lateral chest views. Br J Radiol. 2015;88(1050):20140378.
27. Algın O, Gökalp G, Topal U. Signs in chest imaging. Diagn Interv Radiol. 2011;17:18–29.
28. Hanna TN, Lamoureux C, Krupinski EA, et al. Effect of shift, schedule, and volume on interpretive accuracy: a retrospective analysis of 2.9 million radiologic examinations. Radiology. 2018;287:205–12.
29. Arenson RL. Factors affecting interpretative accuracy: how can we reduce errors ? Radiology. 2018;287:213–4.
30. Kahn CE. From images to actions: opportunities for artificial intelligence in radiology. Radiology. 2018;285:719–20.

3

Approach to Imaging of Mediastinal Conditions in the Adult

Sanjeev Bhalla and Edith Marom

Learning Objectives

- To understand an approach to the adult mediastinum based on localization of lesions within the mediastinum and attenuation/intensity features on cross-sectional imaging.
- To highlight conditions that disregard the compartmental model.
- To use some cases to show the additional value of MR in evaluating the adult mediastinum.

3.1 Introduction

The mediastinum is an anatomic space defined by the thoracic inlet superiorly and the diaphragm inferiorly. It extends from the sternum to the vertebral bodies. Yet, despite its landmarks, there are no structures that completely separate the mediastinum from the neck above or the retroperitoneum below. Imaging of the mediastinum and generating a relevant different diagnosis rest on the principles of localization and characterization.

Once a process or mass can be localized to the mediastinum, it should be localized within the mediastinum. Many of us use an approach first championed by Ben Felson. Using a lateral radiograph or sagittal CT or MR, a line is drawn from the anterior tracheal wall to the posterior inferior vena cava. This line separates the anterior mediastinum from the middle mediastinum. A second line is drawn 1 cm posterior to the anterior margin of the vertebral body. This line separates the middle from the posterior mediastinum. No anatomic structures actually divide the mediastinal compartments, but this approach can be useful in creating concise, meaningful differential diagnoses. Keep in mind certain processes may involve more than one compartment and that a large mass may be hard to localize.

More recently, the International Thymic Malignancy Interest Group (ITMIG) has proposed a modification of lesion localization based on MDCT. In this model, three compartments are used: prevascular, visceral, and paravertebral. The main difference from the modified Felson technique is the inclusion of the heart and aorta in the visceral compartment (middle compartment) (Fig. 3.1).

After localization, cross-sectional imaging (either CT or MR) should be performed for lesion characterization. Knowing whether a lesion has a significant vascular, fluid or fat component can be very helpful in suggesting a more specific diagnosis. PET/CT is used mainly to evaluate lymph node metastases in lung cancer. It is used as well in the evaluation of solid mediastinal masses.

This approach of localization and characterization will provide the interpreting radiologist a solid foundation in imaging the mediastinum.

3.2 Anterior Mediastinum/Prevascular Compartment

Most anterior or prevascular mediastinal masses are thymic in origin. Even lymphomas and germ cell tumors tend to arise in cells within the thymus. A useful differential list should be based on age, as germ cell tumors are almost unheard of in patients older than 45 years. Most anterior mediastinal masses tend to be lymphomas, germ cell tumors, or thymomas. Many texts will include thyroid goiter in the list for anterior mediastinal lesions. We, however, have found that most goiters tend to extend into the middle mediastinum or visceral compartment (Fig. 3.2).

S. Bhalla (✉)
Mallinckrodt Institute of Radiology, Washington University, Saint Louis, MO, USA
e-mail: sanjeevbhalla@wustl.edu

E. Marom
Radiology Department, The Chaim Sheba Medical Center, Tel Aviv University, Ramat Gan, Israel

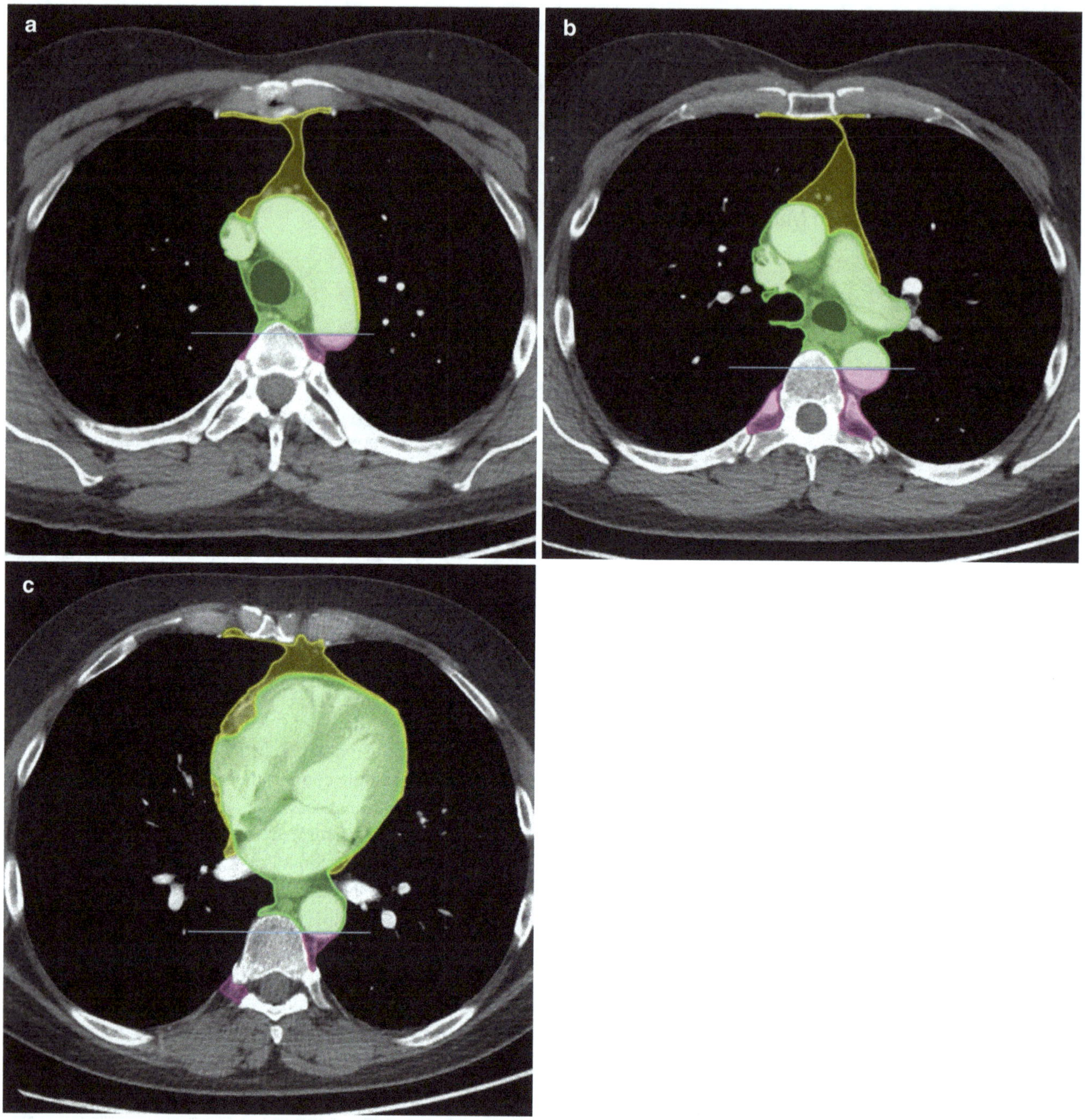

Fig. 3.1 ITMIG definition of the mediastinal compartments at the level of the transverse aorta (**a**), left pulmonary artery (**b**), and heart (**c**). The prevascular compartment is anterior or peripheral to the pericardium (X color), whereas the paravertebral compartment is separated from the visceral compartment by a line (X color) 1 cm posterior to the anterior vertebral body border

Observing fluid attenuation or intensity can be very helpful in approaching anterior mediastinal masses. Pure cystic lesions are benign (usually thymic or pericardial cysts). Separating pericardial from thymic cysts is based on location as thymic cysts tend to be spade-shaped and reside in the thymic bed, while pericardial cysts tend to be rounder and are more commonly found in the right cardiophrenic angle (Fig. 3.3). As the amount of soft tissue within the lesion increases, one should consider the increased likelihood of a malignancy. Both lymphoma and cystic thymoma will tend to have soft tissue elements that will enhance on MR or CT (Fig. 3.4). Germ cell tumors also follow this rule. The classic teaching is that the germ cell tumor should be fat in attenuation. Many teratomas do contain some fat elements, but almost all are cystic (Fig. 3.5). As with the other lesions, if the soft tissue elements dominate, then a malignant germ cell tumor should be favored, such as seminoma. Interestingly, malignant germ cell tumors are quite rare in female patients.

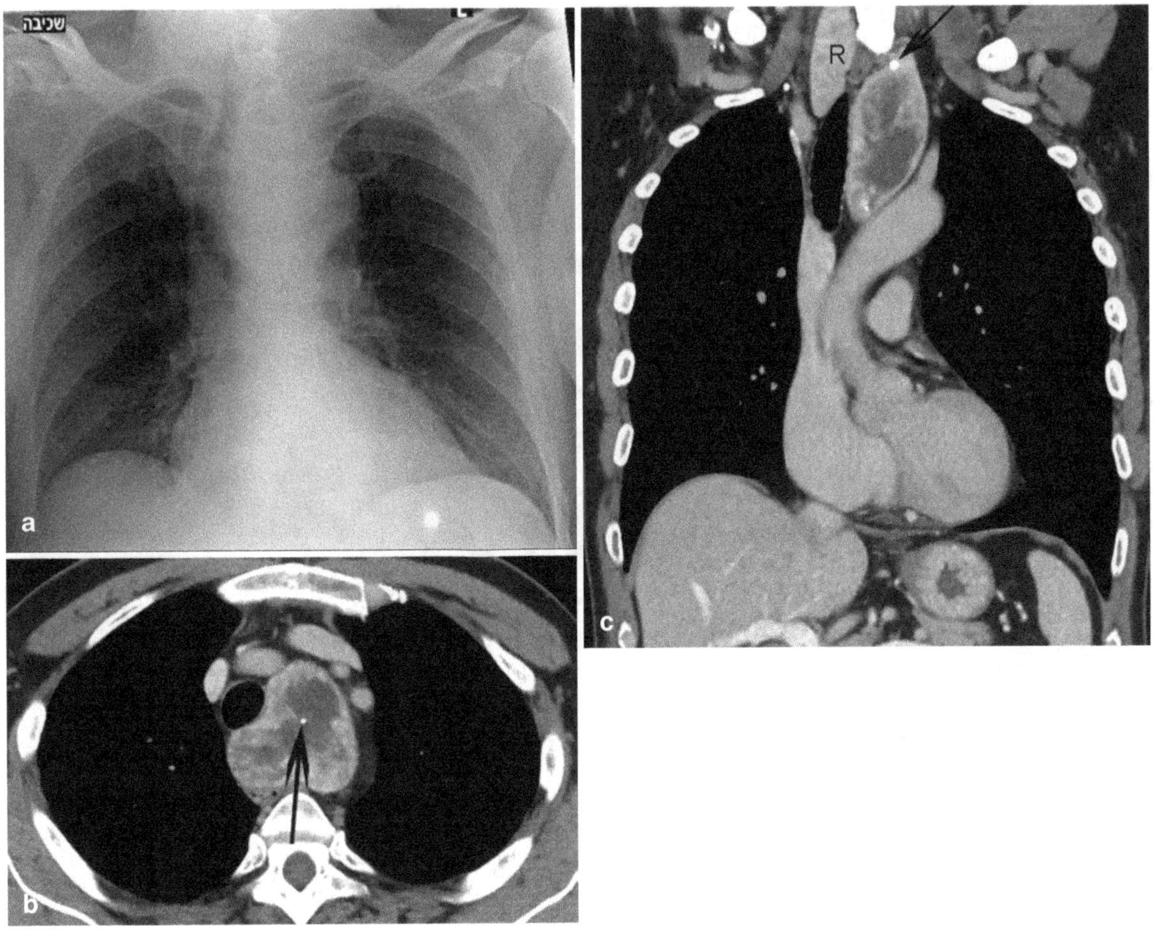

Fig. 3.2 Thyroid goiter. Frontal chest radiograph (**a**) of an asymptomatic 74-year-old man demonstrates a mass in the mediastinum displacing the trachea to the left. Axial (**b**) and coronal reformations (**c**) of a contrast-enhanced CT confirm the mass is in the visceral or middle mediastinum, shows intense enhancement, similar to the enhancement of the right thyroid lobe (R in image C), and contains course calcifications (arrows) and low attenuation regions with it. These findings, of a heterogeneous intensely enhancing mass, with low attenuation regions, and course calcifications, connecting to the thyroid, are typical for intrathoracic extension of a goiter

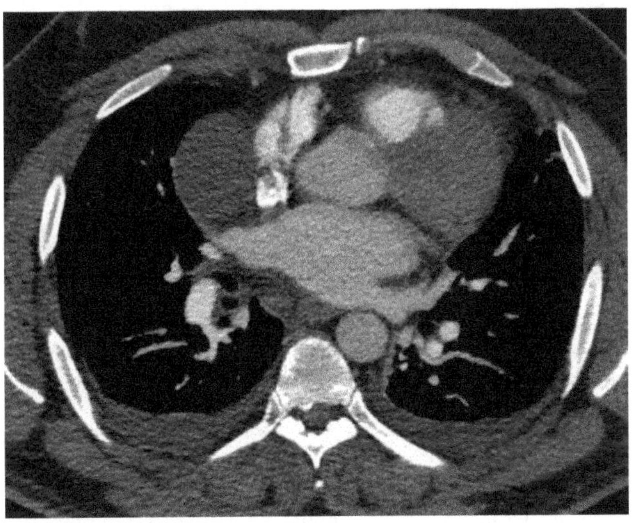

Fig. 3.3 Pericardial cyst. Axial contrast-enhanced CT (**a**) of a 56-year-old man demonstrates a cystic mass abutting the right heart border with imperceptible walls, of water density and no enhancing nodule or septa, typical for a pericardial cyst

The visualization of fat intensity or attenuation can also be very helpful. In the anterior or prevascular mediastinum, most fatty masses are benign. As described above, an anterior mediastinal mass with fat and fluid suggests a teratoma (benign germ cell tumor) (Fig. 3.5). If the mass is purely fat, it may be the very rare thymolipoma but more likely will be a fat pad or anterior hernia (Morgagni hernia). Coronal or sagittal images are quite helpful in depicting vessels originating below the diaphragm. Visualization of these are key in separating hernias from fat pads or fatty tumors. In our practices, infarction of a pericardial fat pad or fat within the Morgagni hernia may present with chest pain. In the era of the frequent use of CT in the evaluation of chest pain, these areas of fat necrosis can simulate a neoplasm. Awareness of this potential pitfall will allow the patients to be treated appropriately.

Calcification can also be helpful. The incidence of calcification in thymomas varies from 10 to 40% (Fig. 3.6). Circular

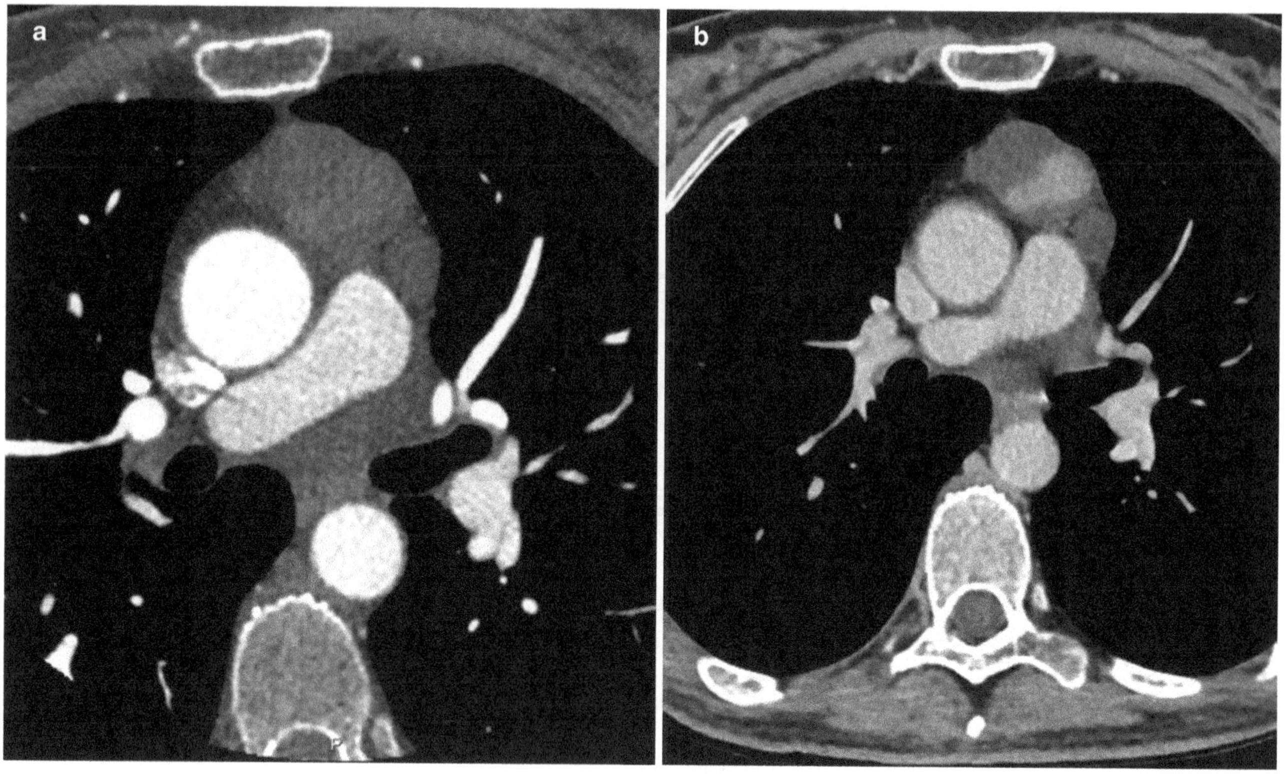

Fig. 3.4 Cystic thymoma. Axial view from a contrast-enhanced coronary artery CT in a 51-year-old woman demonstrated a cystic mass in the prevascular mediastinum. At this phase of early imaging after contrast injection, intralesional nodular enhancement is not readily seen, better demonstrated on a routine contrast-enhanced chest CT (B). Delayed imaging after contrast enhancement or MR imaging with its improved contrast resolution is used to ensure cystic lesions in the prevascular mediastinum do not contain enhancing soft tissue which usually indicated malignancy, as was proven in this cystic type B1 thymoma

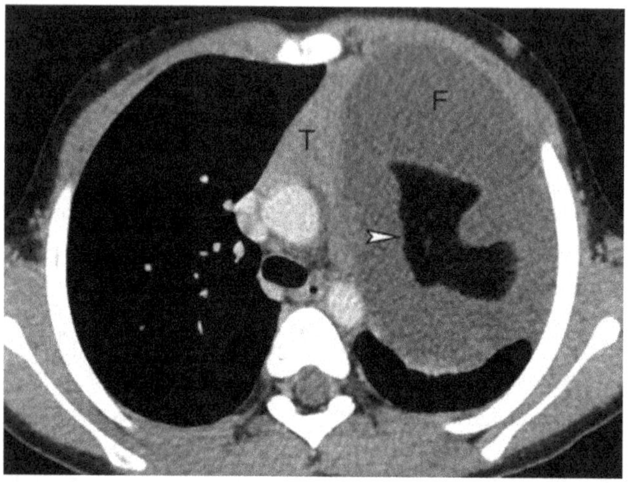

Fig. 3.5 Mature teratoma. Axial view of a contrast-enhanced chest CT at the level of the thymus (T) in a 5-year-old boy. There is a fluid-filled (F) large prevascular mass containing obvious fat

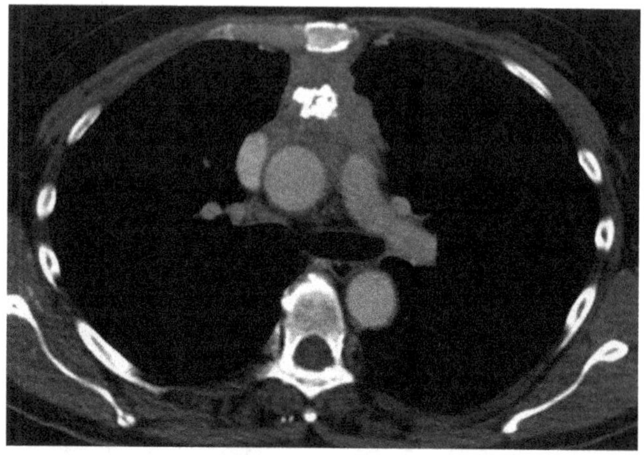

Fig. 3.6 Thymoma with calcifications. Contrast-enhanced chest CT of a 65-year-old woman shows a prevascular mass with dense calcifications proven at resection to represent a type B3 thymoma. Thymoma may present with dense or even curvilinear calcifications

peripheral calcification may occur in solid thymomas. Teratomas contain calcium in about 35% of cases. Untreated lymphomas do not calcify and about 5% of them show calcifications after radiation therapy. Peripheral circular calcification can be a finding of an aneurysm. In this location, many such aneurysms represent bypass graft aneurysms. The presence of mediastinal wires should be a clue to this potential diagnosis.

Vascular or hyperenhancing lesions may present within the anterior or prevascular mediastinum. Often, these are related to the heart, ascending aorta. Rarely, ectopic parathyroid adenomas may present as vigorously enhancing anterior prevascular masses.

> **Key Point**
> - Most anterior mediastinal masses are of thymic origin. Patient age and attenuation characteristics are key in narrowing the differential diagnosis. MR can be helpful in characterizing cystic lesions and in diagnosing thymic hyperplasia.

3.3 Middle Mediastinum/Visceral Compartment

Most middle mediastinal or visceral compartment masses represent lymphadenopathy, foregut duplication cysts, vascular lesion, or esophageal processes. They usually present with right paratracheal widening on a frontal chest radiograph or occasionally the doughnut sign on a lateral examination. As with the anterior mediastinal conditions, assessment of attenuation or intensity can be helpful. In the ITMIG model, the heart is included in this compartment. In our experience, left ventricular and left atrial conditions may occasionally simulate middle mediastinal, visceral masses.

If the mass is fluid in characteristic, the middle mediastinal mass most likely represents a foregut duplication cyst (either bronchogenic or esophageal). These cysts occasionally are higher in attenuation as a result of infection (Fig. 3.7) or hemorrhage and may even contain a fluid-calcium level from milk of calcium. The risk of malignancy in these conditions tends to almost nonexistent. As with anterior mediastinal lesions, the ratio of soft tissue to fluid needs to be considered. A foregut duplication cyst should have no soft tissue, enhancing element. If soft tissue is encountered, one must consider a potentially more significant process, usually low-attenuating lymphadenopathy. Such low-attenuating lymph nodes may be encountered in lung cancer, mucinous

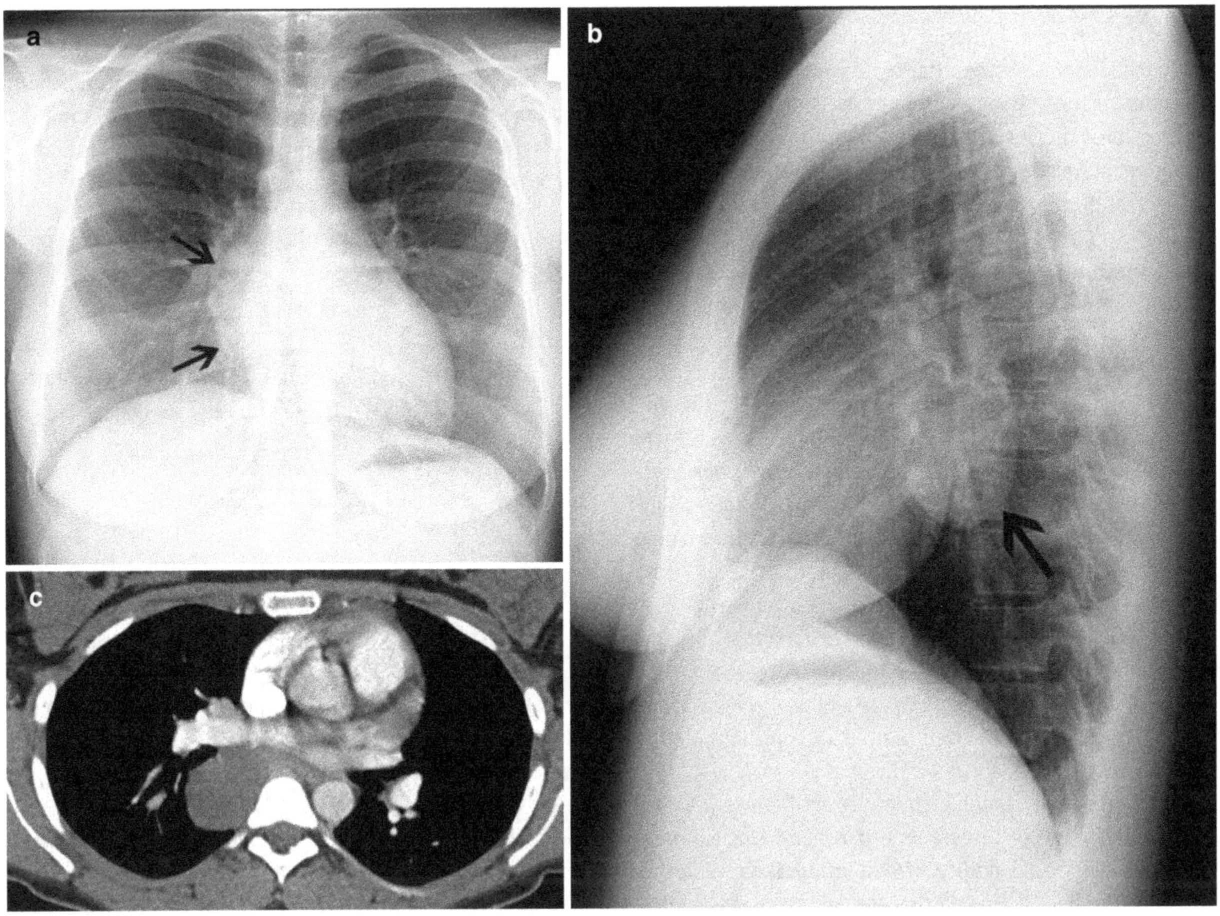

Fig. 3.7 Asymptomatic bronchogenic cyst in a 19-year-old woman incidentally discovered on a preoperative chest radiograph (**a**, **b**). There is a mass posterior to the heart (arrows in A) displacing the right lower lobe bronchovascular structures laterally but best appreciated on the lateral film (arrow in B). Contrast-enhanced chest CT (**b**) demonstrates a homogeneous mass abutting the takeoff of the right lower lobe bronchus and esophagus measuring 41HU, often encountered in duplication cysts which contain proteinaceous material. Note the absence of any thickened or enhancing septa or nodules

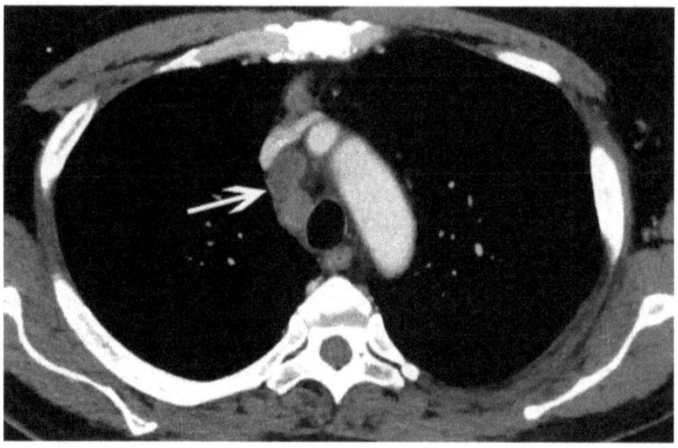

Fig. 3.8 Tuberculosis. Contrast-enhanced chest CT of a 64-year-old febrile new immigrant. Chest radiograph at presentation (**a**) demonstrates loss of the right paratracheal line which was clearly present on a baseline chest radiograph (arrow in **b**) performed 1 year earlier. Contrast-enhanced chest CT (**c**) confirms that indeed there are enlarged right paratracheal lymph nodes, some of which have peripheral enhancement and a low attenuation center (arrow). Such low attenuation lymph nodes in the correct clinical setting are highly suggestive of tuberculosis

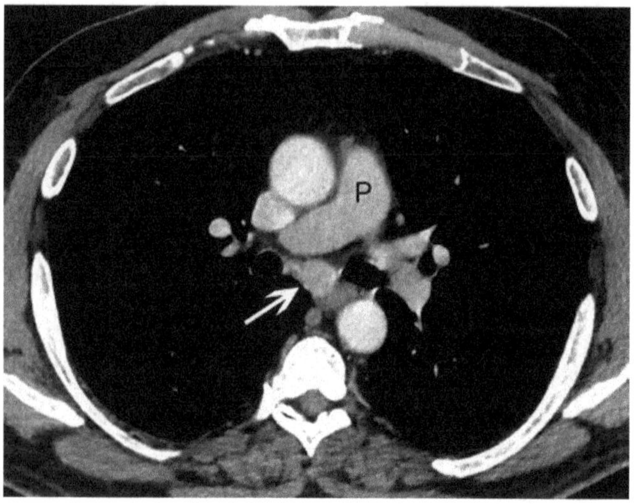

Fig. 3.9 Renal cell enhancing metastasis to the subcarinal lymph node in a 65-year-old man with renal cell carcinoma. Axial contrast-enhanced chest CT demonstrates subcarinal lymphadenopathy (arrow) at the level of the pulmonary artery (P). The subcarinal lymph node shows avid enhancement, measured as 105HU, identical to the contrast within the pulmonary artery

neoplasms, and mycobacterial disease (Fig. 3.8). In the superior mediastinum, papillary thyroid carcinoma can rarely mimic a foregut duplication cyst.

Unlike the anterior mediastinum or visceral compartment, fat cannot be considered benign. Although esophageal or tracheal lipomas and esophageal fibrovascular polyps contain fat, so may mediastinal liposarcomas. Although rare, these lesions may insinuate through the mediastinum and often have a predilection for the middle mediastinum.

Hypervascular lesions in the middle mediastinum or visceral compartment are most often hypervascular lymph nodes, or an intrathoracic extension of a goiter. Rarely a paraganglioma may present in this space. Interestingly, many of these lesions tend to abut the left atrium. The hypervascular lymph nodes (defined as higher in attenuation than skeletal muscle) may be seen with melanoma, plasmacytoma, Castleman's disease, Kaposi sarcoma, and thyroid and renal cell cancer (Fig. 3.9). When the high attenuating structure is tubular, a vessel must be considered. Aortic arch anomalies and azygous vein enlargement often present as a middle mediastinal mass on radiography. Azygous vein variants tend to enlarge on portable radiographs (when the patient is supine) compared with upright radiographs.

Most mediastinal lymphadenopathy will present in the middle mediastinum or visceral compartment. Occasionally, these nodes will be calcified. Most often these calcified nodes are indicative of an old granulomatous process such as healed tuberculosis or histoplasmosis or sarcoidosis, but care must be taken to remember that certain tumors also tend to present with calcified mediastinal lymph nodes, including ovarian serous adenocarcinomas, mucinous colon neoplasms, and osteosarcomas.

Another potential for a perceived middle mediastinal mass on radiography will be a dilated esophagus. Although a distal mass may also result in esophageal dilatation, it is usually only achalasia that results in esophageal widening that can be seen on a chest radiograph.

Key Point

- Most middle mediastinal masses will consist of lymphadenopathy, duplication cysts, vascular lesions, or esophageal masses. Attenuation characteristics of the lymphadenopathy compared to skeletal muscle can be helpful at honing in on the correct diagnosis.

3.4 Posterior Mediastinum/Paravertebral Compartment

A vast majority of posterior mediastinal or paravertebral masses will be neurogenic in origin (Fig. 3.10). In adults, these tend to be benign nerve sheath tumors, usually schwannomas and neurofibromas. In kids and younger adults, these tend to be sympathetic ganglion in origin, such as ganglioneuroblastoma, neuroblastoma, or ganglioneuroma. The key in separating the two groups is to assess the overall shape, comparing Z-axis to the XY-axis. The nerve sheath tumors tend to be spherical (equal in all three axes), while the ganglion lesions are longer in the Z-axis and are more cylindrical (akin to a sausage). Osseous lesions represent the second most common group of posterior mediastinal disease.

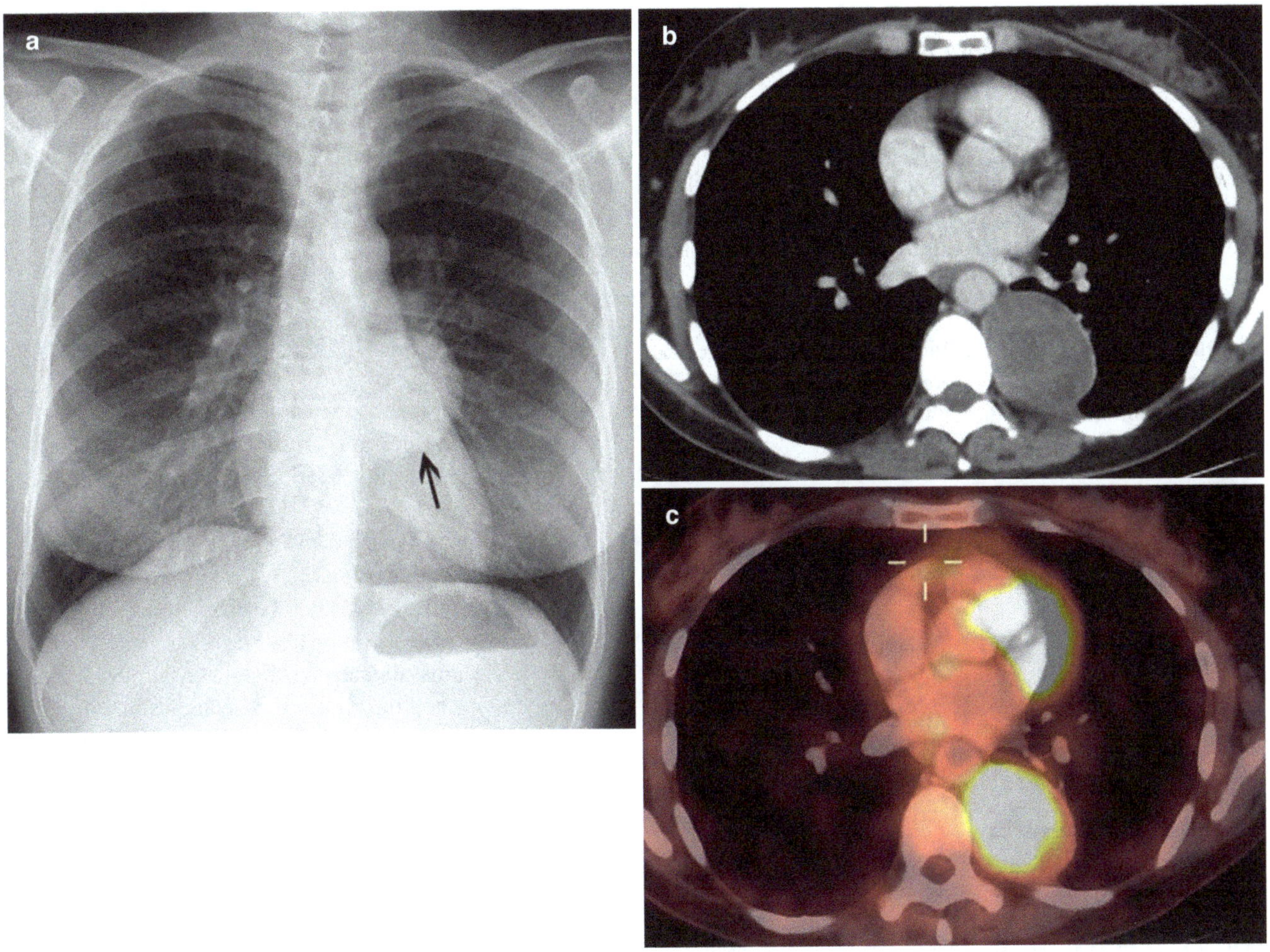

Fig. 3.10 Benign peripheral nerve sheath tumor. Frontal chest radiograph in an asymptomatic 51-year-old woman demonstrates a posterior mediastinal mass (arrow). Contrast-enhanced chest CT (**b**) at the level of the heart demonstrates the mass is centered in the paravertebral mediastinum. FDG PET/CT (**c**) revealed the mass was FDG avid with an SUVmax of 6.8. Most masses in this location represent benign peripheral nerve sheath tumors. Their FDG avidity is variable and may be very high despite being benign

Although metastases are often considered, one cannot forget about diskitis/osteomyelitis. This latter condition can present with insidious back pain and can easily be overlooked.

As with the other compartments, attenuation or intensity can be helpful. On CT, a potential pitfall is that myelin-rich neurogenic lesions may look cystic. For this reason, we often rely on MR with posterior mediastinal/paravertebral lesions. True posterior mediastinal cystic lesions are rare. Although neuroenteric cysts exist, they are often associated with vertebral anomalies and rarely encountered de novo in adults. Instead, a cystic lesion in the posterior mediastinum is much more likely to represent a lateral meningocoele or post-traumatic nerve root avulsion.

Fatty lesions are unusual in the posterior mediastinum but when encountered may invoke extramedullary hematopoiesis. Although rare, in patients with anemia, extramedullary hematopoiesis may develop in this space. The etiology of this condition remains unknown. Some authors have postulated that it develops from extruded marrow, while others have suggested that it develops from totipotent cells in the paravertebral space. When the patient is anemic, extramedullary hematopoiesis will present with bilateral masses that enhance similar to the spleen without a connecting bridge. As the patient returns to normal hematocrit, the yellow marrow will take over. The net effect is bilateral posterior mediastinal fatty masses. In the elderly, Bochladek hernias should be included in the differential diagnosis. Often the diaphragmatic defect can be seen.

Hypervascular lesions in in the posterior mediastinum or paravertebral space are less helpful than with the other compartments. Most often these are related to an aneurysmal aorta or enlarged collateral vessels as with aortic coarctation. As described above, extramedullary hematopoiesis may be seen with bilateral hypervascular paravertebral masses.

Key Point

- Most posterior mediastinal masses are neurogenic in origin. Osseous lesions, however, should not be forgotten. Mutiplanar reconstructions and MR are particularly helpful in this compartment.

3.5 Conditions that Disregard the Compartment Model

Certain conditions tend to disregard the compartment model of the mediastinum. Even with these lesions understanding the attenuation or intensity can be helpful. These include infection and hematoma, which will result in fat stranding and soft tissue attenuation throughout the mediastinum, often in more than one compartment.

Lymphangiomas and hemangiomas also tend to disregard the compartment model. The former tend to be fluid in their attenuation and insinuate throughout, while the latter will be higher in attenuation.

Of course, lung cancer may present with metastases to any compartment and unfortunately and tends to metastasize to more than one region.

Key Point
- Infections, lymphangiomas, and hematomas tend to disregard the compartmental model.

3.6 Conclusion

The mediastinum represents a space that may be impacted by a large number of lesions. Regardless whether one uses the modified Felson technique or the newer ITMIG approach, having an approach based on location and characterization will allow the radiologist the ability to create a useful, targeted differential diagnosis (Table 3.1).

Take-Home Messages
- A solid approach to the adult mediastinum uses the patient's age, lesion cross-sectional attenuation/intensity, and lesion location to generate the differential diagnosis.
- This compartment model is based on certain anatomic landmarks (Fig. 3.1).
- Although most lesions will be characterized by CT, MR may have additional value in characterizing cystic lesions, diagnosing thymic hyperplasia and separating neurogenic from osseous lesions in the posterior mediastinum/paravertebral compartment.

Table 3.1 Location and characteristic approach to mediastinal masses in the adult

Mediastinal compartment	Most common	Fluid	Fat	Hypervascular
Anterior/prevascular	Thymoma Lymphoma Germ cell tumor	Thymic cyst Pericardial cyst Lymphoma	Teratoma Thymolipoma Fat pad Morgagni hernia	Heart* Coronary arteries* Ascending aorta* Parathyroid adenoma
Middle/visceral	Lymphadenopathy Duplication cyst Vascular anomaly	Duplication cyst Lymphadenopathy	Lipoma Liposarcoma Fibrovascular polyp Hiatal hernia	Arch anomaly Azygous vein Lymph nodes Goiter Heart*
Posterior/paravertebral	Neurogenic Osseous met Diskitis	Neurenteric cyst Lateral meningocoele Traumatic	Extramedullary hematopoiesis Bochladek hernia	Aorta or collaterals
More than one	Infection Hematoma Lung cancer	Lymphangioma	Liposarcoma Lipomatosis	Hemangioma

The main difference between the older Felson technique and the newer ITMIG approach is inclusion of the heart in anterior mediastinum vs. visceral compartment. The conditions marked with an asterisk (*) may vary on localization based on technique used

Suggested Readings

Adam A, Hochholzer L. Ganglioneuroblastoma of the posterior mediastinum: a clinicopathologic review of 80 cases. Cancer. 1981;47:373–81.

Baron RL, Sagel SS, Baglan RJ. Thymic cysts following radiation therapy for Hodgkin disease. Radiology. 1981;141:593–7.

Carter BW, Benveniste MF, Madam R, et al. ITMIG classification of mediastinal compartments and multidisciplinary approach to mediastinal masses. RadioGraphics. 2017;37:413–36.

Chen JL, Weisbrod GL, Herman SJ. Computed tomography and pathologic correlations of thymic lesions. J Thorac Imaging. 1988;3:61–5.

Cohen AJ, Thompson LN, Edwards FH, et al. Primary cysts and tumours of the mediastinum. Ann Thorac Surg. 1991;51:378–86.

Do YS, Im JG, Lee BH, et al. CT findings in malignant tumors of thymic epithelium. J Comput Assist Tomogr. 1995;19:192–7.

Erasmus JJ, McAdams HP, Donnelly LF, Spritzer CE. MR imaging of mediastinal masses. Magn Reson Imaging Clin North Am. 2000;8:59–89.

Faul JL, Berry GJ, Colby TV, et al. Thoracic lymphangiomas, lymphangiectasis, lymphangiomatosis, and lymphatic dysplasia syndrome. Am J Respir Crit Care Med. 2000;161:1037–46.

Gaerte SC, Meyer CA, Winer-Muram HT, et al. Fat-containing lesions of the chest. RadioGraphics. 2002;22:615–78.

Hoffman OA, Gillespie DJ, Aughenbaugh GL, Brown LR. Primary mediastinal neoplasms (other than thymoma). Mayo Clin Proc. 1993;68:880–91.

Jeung M-Y, Gasser B, Gangi A, et al. Imaging of cystic masses of the mediastinum. RadioGraphics. 2002;22:S79–93.

Jolles H, Henry DA, Roberson JP, et al. Mediastinitis following median sternotomy: CT findings. Radiology. 1996;201:463–6.

Knapp RH, Hurt RD, Payne WS, et al. Malignant germ cell tumors of the mediastinum. J Thorac Cardiovasc Surg. 1985;89:82–9.

Long JA Jr, Doppman JL, Nienhuis AW. Computed tomographic studies of thoracic extramedullary hematopoiesis. J Comput Assist Tomogr. 1980;4:67–70.

Moeller KH, Rosado-de-Christenson ML, Templeton PA. Mediastinal mature teratoma: imaging features. Am J Roentgenol. 1997;169:985–90.

McAdams HP, Rosado-de-Christenson M, Fishback NF, Templeton PA. Castleman disease of the thorax: radiologic features with clinical and histopathologic correlation. Radiology. 1998;209:221–8.

Miles J, Pennybacker J, Sheldon P. Intrathoracic meningocele. Its development and association with neurofibromatosis. J Neurol Neurosurg Psychiatry. 1969;32:99–110.

Miyake H, Shiga M, Takaki H, et al. Mediastinal lymphangiomas in adults: CT findings. J Thorac Imaging. 1996;11:83–5.

Moran CA, Suster S. Primary germ cell tumors of the mediastinum: I. Analysis of 322 cases with special emphasis on teratomatous lesions and a proposal for histopathologic classification and clinical staging. Cancer. 1997;80:681–90.

Nakata H, Nakayama C, Kimoto T, et al. Computed tomography of mediastinal bronchogenic cysts. J Comput Assist Tomogr. 1982;6:733–8.

Pombo F, Rodriguez E, Mato J, et al. Patterns of contrast enhancement of tuberculous lymph nodes demonstrated by computed tomography. Clin Radiol. 1992;46:13–7.

Riccardo Marano MD, Carlo Liguori MD, Giancarlo Savino MD, et al. Cardiac silhouette findings and mediastinal lines and stripes radiograph and CT scan correlation. Chest. 2011;139:1186–96.

Rosado-de-Christenson ML, Galobardes J, Moran CA. Thymoma: radiologic–pathologic correlation. RadioGraphics. 1992;12:151–68.

Rosado-de-Christenson ML, Pugatch RD, Moran CA, Galobardes J. Thymolipoma: analysis of 27 cases. Radiology. 1994;193:121–6.

Rosado-de-Christenson ML, Templeton PA, Moran CA. From the archives of the AFIP. Mediastinal germ cell tumors: radiologic and pathologic correlation. RadioGraphics. 1992;12:1013–30.

Rossi SE, McAdams HP, Rosado-de-Christenson ML, et al. Fibrosing mediastinitis. RadioGraphics. 2001;21:737–57.

Shaffer K, Rosado-de-Christenson ML, Patz EF Jr, et al. Thoracic lymphangioma in adults: CT and MR imaging features. Am J Roentgenol. 1994;162:283–9.

Spizarny DL, Rebner M, Gross BH. CT evaluation of enhancing mediastinal masses. J Comput Assist Tomogr. 1987;11:990–3.

Strollo DC, Rosado-de-Christenson ML. Tumors of the thymus. J Thorac Imaging. 1999;14:152–71.

Strollo DC, Rosado de Christenson ML, Jett JR. Primary mediastinal tumors. Part 1: tumours of the anterior mediastinum. Chest. 1997;112:511–22.

Strollo DC, Rosado-de-Christenson ML, Jett JR. Primary mediastinal tumors: part II. Tumours of the middle and posterior mediastinum. Chest. 1997;112:1344–57.

Suwatanapongched T, Gierada DS. CT of thoracic lymph nodes. Part II: diseases and pitfalls. Br J Radiol. 2006;79:999–1006.

Takahashi K, Al-Janabi NJ. Computed tomography and magnetic resonance imaging of mediastinal tumors. J Magn Reson Imaging. 2010;32:1325–39.

Thacker PG, Mahani MG, Heider A, Lee EY. Imaging evaluation of mediastinal masses in children and adults practical diagnostic approach based on a new classification system. Thorac Imaging. 2015;30:247–67.

Whitten CR, Khan S, Munneke GJ, Grubnic S. A diagnostic approach to mediastinal abnormalities. RadioGraphics. 2007;27:657–71.

Woodring JH, Loh FK, Kryscio RJ. Mediastinal hemorrhage: an evaluation of radiographic manifestations. Radiology. 1984;151:15–21.

Zylak CJ, Eyler WR, Spizarny DL, Stone CH. Developmental lung anomalies in the adult: radiologic-pathologic correlation. RadioGraphics. 2002;22:S25–43.

Zylak CJ, Pallie W, Jackson R. Correlative anatomy and computed tomography: a module on the mediastinum. RadioGraphics. 1982;2(4):555–92.

4

Plain Film and HRCT Diagnosis of Interstitial Lung Disease

Sujal R. Desai, Helmut Prosch, and Jeffrey R. Galvin

Learning Objectives

- To learn how to systematically approach HRCTs of interstitial lung diseases.
- To become familiar with the most important interstitial lung diseases.

There is little doubt that imaging tests have a central role in the investigation of patients with suspected and established diffuse interstitial lung diseases (DILD). In most cases, physicians who manage patients with DILD will request a plain chest radiograph. However, high-resolution computed tomography (HRCT) is usually indicated, particularly at the initial review. HRCT, for a variety of reasons discussed below, is superior to plain radiography. In many cases where, historically, biopsy might have been considered mandatory, there has been a paradigm shift because of HRCT. For example, in some patients with idiopathic pulmonary fibrosis (characterized by the histological pattern of usual interstitial pneumonia), the HRCT appearance may be characteristic enough to render biopsy unnecessary [4, 22, 58]. In instances where a radiological diagnosis is not possible, HRCT may provide guidance as to the best site for surgical biopsy. More recently, HRCT has moved into the realms of prognostic evaluation and disease staging [11, 16, 56, 59].

S. R. Desai
Royal Brompton Hospital, London, UK
e-mail: s.desai@rbht.nhs.uk

H. Prosch
Department of Biomedical Imaging and Image-guided Therapy, Medical University of Vienna, Vienna, Austria
e-mail: helmut.prosch@meduniwien.ac.at

J. R. Galvin (✉)
University of Maryland, Silver Spring, MD, USA

4.1 The HRCT Technique

In the era of multi-detector row CT machines, a brief reminder of the HRCT technique is pertinent. The two technical features that differentiate HRCT imaging from conventional CT are, first, the narrow x-ray beam collimation that significantly improves spatial resolution and, second, the use of a dedicated reconstruction algorithm [35]. The "high-frequency" algorithm effectively exaggerates the naturally high-contrast milieu of the lungs (i.e., aerated lung versus more solid elements) [35]. The conspicuity of vessels, small bronchi, and interlobular septa is increased compared to conventional (thick-section) CT images [38]. An important downside of high-frequency algorithms is the increased visibility of image noise, although, in practice, this generally does not hamper radiological interpretation.

4.2 HRCT in Diffuse Interstitial Lung Disease

The term DILD is a convenient "catch-all" for a heterogeneous group of disorders (Table 4.1) [4]. The DILDs have been subcategorized as follows: (a) DILDs that have a known etiology (e.g., secondary to exposure to certain drugs or a connective tissue disorder); (b) the idiopathic interstitial pneumonias (which themselves have undergone classification [5] and a more recent update [52]); (c) the granulomatous DILDs; and (d) a group of diffuse lung diseases that include Langerhans cell histiocytosis and lymphangioleiomyomatosis.

In patients with established diffuse lung disease, HRCT will not only detect but also characterize parenchymal abnormalities with greater accuracy than plain chest radiography. One important caveat is that in patients with nodular infiltrates, traditional "interspaced" HRCT images may mislead; on thin-section images, the dimensions of nodules and pulmonary vessels may be comparable, which makes distinction difficult [47]. This is unlikely to be an issue on thin-section

Table 4.1 Classification of diffuse interstitial lung diseases (DILD)

DILD with known cause
• Connective tissue disorders
• Rheumatoid arthritis
• Asbestosis
• Hypersensitivity pneumonitis
• Others
Idiopathic interstitial pneumonias
• Idiopathic pulmonary fibrosis
• Idiopathic non-specific interstitial pneumonia
• Respiratory bronchiolitis interstitial lung disease
• Desquamative interstitial pneumonia
• Acute interstitial pneumonia
• Pleuroparenchymal fibroelastosis
Granulomatous DILD
• Sarcoidosis
• Silicosis
• Hypersensitivity pneumonia
• Drug-induced DILD
• Combined variable immune deficiency syndrome
• Others
Other DILD
• Langerhans cell histiocytosis
• Lymphangioleiomyomatosis
• Lymphoid interstitial pneumonia
• Birt-Hogg-Dubé syndrome
• Alveolar proteinosis
• Others

volumetric acquisitions. In practice, the range of CT features that commonly indicate the presence of ILD is relatively limited. Thus, radiologists will typically encounter some combination of reticulation, ground-glass opacification, honeycombing, dilatation of airways in regions of reticulation and ground-glass opacification ('traction bronchiectasis'), nodules, and thickening of the interlobular septa [17].

Findings at HRCT generally reflect the *macroscopic* abnormalities seen by the pathologist. This was elegantly demonstrated in the very early days of HRCT by Müller and colleagues who showed that morphologic features in patients with idiopathic pulmonary fibrosis—at that time still known by the moniker "cryptogenic fibrosing alveolitis"—reflected the histopathological changes [37]. A reticular pattern was seen in seven of nine patients and corresponded to areas of irregular fibrosis at microscopy.

Not surprisingly, because there is no anatomical superimposition, the sensitivity of HRCT is better than that of chest radiography. However, a more important issue than sensitivity is the confidence and accuracy with which a diagnosis can be made. In the oft-quoted landmark study by Mathieson and colleagues, experienced chest radiologists were asked to independently indicate up to three diagnoses, on chest radiographs and CT, in 118 patients with a variety of biopsy-confirmed ILDs [34]. Importantly, for the first-choice diagnosis, readers were asked to assign a level of confidence. The first important finding of this study (which effectively put HRCT on the map), was that, compared with chest radiography, a confident diagnosis was made nearly *twice* as often with HRCT. The second, and perhaps more striking, message was that when experienced radiologists were confident of the diagnosis on HRCT, they were almost always correct [34]; by contrast, a confident diagnosis on chest x-ray (which, incidentally, was offered in only one-quarter of cases) was associated with a significantly lower rate of correct diagnoses.

The results of subsequent studies have not always mirrored those of the initial study by Mathieson [34, 42]. However, because of study design, the majority of the comparative studies in HRCT likely undervalued its true utility [58]: first, there was no recourse to pretest probabilities for observers in early series, and, therefore, these do not accurately reflect clinical practice. Second, radiologists (and specifically those with an interest in thoracic disease) have become increasingly familiar with the spectrum of HRCT patterns and disease. This, almost certainly, would be associated with a proportionate increase in the confidence of *experienced* observers in making HRCT diagnoses, were such a study to be repeated today. Some justification for this last statement comes from a study that addressed the clinically vexing issue of "end-stage" lung disease [43], in which two experienced thoracic radiologists independently made correct first-choice diagnoses in just under 90% of cases with nearly two-thirds being made with high confidence. On first inspection, these data seem less than impressive. However, the results of open lung biopsy (the supposed "gold-standard" for the diagnosis of DILD) are often inconclusive, in part, no doubt, relating to the degree of observer variability between pathologists [39].

Key Point
- HRCT is the modality of choice for the investigation of patients with a suspected DILD.

4.3 An Approach to HRCT Diagnoses

It may come as some comfort to delegates that HRCT interpretation can be difficult, even for trained thoracic radiologists! This is not surprising given the sheer numbers of documented DILDs. This wide spectrum of disorders manifests with a relatively small number of histopathological patterns (e.g., fibrosis, consolidation, intra-alveolar hemorrhage), which, in turn, are reflected by a similarly select group of HRCT features (i.e., reticulation, ground-glass opacification, nodularity, thickening of interlobular septa). However, with a systematic approach to HRCT interpretation, the observer should, in time, be able to offer a sensible (and manageably short) list of differential diagnoses. To this end, a proposed schema, presented in the form of questions that the observer should ask (in roughly the order given), is provided as follows.

4.3.1 Is There a "Real" Abnormality?

This is a crucial first question: the radiologist must first determine whether what is shown on HRCT represents real disease. CT features attributable to technical factors/normal variation (for instance, caused by a poor inspiratory effort, inadequate mAs, regions of physiologically dependent atelectasis) must not be overinterpreted and reported as "disease." Making the distinction between normality and abnormality can also be difficult when there is apparently minimal disease or, conversely, when there is diffuse abnormality (e.g., subtle but widespread decreased [mosaicism] or increased [ground-glass opacity] attenuation).

4.3.2 If There Is An Abnormality, What Is/Are the Predominant HRCT Pattern(s)?

Having decided that there is a definite abnormality on HRCT, the observer should attempt to identify the dominant pattern(s) using only the standard radiological terms [17]. The use of nonstandard terminology (e.g., patchy opacification, parenchymal opacities), or descriptive terms in which there is an implied pathology (e.g., interstitial pattern or alveolitis) is misleading and best avoided.

4.3.3 What Is the Distribution of Disease?

Many DILDs have a predilection for certain zones. Therefore, an evaluation of dominant distribution is of diagnostic value. For instance, it is known that, in the majority of patients with idiopathic pulmonary fibrosis (IPF), disease tends to be most obvious in the mid- to lower zones. This contrasts with fibrosis in patients with sarcoidosis, which typically has a predilection for the upper lobes. In addition to this, the radiologist should take note of the axial distribution (i.e., central versus peripheral), which, in contrast to CXR, can readily be made on HRCT, is of potential value. Using the example of IPF and sarcoidosis again, the former is commonly peripheral (subpleural), whereas, in the latter, disease tends to be central (and bronchocentric). A final example is seen in patients with organizing pneumonia where consolidation may have a striking perilobular predilection [53].

Table 4.2 Differential diagnosis of micronodular diseases based on the distribution type

Centrilobular distribution
- Bronchial diseases
  - Infections
  - Hypersensitivity pneumonia
  - Respiratory bronchiolitis
  - Follicular bronchiolitis
- Vascular diseases
  - Pulmonary edema
  - Vasculitis
  - Pulmonary hypertension
  - Metastatic calcification

Perilymphatic distribution
- Sarcoidosis
- Lymphangitic carcinomatosis
- Pneumoconiosis

Random distribution
- Miliary TB
- Viral infections
- Metastases

In addition to zonal distribution, the distribution on the level of the secondary pulmonary nodule can also be of diagnostic value. This is particularly true for micronodular diseases in which the allocation of nodules to one of the three distribution types (centrilobular, perilymphatic, random) is of use to narrow the differential diagnosis (Table 4.2).

4.3.4 Are There Any Ancillary Findings?

Ancillary HRCT features may suggest or, indeed, exclude certain diagnoses. Thus, the presence or absence of the following may be of diagnostic value in specific cases:

1. *Pleural thickening/effusions/plaques (± calcification)*—may suggest asbestos-related lung disease as opposed to IPF as a possible cause of lung fibrosis.
2. *Lymph node enlargement (hilar/mediastinal)*—reactive intrathoracic nodal enlargement is a recognized "normal" in fibrotic DILDs. However, symmetrical hilar nodal enlargement may suggest a diagnosis of sarcoidosis or occupational lung disease. Intrathoracic nodal enlargement is uncommon in pulmonary vasculitis (e.g., Wegener's granulomatosis).
3. *Bronchiectasis*—coexistent suppurative airway disease in a patient who has established pulmonary fibrosis may point to a diagnosis of an underlying connective tissue disease, such as rheumatoid arthritis.
4. *A dilatation of the esophagus in a patient with CT findings suggesting a non-*specific interstitial pneumonia points toward scleroderma as the underlying disease.

4.3.5 What Is the Likely Pathology?

A knowledge of the relationships between HRCT appearance and the possible histopathological correlates is crucial. Thus, in a patient with predominant consolidation, it is reasonable to conclude that the dominant pathology involves the air spaces, whereas, with reticulation, the pathological process likely affects the interstitium.

4.3.6 What Is the Clinical Background?

Clinical data must always be integrated when formulating a radiological opinion. However, it is often advisable to review the clinical information *after* the evaluation of radiological features. This is particularly true at the very start of HRCT interpretation when the radiologist is deciding whether or not there is a "real" abnormality (see above). Specific clinical features that may be of importance in HRCT interpretation include basic demographic data (age, gender, ethnicity), potential exposures (smoking history, contact with animals, occupation), the time course of the illness (i.e., have symptoms developed over hours and days or weeks and months?), and any relevant past medical history.

4.4 HRCT Appearances in Select DILDs

A working knowledge of the relationship between histopathological changes and HRCT patterns and the typical appearance of common DILDs is of value in day-to-day practice. The following section briefly considers the HRCT appearance in a few DILDs.

4.4.1 Usual Interstitial Pneumonia/Idiopathic Pulmonary Fibrosis

Usual interstitial pneumonia (UIP) is the most common form of chronic fibrosing lung diseases. At low-power microscopy, there is temporally heterogeneous fibrosis admixed with areas of unaffected lung [4]. In areas of fibrosis, there will be characteristic honeycombing. The disease has a striking basal and subpleural predilection. UIP can be caused by a variety of diseases, including connective tissue diseases, chronic hypersensitivity pneumonia, pneumoconiosis, and, in rare cases, also by sarcoidosis. The most common cause of UIP, however, is idiopathic pulmonary fibrosis (IPF), in which no underlying diseases can be diagnosed [45]. IPF is the most common IIP, and, with a median survival from time-to-diagnosis between 2 and 3 years, the one with the worst prognosis [45]. As current treatments are considered to prolong survival, a timely and confident diagnosis of IPF is of paramount importance.

To make a diagnosis of a 'UIP pattern' on HRCT, the radiologist must, therefore, look for the following: i) a reticular pattern; ii) honeycombing (with or without traction bronchiectasis); and iii) a subpleural, basal distribution of disease [45]. The radiologist must also ensure that there are no changes to suggest other diagnoses (i.e., mid/upper zone predominance, a peribronchovascular predominance with subpleural sparing, extensive pure ground-glass, widespread micronodularity, multiple cysts [away from areas of honeycombing], and extensive mosaic attenuation with extensive sharply defined lobular air-trapping on expiration and consolidation) [31] (Fig. 4.1). In the absence of honeycombing (but with the other features listed above), an HRCT diagnosis of 'probable UIP' can be made.

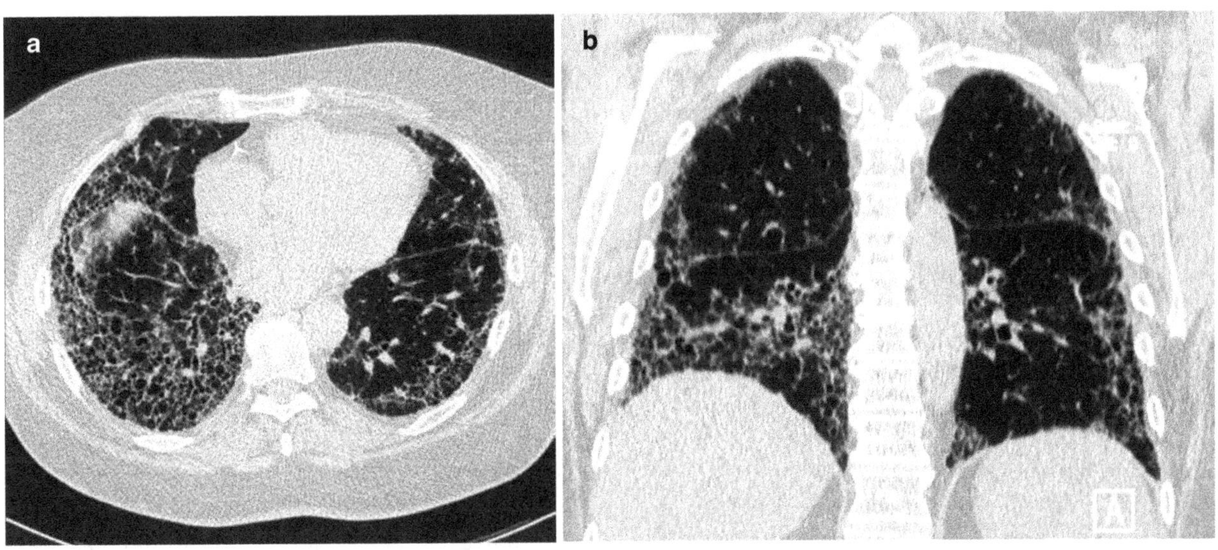

Fig. 4.1 Axial (**a**) and coronal (**b**) reformations of a 72-year-old female patient with progressive dyspnea on exertion. There are reticular abnormalities and honeycombing with basal and subpleural abnormalities. As there are no changes to suggest other diagnoses, the diagnosis of UIP can be made without histological confirmation

The presence of a UIP pattern on HRCT is accurate and obviates histologic confirmation [22, 31, 44, 46]. In patients with a CT pattern of a "probable UIP" and a high clinical likelihood of IPF (age >60 years, current or former smoker, no other potential causes of fibrosis), a confident diagnosis of IPF can be made without a biopsy [31]. However, atypical appearances may be present in over half of patients with biopsy-proven disease [13, 50].

Key Point

- Idiopathic pulmonary fibrosis is the most common IIP and a specific chronic, progressive, fibrosing interstitial pneumonia.

4.4.2 (Cryptogenic) Organizing Pneumonia

Organization is a common response to lung injury and is part of the normal process of lung repair. It is represented on histology by plugs of fibroblastic tissue that fill the alveolar spaces. This same fibroblastic tissue may be identified in respiratory and terminal bronchioles, explaining the use of the older term "bronchiolitis obliterans organizing pneumonia" (BOOP), but which has been replaced by organizing pneumonia (OP) [5]. Organizing pneumonia was first recognized in 1923 as a response to unresolved pneumonia [51]. Most cases are likely to be post-infectious; however, the pathogen is rarely recovered. The OP pattern is also a common feature in a wide range of other diseases including collagen vascular disease, hypersensitivity pneumonitis, chronic eosinophilic pneumonia, drug reaction, and radiation-induced lung injury. The appearance of OP on imaging is highly variable depending on the prior injury and the stage at which it is imaged [26]. A minority of cases present as solitary pulmonary nodules or focal areas of consolidation. However, the dominant finding in OP is bilateral consolidation that is peripheral, often with sparing of the subpleural portion of the lung (Fig. 4.2). Opacities are often perilobular and may be associated with septal lines. In some patients, OP may progress to an NSIP pattern of fibrosis. Although many patients with OP will clear with steroids, a substantial minority are left with significant disability due to pulmonary fibrosis [3, 26, 29].

Most cases of OP respond quite rapidly to steroid treatment. Recurrences are frequently observed, particularly in patients subsequent to a too-short steroid treatment.

Key Point

- Organizing pneumonia is a non-specific response to lung injury and is characterized by a filling of the alveolar space with fibroblastic tissue.

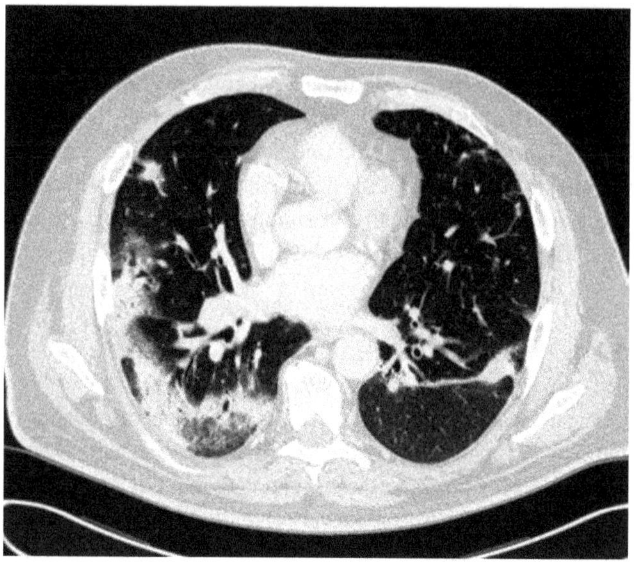

Fig. 4.2 Axial CT scan of a 64-year-old male patient with a treatment-resistant pneumonia. The CT scan shows bilateral peripheral consolidation, with sparing of the subpleural portion of the lung. The findings are suggestive of an organizing pneumonia

4.4.3 Non-specific Interstitial Pneumonia

After UIP, non-specific interstitial pneumonia (NSIP) is the most common pattern of idiopathic interstitial pneumonias (IIP) and is associated with a better rate of survival [12, 13, 52]. This pattern of IIP may be idiopathic but, more commonly, is seen in a variety of clinical contexts, including connective tissue disorders (especially systemic sclerosis) and as a consequence of drug-related toxicity. At a histologic level, there are varying amounts of interstitial inflammation and fibrosis, which, in stark contrast to what is seen in UIP, have a temporally and spatially uniform appearance.

On HRCT, one of the key findings is ground-glass opacification, which is typically bilateral and symmetrically distributed in the lower zones [12, 33] (Fig. 4.3). A (relative) sparing of the subpleural space is seen in up to 43% of the cases [49]. In some patients, over time, the extent of ground-glass may decrease and become replaced by reticulation (i.e., with UIP-like features) [49]. Reticulation (generally without significant honeycombing) is usually also present.

Key Point

- NSIP is most commonly seen in patients with connective tissue disorders and, on HRCT, is characterized by symmetrical, bilateral ground-glass opacification with a basal predominance.

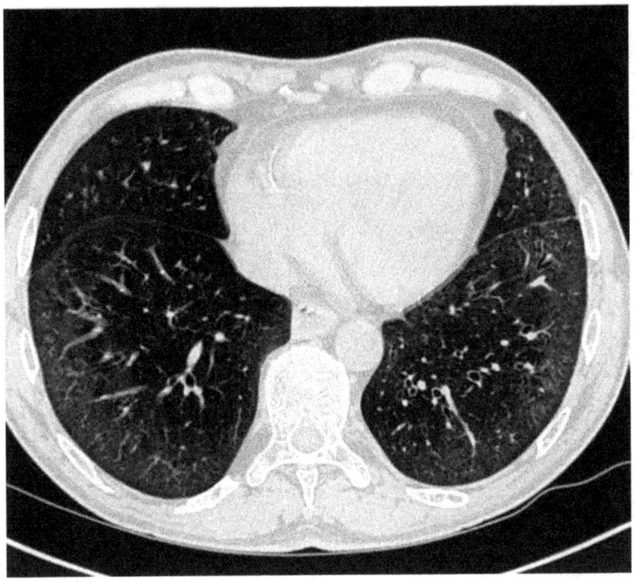

Fig. 4.3 Axial CT scan of a 61-year-old female patient with known scleroderma. The CT scan shows symmetrical, peripheral, extensive ground-glass opacities, with a relative sparing of the subpleural space. The findings are highly suggestive of a non-specific interstitial pneumonia (NSIP)

4.4.4 Smoking-Related Lung Diseases

Respiratory bronchiolitis (RB), of variable severity, is an almost invariable pathologic finding in all smokers [41]. Importantly, this pathologic lesion is asymptomatic and not associated with physiologic impairment in the vast majority of cases. However, in a small minority of cases, there will be the clinical manifestations of an interstitial lung disease—it is this clinico-pathologic/radiologic entity that has been called respiratory bronchiolitis interstitial lung disease (RBILD). The cardinal HRCT signs of RB/RBILD include "soft" centrilobular nodules, ground-glass opacification, smooth thickening of the interlobular septa, and lobular foci of decreased attenuation [10, 21, 36].

Desquamative interstitial pneumonia (DIP) was first described by Liebow in 1965. Dyspneic patients with DIP were found to have numerous inflammatory cells in the alveolar spaces [30]. The cells were thought to be desquamated pneumocytes but are now recognized as the same macrophages identified in patients with RB and RB-ILD; the majority of patients with DIP are heavy smokers, and it is now considered part of the spectrum of inflammatory lung disease related to the inhalation of cigarette smoke [21]. Patients with DIP suffer an increased incidence of pulmonary fibrosis that fits the histologic pattern of NSIP [9, 60]. Imaging in patients with DIP is typified by homogeneous or patchy areas of ground-glass opacity in the mid and lower lung zones [9, 20].

In adults, Langerhans cell histiocytosis (LCH) is isolated to the lungs in approximately 90% of cases. Although the pathogenesis is unknown, almost all of the patients are cigarette smokers. PLCH is characterized by bronchiocentric collections of Langerhans cells admixed with a variety of other inflammatory cells, forming a stellate nodule [55]. Over time, infiltration of the airway wall results in damage to the airway wall and subsequent dilatation of the airway [23]. In the late stage of PLCH, small stellate scars are surrounded by emphysematous spaces. The imaging reflects the histologic progression with early bronchiocentric nodules in the upper lobes, progressing to a combination of bizarre-shaped cysts and nodules [1, 28] (Fig. 4.4). In the final stages, the appearance may be indistinguishable from severe bullous emphysema.

It is important to recognize that findings of RB, DIP, pulmonary LCH, and the NSIP pattern of fibrosis commonly coexist in biopsies of dyspneic smokers. Some of the histologic changes are reflected on imaging, while others are below the resolution of chest computed tomography.

The relationship between cigarette smoke and fibrosis remains contentious [8, 10, 15, 24, 25, 61, 62]. Niewoehner's original description of RB did not include fibrosis of the alveolar wall [41]. However, there is substantial support for a relationship between cigarette smoke exposure and a pattern of alveolar wall fibrosis other than UIP [2, 6, 14, 24, 27, 40, 57]. In our experience, there is a group of dyspneic cigarette smokers who present with a combination of well-formed cystic spaces on computed tomography that follow the typical, upper lobe-predominant distribution of smoking-related emphysema, with variable surrounding ground-glass opacity and reticulation that may extend into the lower lung zones [15]. The patients commonly present with strikingly normal flows and volumes on pulmonary function testing and a low diffusing capacity. The unexpectedly normal flows and volumes are the result of the opposing effects of emphysema and fibrosis [57].

4.4.5 Sarcoidosis

Noncaseating, epithelioid cell granulomata are the histopathological hallmark of sarcoidosis. Granulomata distribute along the lymphatics. Thus, the lymphatic pathways that surround the axial interstitium, which invests bronchovascular structures, and those that exist subpleurally (including the subpleural lymphatics along the fissures) are typically involved (Fig. 4.4). Not surprisingly, a nodular infiltrate (presumably reflecting conglomerate granulomata) with a propensity to involve the bronchovascular elements is a characteristic CT finding [7, 32]. Subpleural nodularity is also commonly seen. In the later stages of the disease, there

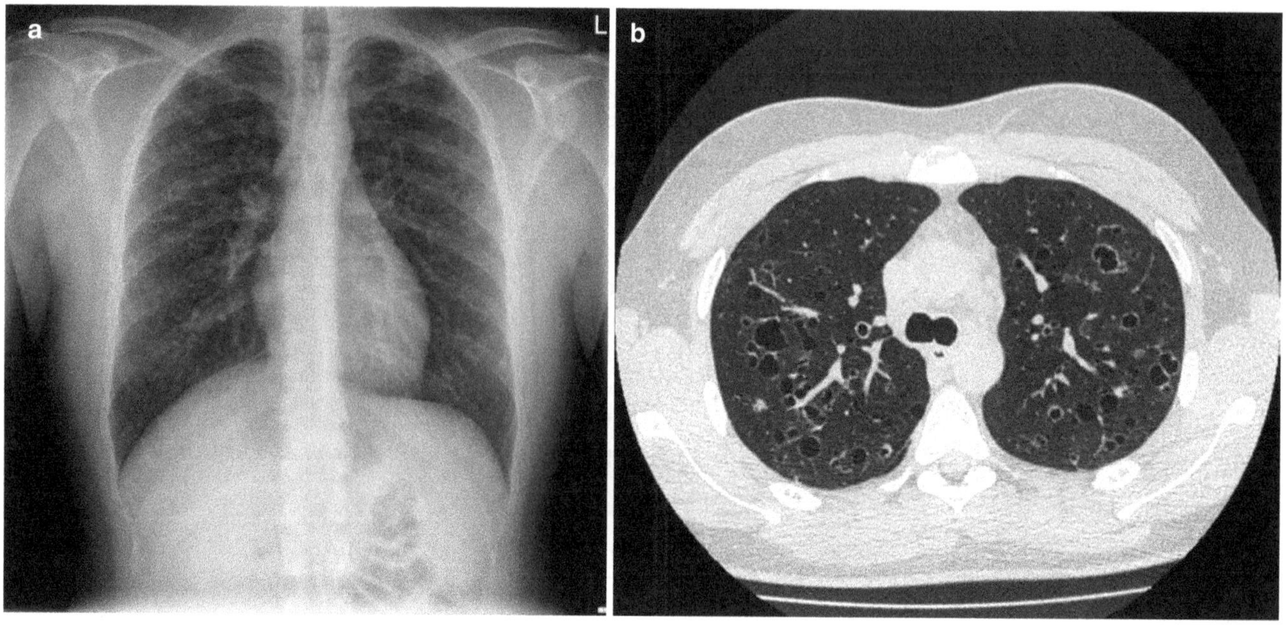

Fig. 4.4 Chest radiograph (**a**) and axial CT scan (**b**) of a 23-year-old male patient with coughing and dyspnea on exertion, which shows thin- and thick-walled cysts with an upper lobe predominance. In addition to the cysts, the CT scans also show some ill-defined nodules. The findings are highly suggestive of a Langerhans cell histiocytosis (LCH)

may be obvious signs of established lung fibrosis with upper zone volume loss, parenchymal distortion, and traction bronchiectasis. Because of the bronchocentric nature of the disease, signs of small airways disease are seen at CT in some patients with sarcoidosis [18].

Key Point

- Sarcoidosis is a systemic granulomatous disease that most frequently manifests in the chest. Granulomata in sarcoidosis tend to follow a perilymphatic distribution pattern, with a predominance in the upper lung zones.

4.4.6 Hypersensitivity Pneumonitis

Exposure to a range of organic antigens will cause lung disease in some patients, probably due to an immunologically mediated response. In the subacute stage, there is an interstitial infiltrate comprising lymphocytes and plasma cells, with a propensity for small airways (bronchioles) involvement. Scattered noncaseating granulomata may be seen. Predictably, at CT, there is diffuse ground-glass opacification, ill-defined centrilobular nodules and lobular areas of decreased attenuation on images performed at end-expiration [19, 48] (Fig. 4.5). The CT appearance in subacute hypersensitivity pneumonitis may be identical to that in patients with respiratory bronchiolitis-associated interstitial lung disease (RBILD) [10]. However, consideration of the smoking history may help in differentiation: a history of smoking is the norm in the vast majority of patients with RBILD, whereas cigarette smoke appears to lead to a relative protection against the development of hypersensitivity pneumonitis.

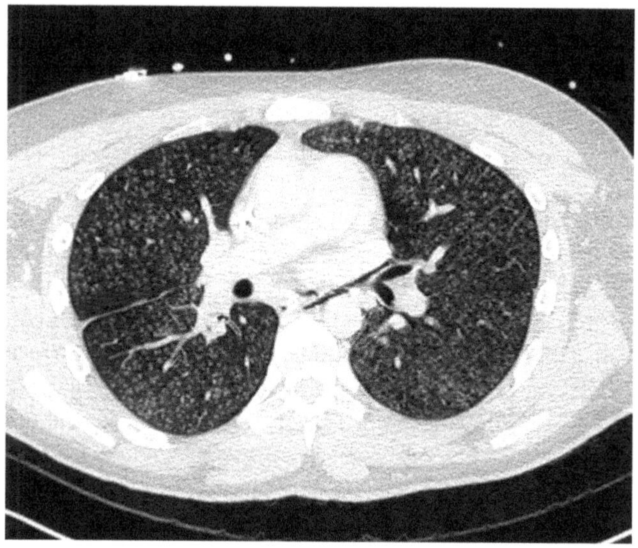

Fig. 4.5 Axial CT scan of a 19-year-old male patient with flu-like symptoms for some weeks. The CT scan shows countless ill-defined centrilobular nodules. The suspicion of an acute hypersensitivity pneumonia could be confirmed by a high lymphocyte count at bronchoscopy and by the history of exposure to mold

Chronic hypersensitivity pneumonia (CHP) is the consequence of a prolonged or repetitive course of acute HP and is characterized by fibrotic changes on HRCT and/or histology [54]. On HRCT, CHP is characterized by the presence of reticular abnormalities and traction bronchiectasis, with a predominance in the upper and middle lung fields, and frequently shows a peribronchovascular accentuation with subpleural sparing [54]. Honeycombing is observed in up to 69% of the cases [54]. Centrilobular nodules, air trapping, and/or a mosaic pattern in a patient with a fibrosing lung disease is a good clue to the diagnosis of CHP.

4.5 Concluding Remarks

HRCT plays a central role in the differential diagnosis of DILD. The final diagnosis requires a combination of radiological, clinical, and serological information, which is best accomplished in an interdisciplinary discussion. In many cases, the diagnosis achieved in this way is so confident that a histopathological confirmation is not necessary.

Take-Home Messages

- DILDs require a systematic analysis of the HRCT.
- The HRCT differential diagnosis of DILD is based on a systematic analysis of the predominant CT pattern, the ancillary CT findings, and the distribution of the findings.
- The final diagnosis of DILDs should be made in an interdisciplinary discussion.

References

1. Abbott GF, Rosado-De-Christenson ML, Franks TJ, et al. From the archives of the AFIP: pulmonary Langerhans cell histiocytosis. Radiographics. 2004;24:821–41.
2. Adesina AM, Vallyathan V, Mcquillen EN, et al. Bronchiolar inflammation and fibrosis associated with smoking. A morphologic cross-sectional population analysis. Am Rev Respir Dis. 1991;143:144–9.
3. Akira M, Inoue Y, Arai T, et al. Long-term follow-up high-resolution CT findings in non-specific interstitial pneumonia. Thorax. 2011;66:61–5.
4. Anonymous. American Thoracic Society. Idiopathic pulmonary fibrosis: diagnosis and treatment. International consensus statement. American Thoracic Society (ATS), and the European Respiratory Society (ERS). Am J Respir Crit Care Med. 2000;161:646–64.
5. Anonymous. American Thoracic Society/European Respiratory Society international multidisciplinary consensus classification of the idiopathic interstitial pneumonias. This joint statement of the American Thoracic Society (ATS), and the European Respiratory Society (ERS) was adopted by the ATS board of directors, June 2001 and by the ERS executive committee, June 2001. Am J Respir Crit Care Med. 2002;165:277–304.
6. Auerbach O, Garfinkel L, Hammond EC. Relation of smoking and age to findings in lung parenchyma: a microscopic study. Chest. 1974;65:29–35.
7. Brauner MW, Grenier P, Mompoint D, et al. Pulmonary sarcoidosis: evaluation with high-resolution CT. Radiology. 1989;172:467–71.
8. Churg A, Muller NL, Wright JL. Respiratory bronchiolitis/interstitial lung disease: fibrosis, pulmonary function, and evolving concepts. Arch Pathol Lab Med. 2010;134:27–32.
9. Craig PJ, Wells AU, Doffman S, et al. Desquamative interstitial pneumonia, respiratory bronchiolitis and their relationship to smoking. Histopathology. 2004;45:275–82.
10. Desai SR, Ryan SM, Colby TV. Smoking-related interstitial lung diseases: histopathological and imaging perspectives. Clin Radiol. 2003;58:259–68.
11. Edey AJ, Devaraj AA, Barker RP, et al. Fibrotic idiopathic interstitial pneumonias: HRCT findings that predict mortality. Eur Radiol. 2011;21:1586–93.
12. Flaherty KR, Martinez FJ, Travis W, et al. Nonspecific interstitial pneumonia (NSIP). Semin Respir Crit Care Med. 2001;22:423–34.
13. Flaherty KR, Thwaite EL, Kazerooni EA, et al. Radiological versus histological diagnosis in UIP and NSIP: survival implications. Thorax. 2003;58:143–8.
14. Frasca JM, Auerbach O, Carter HW, et al. Morphologic alterations induced by short-term cigarette smoking. Am J Pathol. 1983;111:11–20.
15. Galvin JR, Franks TJ. Smoking-related lung disease. J Thorac Imaging. 2009;24:274–84.
16. Goh NS, Desai SR, Veeraraghavan S, et al. Interstitial lung disease in systemic sclerosis: a simple staging system. Am J Respir Crit Care Med. 2008;177:1248–54.
17. Hansell DM, Bankier AA, Macmahon H, et al. Fleischner society: glossary of terms for thoracic imaging. Radiology. 2008;246:697–722.
18. Hansell DM, Milne DG, Wilsher ML, et al. Pulmonary sarcoidosis: morphologic associations of airflow obstruction at thin-section CT. Radiology. 1998;209:697–704.
19. Hansell DM, Wells AU, Padley SP, et al. Hypersensitivity pneumonitis: correlation of individual CT patterns with functional abnormalities. Radiology. 1996;199:123–8.
20. Hartman TE, Primack SL, Kang EY, et al. Disease progression in usual interstitial pneumonia compared with desquamative interstitial pneumonia. Assessment with serial CT. Chest. 1996;110:378–82.
21. Heyneman LE, Ward S, Lynch DA, et al. Respiratory bronchiolitis, respiratory bronchiolitis-associated interstitial lung disease, and desquamative interstitial pneumonia: different entities or part of the spectrum of the same disease process? AJR Am J Roentgenol. 1999;173:1617–22.
22. Hunninghake GW, Zimmerman MB, Schwartz DA, et al. Utility of a lung biopsy for the diagnosis of idiopathic pulmonary fibrosis. Am J Respir Crit Care Med. 2001;164:193–6.
23. Kambouchner M, Basset F, Marchal J, et al. Three-dimensional characterization of pathologic lesions in pulmonary langerhans cell histiocytosis. Am J Respir Crit Care Med. 2002;166:1483–90.
24. Katzenstein AL, Mukhopadhyay S, Zanardi C, et al. Clinically occult interstitial fibrosis in smokers: classification and significance of a surprisingly common finding in lobectomy specimens. Hum Pathol. 2010;41:316–25.
25. Kawabata Y, Hoshi E, Murai K, et al. Smoking-related changes in the background lung of specimens resected for lung cancer: a semiquantitative study with correlation to postoperative course. Histopathology. 2008;53:707–14.
26. Kligerman SJ, Franks TJ, Galvin JR. From the radiologic pathology archives: organization and fibrosis as a response to lung injury in diffuse alveolar damage, organizing pneumonia, and acute fibrinous and organizing pneumonia. Radiographics. 2013;33:1951–75.

27. Lang MR, Fiaux GW, Gillooly M, et al. Collagen content of alveolar wall tissue in emphysematous and non-emphysematous lungs. Thorax. 1994;49:319–26.
28. Leatherwood DL, Heitkamp DE, Emerson RE. Best cases from the AFIP: pulmonary Langerhans cell histiocytosis. Radiographics. 2007;27:265–8.
29. Lee JW, Lee KS, Lee HY, et al. Cryptogenic organizing pneumonia: serial high-resolution CT findings in 22 patients. AJR Am J Roentgenol. 2010;195:916–22.
30. Liebow AA, Steer A, Billingsley JG. Desquamative interstitial pneumonia. Am J Med. 1965;39:369–404.
31. Lynch DA, Sverzellati N, Travis WD, et al. Diagnostic criteria for idiopathic pulmonary fibrosis: a Fleischner society white paper. In: Lancet Respir Med; 2017.
32. Lynch DA, Webb WR, Gamsu G, et al. Computed tomography in pulmonary sarcoidosis. J Comput Assist Tomogr. 1989;13:405–10.
33. Macdonald SL, Rubens MB, Hansell DM, et al. Nonspecific interstitial pneumonia and usual interstitial pneumonia: comparative appearances at and diagnostic accuracy of thin-section CT. Radiology. 2001;221:600–5.
34. Mathieson JR, Mayo JR, Staples CA, et al. Chronic diffuse infiltrative lung disease: comparison of diagnostic accuracy of CT and chest radiography. Radiology. 1989;171:111–6.
35. Mayo JR, Webb WR, Gould R, et al. High-resolution CT of the lungs: an optimal approach. Radiology. 1987;163:507–10.
36. Moon J, Du Bois RM, Colby TV, et al. Clinical significance of respiratory bronchiolitis on open lung biopsy and its relationship to smoking related interstitial lung disease. Thorax. 1999;54:1009–14.
37. Muller NL, Miller RR, Webb WR, et al. Fibrosing alveolitis: CT-pathologic correlation. Radiology. 1986;160:585–8.
38. Murata K, Khan A, Rojas KA, et al. Optimization of computed tomography technique to demonstrate the fine structure of the lung. Investig Radiol. 1988;23:170–5.
39. Nicholson AG, Addis BJ, Bharucha H, et al. Inter-observer variation between pathologists in diffuse parenchymal lung disease. Thorax. 2004;59:500–5.
40. Niewoehner DE, Hoidal JR. Lung fibrosis and emphysema: divergent responses to a common injury? Science (New York, NY). 1982;217:359–60.
41. Niewoehner DE, Kleinerman J, Rice DB. Pathologic changes in the peripheral airways of young cigarette smokers. N Engl J Med. 1974;291:755–8.
42. Padley SP, Hansell DM, Flower CD, et al. Comparative accuracy of high resolution computed tomography and chest radiography in the diagnosis of chronic diffuse infiltrative lung disease. Clin Radiol. 1991;44:222–6.
43. Primack SL, Hartman TE, Hansell DM, et al. End-stage lung disease: CT findings in 61 patients. Radiology. 1993;189:681–6.
44. Raghu G. Idiopathic pulmonary fibrosis: guidelines for diagnosis and clinical management have advanced from consensus-based in 2000 to evidence-based in 2011. Eur Respir J. 2011;37:743–6.
45. Raghu G, Collard HR, Egan JJ, et al. An official ATS/ERS/JRS/ALAT statement: idiopathic pulmonary fibrosis: evidence-based guidelines for diagnosis and management. Am J Respir Crit Care Med. 2011;183:788–824.
46. Raghu G, Remy-Jardin M, Myers JL, et al. Diagnosis of idiopathic pulmonary fibrosis. An official ATS/ERS/JRS/ALAT clinical practice guideline. Am J Respir Crit Care Med. 2018;198:e44–68.
47. Remy-Jardin M, Remy J, Deffontaines C, et al. Assessment of diffuse infiltrative lung disease: comparison of conventional CT and high-resolution CT. Radiology. 1991;181:157–62.
48. Remy-Jardin M, Remy J, Wallaert B, et al. Subacute and chronic bird breeder hypersensitivity pneumonitis: sequential evaluation with CT and correlation with lung function tests and bronchoalveolar lavage. Radiology. 1993;189:111–8.
49. Silva CI, Muller NL, Hansell DM, et al. Nonspecific interstitial pneumonia and idiopathic pulmonary fibrosis: changes in pattern and distribution of disease over time. Radiology. 2008;247:251–9.
50. Sverzellati N, Wells AU, Tomassetti S, et al. Biopsy-proved idiopathic pulmonary fibrosis: Spectrum of nondiagnostic thin-section CT diagnoses. Radiology. 2010;254:957–64.
51. Symmers D, Hoffman AM. The increased incidence of organizing pneumonia: preliminary communication. J Am Med Assoc. 1923;81:297–8.
52. Travis WD, Costabel U, Hansell DM, et al. An official American thoracic society/European respiratory society statement: update of the international multidisciplinary classification of the idiopathic interstitial pneumonias. Am J Respir Crit Care Med. 2013;188:733–48.
53. Ujita M, Renzoni EA, Veeraraghavan S, et al. Organizing pneumonia: perilobular pattern at thin-section CT. Radiology. 2004;232:757–61.
54. Vasakova M, Morell F, Walsh S, et al. Hypersensitivity pneumonitis: perspectives in diagnosis and management. Am J Respir Crit Care Med. 2017;196:680–9.
55. Vassallo R, Ryu JH, Colby TV, et al. Pulmonary Langerhans'-cell histiocytosis. N Engl J Med. 2000;342:1969–78.
56. Walsh SL, Wells AU, Sverzellati N, et al. An integrated clinicoradiological staging system for pulmonary sarcoidosis: a case-cohort study. Lancet Respir Med. 2014;2:123–30.
57. Washko GR, Hunninghake GM, Fernandez IE, et al. Lung volumes and emphysema in smokers with interstitial lung abnormalities. N Engl J Med. 2011;364:897–906.
58. Wells A. Clinical usefulness of high resolution computed tomography in cryptogenic fibrosing alveolitis. Thorax. 1998;53:1080–7.
59. Wells AU, Antoniou KM. The prognostic value of the GAP model in chronic interstitial lung disease: the quest for a staging system. Chest. 2014;145:672–4.
60. Wells AU, Nicholson AG, Hansell DM. Challenges in pulmonary fibrosis. 4: smoking-induced diffuse interstitial lung diseases. Thorax. 2007;62:904–10.
61. Wright JL, Tazelaar HD, Churg A. Fibrosis with emphysema. Histopathology. 2011;58:517–24.
62. Yousem SA, Colby TV, Gaensler EA. Respiratory bronchiolitis-associated interstitial lung disease and its relationship to desquamative interstitial pneumonia. Mayo Clin Proc. 1989;64:1373–80.

5

CT Diagnosis and Management of Focal Lung Disease

Gerald F. Abbott and Ioannis Vlahos

Learning Objectives

- To learn the imaging features of benign and malignant pulmonary nodules
- To learn the 2017 revised Fleischner Society guidelines for management of CT detected pulmonary nodules
- To understand the spectrum of subsolid pulmonary nodules, the serial evolution of ground-glass nodules to mixed attenuation nodules, and the significance of their solid components

The diagnosis of focal lung disease has progressed in accuracy in recent decades, paralleling the technological advances of computed tomography (CT). In contrast to chest radiography, the utilization of thin-section CT (HRCT) has enabled radiologists to more accurately determine the imaging characteristics of individual lung lesions and guide patient management in a more precise manner.

Focal pulmonary opacities can be broadly categorized as nodules, masses, or focal parenchymal airspace disease. Nodules are characterized as spherical well-defined opacities measuring up to 3 cm. In practice, this definition also includes more ill-defined or irregular nodules that might be more appropriately considered "nodular opacities." A mass is defined as an opacity (solid or partly solid) measuring >3 cm [1]. With its ability to evaluate the density and contour morphometry of nodules and masses, CT allows better characterization of these findings, and the resulting CT densitometry data may be supplemented by more specific CT techniques to determine enhancement (e.g., dual-energy CT), verify the evolution of findings by follow-up CT imaging, assess physiologic activity (PET/CT), and ultimately guide fine-needle aspiration or biopsy.

G. F. Abbott (✉)
Thoracic Imaging FND-202, Massachusetts General Hospital, Boston, MA, USA

St George's Medical School, University of London, London, UK

I. Vlahos
Department of Radiology, St. George's Hospital and NHS Trust, St George's Medical School, University of London, London, UK
e-mail: Johnny.vlahos@stgeorges.nhs.uk

5.1 Benign Solid Nodule Features

CT evaluation may reveal specific benign characteristics of a solitary pulmonary nodule including the identification of calcification or fat within the nodule, aided by the utilization of thin-section contiguous images (1–3 mm) through nodules of interest. Although fat may be evident on visual inspection alone, measurements of fat with such technique should be less than −30 to −40HU and often are as low as −150HU (Fig. 5.1). Measurements should be performed using a suitable sized region of interest (ROI) that encompasses an area that is still within the nodule on the slices above and below the measured slice. This reduces the risk of an erroneously low measurement due to partial volume average effects of any adjacent low-density lung parenchyma.

There is no absolute Hounsfield unit (HU) measurement that confirms calcification although measurements of >200 are usually related to pixels occupied by calcific material. Visual comparison to other thoracic osseous structures is considered sufficient for determining the calcific nature of lesions. The identification of diffuse, central, lamellated, or popcorn-type calcification in a pulmonary nodule is diagnostic of a benign lesion—and all but the latter may be indicative of healed granulomatous disease. Popcorn-type calcification is considered characteristic of a pulmonary hamartoma and when found in combination with intralesional fat is considered diagnostic of that entity. Eccentric calcification is indeterminate—sometimes benign and related to granulomatous disease—but also occurring in malignant lesions such as bronchial carcinoid tumors. Occasionally, eccentric calcification within a lung nodule or mass may reflect a small granu-

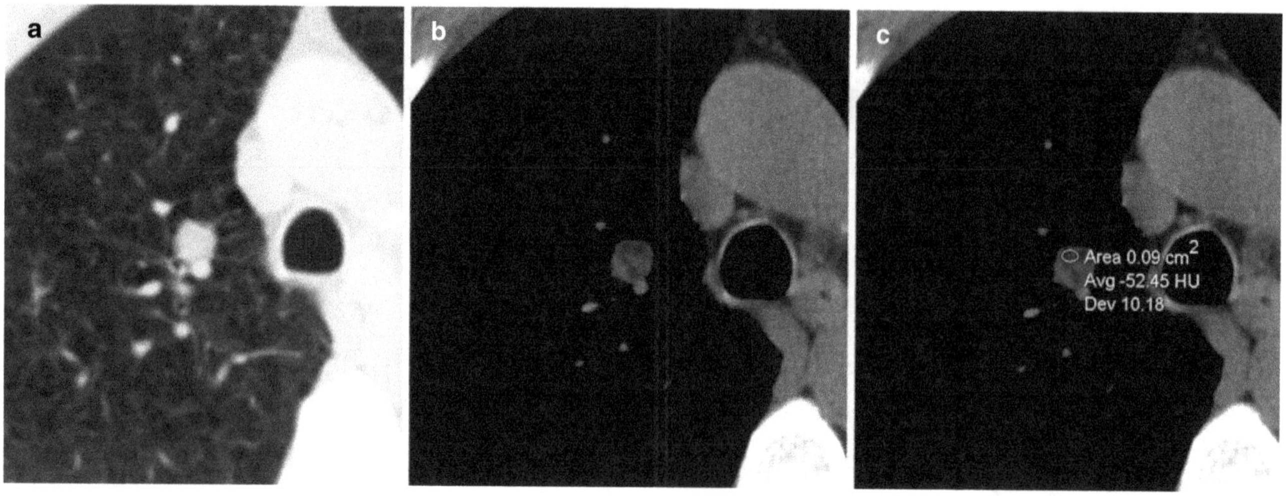

Fig. 5.1 Hamartoma. Composite CT image of a pulmonary nodule in lung window (**a**) and soft-tissue window (**b**) shows a well-circumscribed nodule in the right upper lobe that appears heterogeneous on soft-tissue window (**b**). Region-of-interest (ROI) evaluation of Hounsfield units (HU) reveals intralesional tissue within the range of fat (-52HU)

loma that has been engulfed within an enlarging adjacent neoplasm. Dystrophic or stippled calcifications are also indeterminate—sometimes benign—but well recognized to occur within bronchial carcinoid tumors, non-small cell lung cancer, and small cell carcinoma and are thus not a helpful discriminator between benign and malignant nodules. It is important for radiologists to be familiar with these patterns of calcification that may occur within pulmonary nodules and mass lesions (Fig. 5.2). Furthermore, it is recommended that pulmonary nodules and masses be inspected on coronal and sagittal images in addition to routine axial images. This practice enables not just the verification of maximal lesion dimensions but also clarifies such features as central versus eccentric calcification since the eccentric location of calcification may only be evident in those planes [2].

Other morphological features that are associated with benign lesions include a polygonal, elongated, elliptical, linear, or plaque-like shape, particularly when related to the fissures or pleural surfaces. Indeed such lesions are not all by definition strictly nodules. Some might be best characterized as scars, whereas triangular or elliptoid nodules may represent normal intrapulmonary lymph nodes. These findings are reported with variable incidence by pathologists and similarly with variable incidence and confidence by radiologists.

On CT images, intrapulmonary lymph nodes manifest as perifissural nodules (PFNs) and are routinely demonstrated on thin-section chest CT. Typical PFNs are small (<10 mm) and more often located in the lower lobes, below the level of the carina. They characteristically have a lentiform, triangular, or polygonal shape with 1–3 interlobular septal extensions and are located on or within 10 mm of the visceral

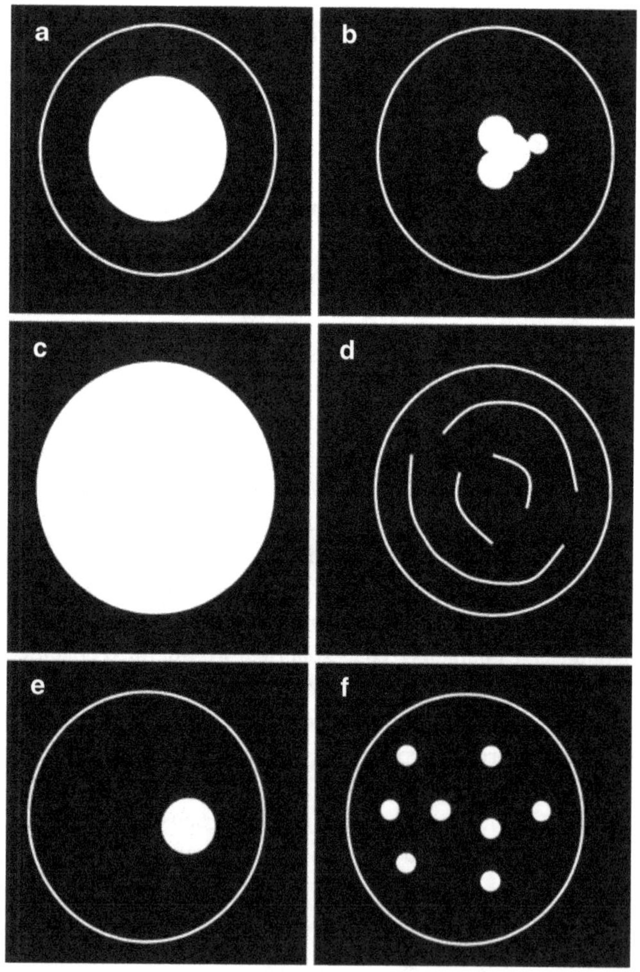

Fig. 5.2 Patterns of calcification. Benign patterns of calcification: (**a**) (central), (**b**) (popcorn), (**c**) (diffuse), and (**d**) (lamellated/concentric); and indeterminate patterns: (**e**) (eccentric) and (**f**) (stippled)

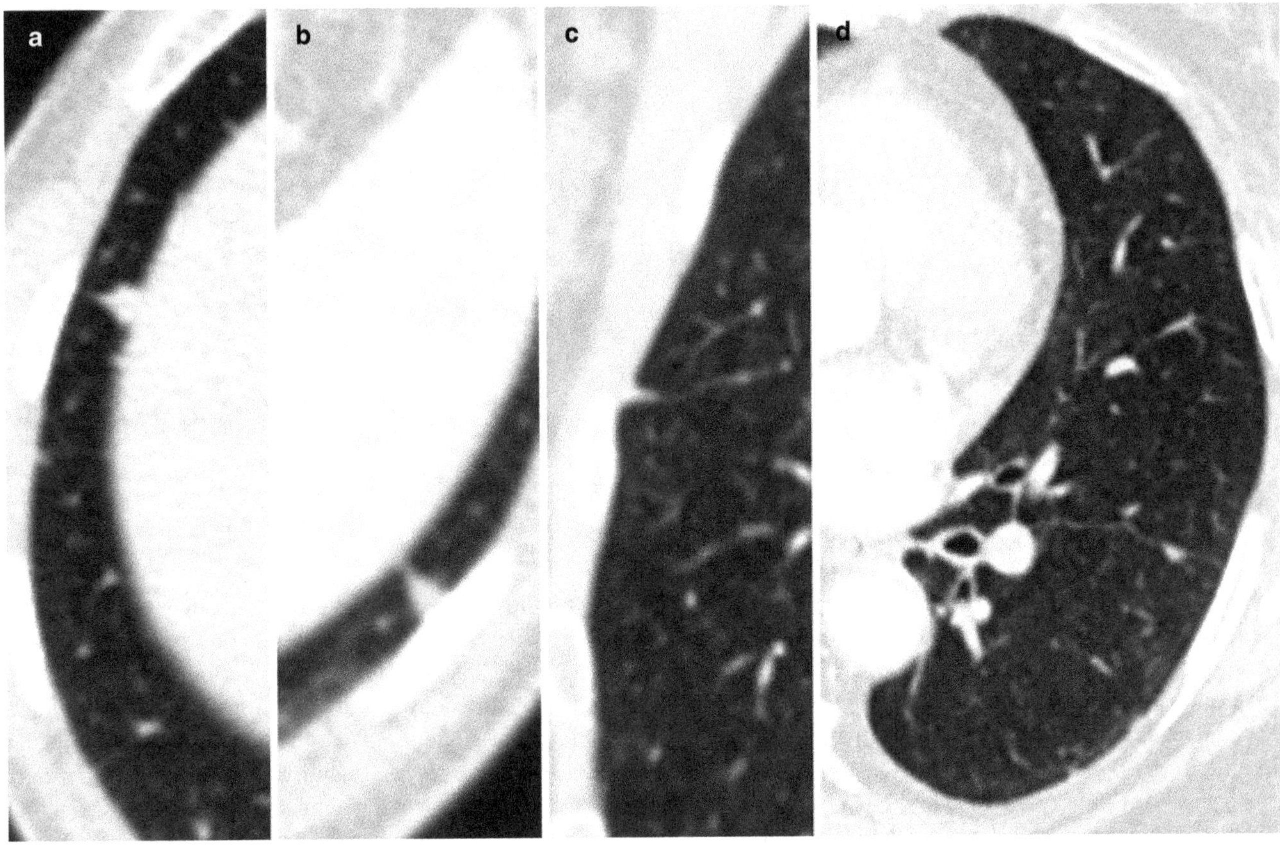

Fig. 5.3 Perifissural nodule (PFN) morphology. Intrapulmonary lymph nodes (**a**–**d**) typically manifest as small perifissural nodules (<10 mm), more often in the lower lobes, with a lentiform, triangular, or polygonal shape with 1–3 interlobular septal extensions, and are located on or within 10 mm of the visceral pleura or a lung fissure (major, minor, or accessory). Their characteristic morphology may be more apparent on coronal or sagittal reformatted images

pleura or a lung fissure (major, minor, or accessory) (Fig. 5.3) [3]. In a recent study, there was moderate inter-reader agreement when classifying nodules as perifissural nodules [4]. Under the revised 2017 Fleischner Society guidelines for management of incidentally detected pulmonary nodules on CT, a PFN with a morphology consistent with an intrapulmonary lymph node does not require follow-up CT, even if the average dimension exceeds 6 mm [5].

5.2 Malignant Solid Nodule Features

Specific features of malignancy are more common in larger pulmonary nodules but relatively uncommon in nodules <1 cm. Such imaging features as spiculation, microlobulation, pleural tags, satellite nodules, and the presence of a bronchus leading directly into a nodule ("CT bronchus sign") are associated with a higher probability of neoplastic disease although this finding may sometimes occur in inflammatory and infectious diseases, including mycobacterial infection. Cavitation may be an imaging manifestation of neoplastic or infectious disease (including bacterial, mycobacterial, and fungal infections) as well as inflammatory disease (e.g., vasculitides, pulmonary Langerhans cell histiocytosis). The detection of thicker-walled cavities on chest radiographs has historically been described as a feature favoring neoplasia, but CT evaluation of the wall thickness of nodules or masses does not corroborate this earlier radiographic interpretation [6, 7].

5.3 Subsolid Nodules

Subsolid nodules include lesions that are of pure ground-glass attenuation on CT as well as those of mixed attenuation—i.e., a combination of ground-glass and solid components. It is well recognized that subsolid lesions with these characteristics are associated with higher prevalence rates of malignancy than solid lesions, particularly when the lesion is of mixed attenuation [8]. Malignant subsolid nodules lie along a spectrum of disease that extends from the small (likely malignant precursor) lesion

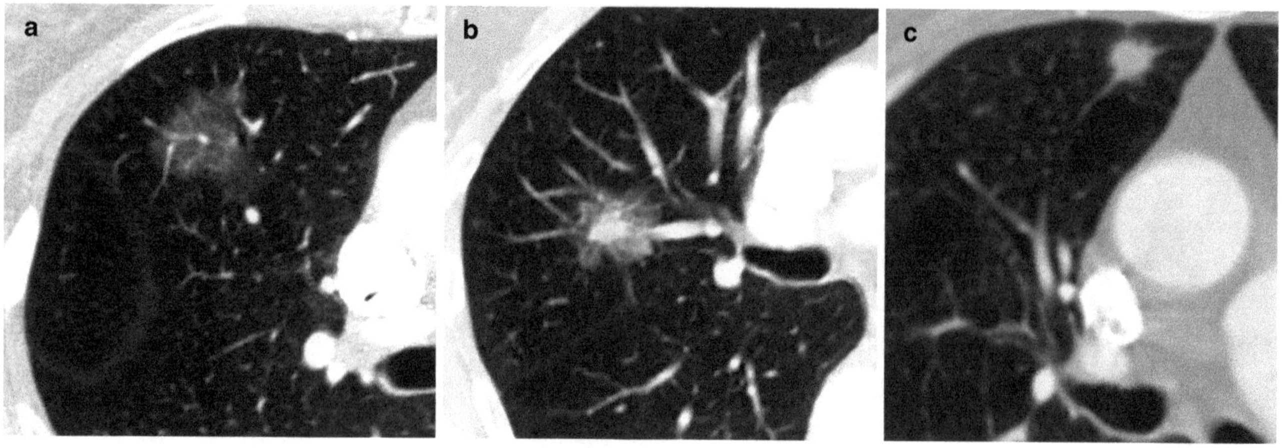

Fig. 5.4 Nodule attenuation patterns. Composite CT image showing a spectrum of attenuation in three pulmonary nodules, ranging from pure ground-glass attenuation (**a**) to mixed attenuation (**b**) to solid (**c**). The solid components in nodules (**b**) and (**c**) correspond with areas of tumor invasion

of atypical adenomatous hyperplasia (AAH) through larger ground-glass nodules and mixed attenuation nodules to solid nodules of invasive adenocarcinoma (Fig. 5.4). This spectrum was elucidated by a reclassification of pulmonary adenocarcinoma introduced jointly in 2011 by the International Association for the Study of Lung Cancer, the American Thoracic Society, and the European Respiratory Society [9]. This new classification was based on observations regarding the heterogeneity of subsolid neoplastic lesions, their characteristics of progression, and their clinical impact. These included the demonstration by Aoki and colleagues that AAH and the lower-stage lesions of what was previously termed bronchioloalveolar carcinoma (BAC, Noguchi subtype A, B, C) were associated with lesions that were almost exclusively ground glass in nature. Conversely, the higher-grade lesions (Noguchi D, E, F) were associated with lesions that became progressively more reticular, demonstrated traction bronchiolectasis, and eventually developed increasing solid components [10, 11].

The current 2011 histopathologic classification replaces the lesion previously termed bronchioloalveolar carcinoma (BAC). Preinvasive lesions—AAH and adenocarcinoma in situ (AIS)—are typically pure ground-glass lesions less than 5 mm and 3 cm, respectively, in size. Minimally invasive adenocarcinoma (MIA) is typically a part-solid lesion where the invasive component measures <5 mm. Larger subsolid lesions with more extensive solid invasive tumor are now termed lepidic predominant adenocarcinoma (LPA). Invasive multifocal mucinous adenocarcinoma replaces the entity previously termed multicentric BAC.

Multiple observers have documented that nodules of pure ground glass or those with minimal solid components typically progress at a very slow growth rate. In one study a comparison of mean volume doubling times in lung cancer patients with solid, part-solid, or pure ground-glass lesions demonstrated a stepwise increase in CT calculated volume doubling times (853 vs 457 vs 158 days) [12]. Therefore, the demonstration of 2-year stability of a subsolid lesion may not be enough to rule out malignancy. In such cases an initial follow-up CT at 3 months may be performed to demonstrate that the lesion persists and is not inflammatory. Follow-up may then be performed at more prolonged time intervals (1–2 years). When comparing these irregular ill-defined lesions, it can be difficult to measure incremental size, and evaluation should include comparison of comparable contiguous thin-section images and evaluation of whether the ground glass or solid component geographically extends around more vessels or airways. It is also important to note that the natural evolution of these lesions may on occasion include a transient reduction in size, likely related to underlying alveolar collapse.

The definitive determination that a subsolid lesion is malignant can be problematic. A progressive increase in overall size or increase in size of the solid component favors malignancy. PET/CT imaging in these cases is often noncontributory as it is well recognized that these lesions may have low SUV-max activity. Additionally, the evaluation of predominantly ground-glass lesions by CT-guided fine-needle aspiration or biopsy should be treated with caution. The results may be subject to significant sampling error and may vary significantly from those discovered in the excised specimen. The extent of invasive adenocarcinoma in particular can be significantly underestimated by percutaneous needle sampling even if this is directed to the more solid components of a lesion.

Key Points

- CT evaluation may reveal specific benign characteristics of a solitary pulmonary nodule including the identification of calcification or fat within the nodule.
- The identification of diffuse, central, lamellated, or popcorn-type calcification in a pulmonary nodule is diagnostic of a benign lesion.
- Subsolid nodules include lesions that are of pure ground-glass attenuation on CT as well as those of mixed attenuation—i.e., a combination of ground-glass and solid components.
- Subsolid nodules are associated with higher prevalence rates of malignancy than solid lesions when the lesion is of mixed attenuation.

5.4 Indeterminate Pulmonary Nodules

The majority of nodules detected on CT imaging are indeterminate and do not manifest with imaging features that can be definitively categorized as benign or malignant. In a 2005 Mayo Clinic screening series of over 1500 patients, over 3300 indeterminate non-calcified nodules were identified, the vast majority of which were small (4 mm or less) and benign [13]. Even in established smokers, the risk of malignancy in nodules of this size is less than 1% [14].

In recent years, evidence-based guidelines published by the Fleischner Society have greatly transformed the management of incidental pulmonary nodules detected on CT. The initial Fleischner guidelines, published in 2005, focused on solid pulmonary nodules and were followed by specific guidelines for subsolid nodules in 2013. Those have been supplanted by revised guidelines published in 2017 that encompass both solid and subsolid pulmonary nodules [5]. The recommended changes are based on new data and accumulated experience. For solid nodules, the minimum threshold size prompting routine follow-up CT has been increased to 6 mm, and fewer follow-up examinations are recommended for stable nodules. Time intervals for recommended follow-up are now given as a range rather than a precise time period (Table 5.1). Patient risk factors have also been expanded beyond the previous parameters based on subject characteristics (smoking history, lung cancer in a first-degree relative, exposure to asbestos, radon, or uranium) to include factors related to gender, race, lesion characteristics (size, attenuation, spiculation, upper lobe location), multiplicity, and the presence of emphysema and/or pulmonary fibrosis (IPF).

Table 5.1 Revised Fleischner guidelines (2017) for solid nodules

Nodule type	Low risk	High risk
Single <6 mm	No routine follow-up	Optional CT at 12 months
Single 6–8 mm	CT at 6–12 months, then consider CT at 18–24 months	CT at 6–12 months, then CT at 18–24 months
Single >8 mm	Consider CT, PET/CT or tissue sampling at 3 months	Consider CT, PET/CT, or tissue sampling at 3 months
Multiple <6 mm	No routine follow-up	Optional CT at 12 months
Multiple 6–8 mm	CT at 3–6 months, then consider CT at 18–24 months	CT at 3–6 months, then CT at 18–24 months
Multiple >8 mm	CT at 3–6 months, then consider CT at 18–24 months	CT at 3–6 months, then CT at 18–24 months

MacMahon H, Naidich DP, Goo JM et al. (2017) Guidelines for Management of Incidental Pulmonary Nodules Detected on CT Images: From the Fleischner Society. Radiology 284:228–243.

Table 5.2 Revised Fleischner guidelines (2017) for subsolid nodules

Nodule type	<6 mm	≥6 mm
Single Ground glass	No routine follow-up	CT at 6–12 months to confirm persistence, then CT every 2 years until 5 years
Single Part solid	No routine follow-up	CT at 3–6 months to confirm persistence. If unchanged and solid component remains <6 mm, annual CT should be performed for 5 years
Multiple	CT at 3–6 months. If stable, consider CT at 2 and 4 years	CT at 3–6 months. Subsequent management based on the most suspicious nodule(s)

MacMahon H, Naidich DP, Goo JM et al. (2017) Guidelines for Management of Incidental Pulmonary Nodules Detected on CT Images: From the Fleischner Society. Radiology 284:228–243.

For subsolid nodules, a longer time period is now recommended before initial CT follow-up, and the total length of follow-up has been extended to 5 years (Table 5.2). The revised Fleischner guidelines specify the use of contiguous thin-section CT (≤1.5 mm) and also stress the importance of utilizing axial, coronal, and sagittal images to facilitate the distinction between nodules and linear opacities that can be misleading when only axial images are evaluated (Fig. 5.5).

It is important to note that these guidelines apply to the management of incidentally detected solid and subsolid pulmonary nodules but do not apply to patients younger than 35 years, immunocompromised patients, or patients with cancer. The revised Fleischner guidelines are also not intended for use in lung cancer screening programs. For screening purposes, adherence to the existing American College of Radiology Lung CT Screening Reporting and Data System (Lung-RADS) guidelines is recommended.

In a separate published statement from the Fleischner Society, recommendations were made regarding the measurement of pulmonary nodules detected on CT images [15]. Those recommendations specify that measurements should be performed on axial sections unless the maximal dimensions lie in the coronal or sagittal plane. In those instances, the measurements should be made on the respective plane and that information should be documented in the radiologic report. Detected lung nodules—including the solid portion of part-solid nodules—should be measured on lung window images, and the dimension of small pulmonary nodules (<10 mm) should be expressed as the average of maximal long-axis and perpendicular maximal short-axis measurements obtained in the same plane (Fig. 5.6a). Both long- and short-axis measurements should be recorded for larger nodules and masses. Part-solid nodules should be measured in a similar fashion (average of long and short dimensions) including ground-glass and cystic components, and the maximum diameter of a solid component should also be recorded if >3 mm (Fig. 5.6b). It is also recommended that a pulmonary nodule be determined to have changed in size when its average diameter has increased or decreased by at least 2 mm, as smaller changes can be spurious—especially for ill-defined nodules.

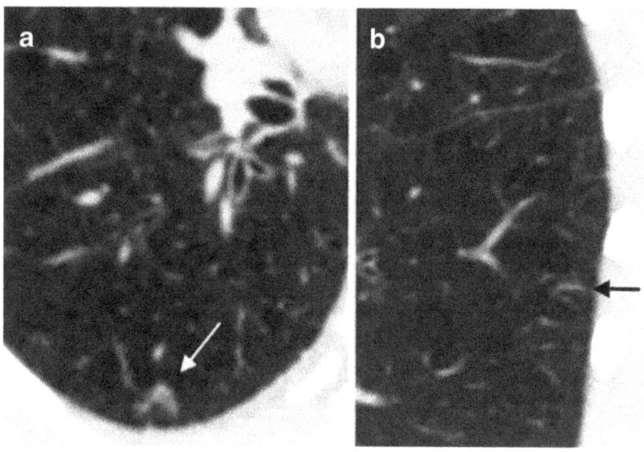

Fig. 5.5 Linear structure misinterpreted as a semisolid nodule. A heterogeneous focal opacity on axial CT ((**a**), arrow) was reported as a "mixed attenuation nodule," described as "suspicious for lung cancer," and a 3-month follow-up CT was recommended. On sagittal imaging (**b**), the corresponding finding is a linear opacity (arrow), likely an interlobular septum or small vessel

5.5 Role of Computer-Assisted Diagnosis for Solid Nodules

Computer-aided detection (CAD) is known to improve the detection of pulmonary nodules, although sensitivity is known to be dependent on lesion characteristics including size, density, and location. Technical parameters also affect sensitivity including the thickness of evaluated CT images and vendor-specific issues related to CT algorithm optimization to effect high detection rates with acceptable false-positive detection rates. Most CAD systems are also accompanied by computer-aided diagnosis (CADx) features for the evaluation of pulmonary nodules.

One of the most useful CADx tools is the ability to perform segmentation of individual nodules, enabling a three-dimensional evaluation of the size and shape of nodular lesions that can be compared with follow-up examinations to determine volumetric growth. This is based upon the observation that the doubling time of benign lesions is far longer than that of malignant lesions [16]. Volumetric evaluation of growth is also more reliable than reader applied uni- or bidimensional measurements of size [17]. Moreover, volumetric evaluation may be more sensitive to the detection of asymmetric growth, a feature that is characteristic of malignant lesions (Fig. 5.7). A commonly utilized threshold for solid lesion volume

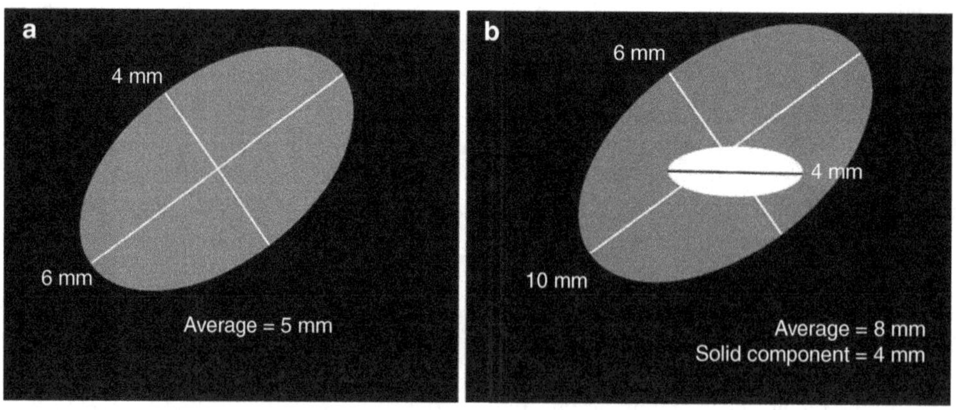

Fig. 5.6 Nodule measurement technique. The size of a solid nodule should be expressed as the average of maximal long-axis and perpendicular maximal short-axis measurements obtained in the same plane (**a**). Subsolid nodules should be measured in a similar fashion (average of long and short dimensions) including ground-glass and cystic components, and the maximum diameter of a solid component should also be recorded if >3 mm (**b**)

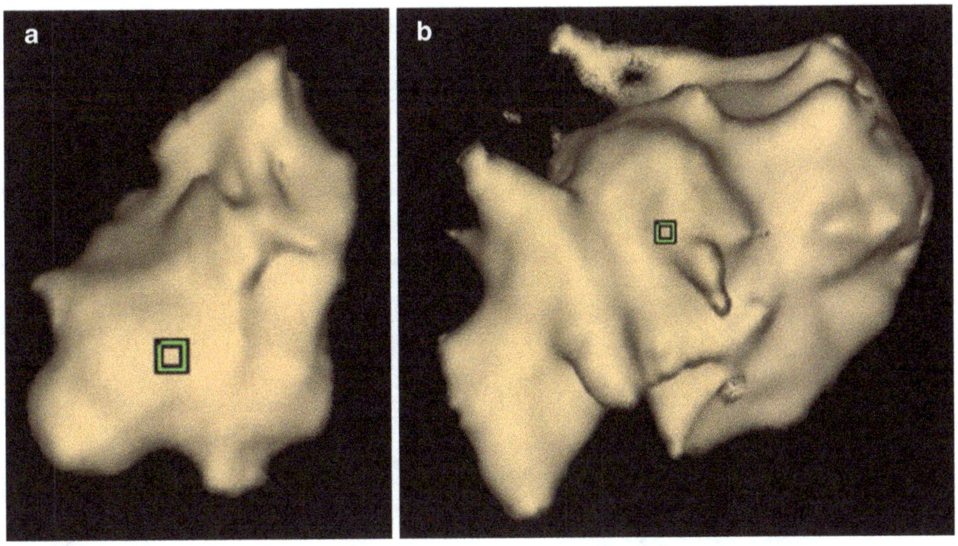

Fig. 5.7 Adenocarcinoma of the lung. Composite image of computer-aided 3-D volumetric evaluation of an irregular pulmonary nodule at baseline (**a**) and 11 months later (**b**) demonstrating asymmetric growth

doubling time is 400 days although several authors have advocated a more stringent threshold of 500 days [18–20]. The accuracy and reproducibility of lung nodule segmentation has been confirmed in artificial and porcine models. However, the reproducibility of in vivo human nodule measurements can be demonstrated to vary by up to 15% when evaluating the same nodule in different phases of inspiration or by utilizing different thickness CT data or software packages [21]. Lesser changes may occur as a result of different reconstruction algorithms or dose variation. The presence or absence of intravenous contrast appears to play a largely inconsequential role. Nonetheless, by ensuring that a similar technique is employed on initial and follow-up examinations, lung nodule volumetry shows great promise and may further reduce the need for follow-up examinations.

5.6 Focal Parenchymal Airspace Disease

A variety of disease entities may manifest on CT as focal airspace opacities. The majority of these will be multifocal and infectious or inflammatory in nature, and the diagnosis is often impossible to determine on the basis of imaging findings alone unless there are uncommon specific features present (e.g., ground-glass halo in invasive aspergillosis). However, the differential diagnosis may be narrowed by referring to a combination of imaging features, disease chronicity or progression, response to treatment, and the immune status of the patient.

The presence of cavitation in airspace disease can be helpful although the differential can again be broad incorporating staphylococcal or gram-negative bacterial infections, mycobacterial disease, or fungal infection. Rounded pneumonia is commoner in children but also occurs in adults, usually due to S. pneumoniae. Appearances are mass-like without air bronchograms resulting from propagation of disease through the collateral air-drift mechanisms of the pores of Kohn and the canals of Lambert. Focal consolidative opacity that is chronic may be characterized by associated findings of mild volume loss and traction bronchiectasis, these features being more common in patients with chronic eosinophilic lung disease or organizing pneumonia. The latter may also present with a "reverse halo" appearance (i.e., central ground-glass opacity with peripheral consolidation) although this appearance is not specific to organizing pneumonia and may be a manifestation of other disease processes, including pulmonary infarction. At times, progressive focal airspace disease may be manifestation of neoplastic disease including lepidic adenocarcinoma, lymphoma, or occasionally mucinous metastases from a gastrointestinal primary tumor. Calcification may be present in mycobacterial disease and occasionally amyloidosis.

5.7 Dual-Energy CT (DECT)

Recent advances in technology have enabled the clinical implementation of dual-energy CT (DECT)—a technique that utilizes the near-simultaneous acquisition of CT images at two x-ray energy levels—high and low kilovoltages. Modern CT scanners, especially those with tube-current modulation capabilities, have resolved earlier concerns about DECT regarding increased radiation dose. The capabilities of DECT include the creation of virtual unenhanced images (allowing differentiation of calcifications, talc, and enhanced thoracic structures) and the acquisition of pulmonary blood volume (PBV) images that allow differentiation of various parenchymal abnormalities including infarcts, atelectasis,

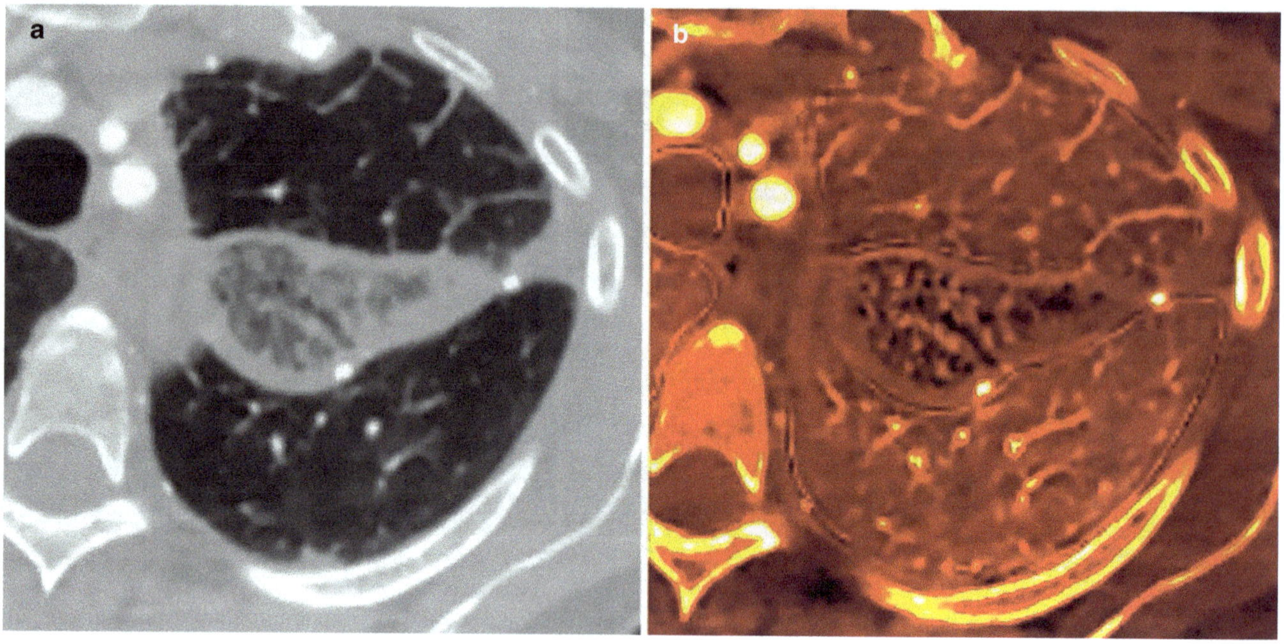

Fig. 5.8 Pulmonary infarction on dual-energy CT. A focal area of consolidation in the left apical region (**a**) represents lingular infarction (following lingula-sparing left upper lobectomy) and manifests with decreased blood flow on a pulmonary blood volume (PBV) image obtained by dual-energy CT (**b**). The lack of blood flow is in contrast to the normally perfused surrounding lung

and pneumonia (Fig. 5.8). Other applications include enhanced capabilities in pulmonary arterial enhancement and diagnosis of pulmonary embolism with a reduced volume of contrast material [22].

Take-Home Message

- The identification of diffuse, central, lamellated, or popcorn-type calcification in a pulmonary nodule is diagnostic of a benign lesion.
- Subsolid nodules are associated with higher prevalence rates of malignancy than solid lesions, particularly when the lesion is of mixed attenuation.
- Under the revised 2017 Fleischner Society guidelines for solid pulmonary nodules, the minimum threshold size prompting routine follow-up CT has been increased to 6 mm.

References

1. Hansell DM, Bankier AA, MacMahon H, et al. Fleischner Society: glossary of terms for thoracic imaging. Radiology. 2008;246:697–722.
2. Ridge CA, Huang J, Cardoza S, et al. Comparison of multiplanar reformatted CT lung tumor measurements to axial tumor measurement alone: impact on maximal tumor dimension and stage. AJR Am J Roentgenol. 2013;2013:959–63.
3. Wang CW, Teng YH, Huang CC. Intrapulmonary lymph nodes: computed tomography findings with histopathologic correlations. Clin Imaging. 2013;37:487–92.
4. Schreuder A, vanGinneken B, Scholten ET, et al. Classification of CT pulmonary opacities as perifissural nodules: reader variability. Radiology. 2018;288:867–75.
5. MacMahon H, Naidich DP, Goo JM, et al. Guidelines for management of incidental pulmonary nodules detected on CT images: from the Fleischner Society. Radiology. 2017;284:228–43.
6. Woodring JH, Fried AM, Chuang VP. Solitary cavities of the lung: diagnostic implications of cavity wall thickness. AJR Am J Roentgenol. 1980;135:1269–71.
7. Honda O, Tsubamoto M, Inoue A, et al. Pulmonary cavitary nodules on computed tomography: differentiation of malignancy and benignancy. J Comput Assist Tomogr. 2007;31:943–9.
8. Henschke CI, Yankelevitz DF, Mirtcheva R, et al. CT screening for lung cancer: frequency and significance of part-solid and nonsolid nodules. AJR Am J Roentgenol. 2002;178(5):1053–7.
9. Travis WD, Brambilla E, Noguchi M, et al. International Association for the Study of Lung Cancer/American Thoracic Society/European Respiratory Society international multidisciplinary classification of lung adenocarcinoma. J Thorac Oncol. 2011;6:244–85.
10. Noguchi M, Morikawa A, Kawasaki M, et al. Small adenocarcinoma of the lung. Histologic characteristics and prognosis. Cancer. 1995;75(12):2844–52.
11. Aoki T, Nakata H, Watanabe H, et al. Evolution of peripheral lung adenocarcinomas: CT findings correlated with histology and tumor doubling time. AJR Am J Roentgenol. 2000;174(3):763–8.
12. Hasegawa M, Sone S, Takashima S, et al. Growth rate of small lung cancers detected on mass CT screening. Br J Radiol. 2000;73(876):1252–9.
13. Swensen SJ, Jett JR, Hartman T. E.et al. CT screening for lung cancer: five-year prospective experience. Radiology. 2005;235(1):259–65.
14. Piyavisetpat N, Aquino SL, Hahn PF, et al. Small incidental pulmonary nodules: how useful is short-term interval CT follow-up? J Thorac Imaging. 2005;20(1):5–9.
15. Bankier AA, MacMahon H, Goo JM, et al. Recommendations for measuring pulmonary nodules at CT: a statement from the Fleischner Society. Radiology. 2017;285:584–600.

16. Yankelevitz DF, Reeves AP, Kostis WJ, et al. Small pulmonary nodules: volumetrically determined growth rates based on CT evaluation. Radiology. 2000;217:251–6.
17. Jennings SG, Winer-Muram HT, Tarver RD, Farber MO. Lung tumor growth: assessment with CT—comparison of diameter and cross-sectional area with volume measurements. Radiology. 2004;231(3):866–71.
18. Jennings SG, Winer-Muram HT, Tann M, Ying J, Dowdeswell I. Distribution of stage I lung cancer growth rates determined with serial volumetric CT measurements. Radiology. 2006;241(2):554–63.
19. Revel MP, Merlin A, Peyrard S, et al. Software volumetric evaluation of doubling times for differentiating benign versus malignant pulmonary nodules. AJR Am J Roentgenol. 2006;187(1):135–42.
20. Honda O, Kawai M, Gyobu T, et al. Reproducibility of temporal volume change in CT of lung cancer: comparison of computer software and manual assessment. Br J Radiol. 2009;82(981):742–7.
21. Bolte H, Riedel C, Muller-Hulsbeck S, et al. Precision of computer-aided volumetry of artificial small solid pulmonary nodules in ex vivo porcine lungs. Br J Radiol. 2007;80(954):414–21.
22. Otrakji A, Digumarthy SR, Lo Gullo R, et al. Dual-energy CT: spectrum of thoracic abnormalities. Radiographics. 2016;36:38–52.

6

Current Approach to Acute and Chronic Airway Disease

Philippe A. Grenier and Jeffrey P. Kanne

Learning Objectives

- To remind the basic principles of volumetric thin-collimation CT technique permitting to obtain an optimized evaluation of central and peripheral airway
- To know the CT features of most of the diseases involving the trachea and central bronchi
- To know the diagnostic criteria to identify the presence, distribution, and extent of bronchiectasis
- To know the direct and indirect CT features suggestive of inflammation, infection, and obstruction of small airways

6.1 CT Acquisition and Post-processing Techniques [1, 2]

MDCT acquisition is performed through the entirety of the lungs at full-suspended inspiration, using thin collimation (0.6–1.5 mm) without administration of contrast material. Axial images are reconstructed with thin-slice thickness (0.8–1.5 mm) and overlap (50% overlap is optimal). Complementary MDCT acquisition at full continuous forced expiration using reduced technique (120 Kv–20–40 mAs) is often recommended and particularly useful for assessing tracheobronchial collapsibility and expiratory air trapping.

Interpretation is best performed on a PACS workstation. Evaluation of the overlapped thin-section axial images in cine-mode allows the bronchial divisions to be easily followed from the carina to the smallest peripheral bronchi visible on CT. Real-time manipulation of the data set allows the radiologist to select the optimal plane to better depict the distribution and extent of airway abnormalities. Furthermore, multiplanar reformations with use of minimum and maximum intensity projections can be helpful to display airway abnormalities. Minimum intensity projection (minIP) can highlight airway dilation, diverticula, fistulas, and the extent of expiratory air trapping and emphysema. Maximum intensity projection (MIP) accentuates foci of mucoid impaction and small centrilobular nodules and tree-in-bud opacities. Volume rendering techniques (CT bronchography) can segment the airway lumen-wall interface and can be useful to detect subtle changes in airway calibre and to facilitate understanding of complex tracheobronchial abnormalities. Virtual bronchoscopy provides an internal rendering of the tracheobronchial inner surface and can better depict subtle mucosal abnormalities such as neoplasia and granulomatous disease.

P. A. Grenier (✉)
Department Radiology, Sorbonne Université - Hôpital Pitié-Salpêtrière, Paris, France

J. P. Kanne
Department of Radiology, University of Wisconsin School of Medicine and Public Health, Madison, WI, USA
e-mail: kanne@wisc.edu

6.2 Tracheobronchial Tumours (Tables 6.1, 6.2, 6.3, and 6.4) [3–6]

6.2.1 Primary Malignant Neoplasms

Primary malignant neoplasms are rare in the trachea compared to the laryngeal or bronchial cancers. The most frequent histological types are squamous cell carcinoma and adenoid cystic carcinoma, accounting for nearly 80% of all tracheal neoplasms. Adenoid cystic carcinoma (sialadenoid neoplasm) is a low-grade malignancy that is not associated with cigarette smoking. It occurs in patients in their 40s without any sex predilection. In the central airways, adenoid cystic carcinoma has a propensity to infiltrate the wall of the airways with submucosal extension manifesting as a sessile, polypoid, annular, or diffuse infiltration. The inner surface is smooth and regular. An extraluminal growth, visible on CT scan, is a common feature. Squamous cell carcinoma is the most common primary malignancy of the trachea primarily occurring in older men with a history of cigarette smoking.

Table 6.1 Luminal filling defect

- Benign tracheobronchial neoplasm
- Malignant primary tracheobronchial neoplasm
- Metastasis
- Mucus secretions
- Foreign body
- Broncholithiasis

Table 6.2 Multinodular appearance of the inner surface of the airway

- Granulomatosis with polyangiitis
- Tracheobronchial metastases (haematogenous spread)
- Respiratory papillomatosis
- Adenoid cystic carcinoma (multicentric)
- Tracheobronchial amyloidosis
- Tracheobronchopathia osteochondroplastica

Table 6.3 Focal tracheobronchial narrowing

- Posttraumatic strictures
- Postinfectious stenoses (e.g. tuberculosis)
- Tracheobronchial neoplasms (primary and secondary malignant)
- Granulomatosis with polyangiitis (can be multifocal)
- Sarcoidosis
- Inflammatory bowel disease
- Extrinsic compression

Table 6.4 Diffuse tracheobronchial wall thickening

- Infectious tracheobronchitis (TB, aspergillosis)
- Relapsing polychondritis[a]
- Tracheobronchial amyloidosis
- Tracheobronchopathia osteochrondroplastica[a]
- Tracheobronchitis associated with inflammatory bowel disease
- Sarcoidosis (rare manifestation)

[a]*Calcification frequently present and posterior membrane characteristically spared*

On CT, the tumour appears as a polypoid intraluminal mass or as an eccentric irregular wall thickening with an irregular surface. The tumour has a tendency to spread to adjacent mediastinal lymph nodes and to directly invade the mediastinum. Carcinoid tumour is a low-grade malignant neuroendocrine neoplasm representing 1–2% of primary lung neoplams. It appears on CT scan as a well-circumscribed polypoid mass that protrudes into the airway lumen. Segmental or lobar atelectasis and obstructive pneumonitis, as well as foci of calcification are present in 30% of cases. Marked homogeneous early contrast enhancement of an endobronchial nodule reflecting the high vascularity of this neoplasm may be present. Mucoepidermoid carcinoma is a rare neoplasm that originates from the minor salivary glands lining the tracheobronchial tree, occurring in young patients (<40 years old), found mainly in the segmental bronchi and resulting in airway obstruction. The typical CT appearance is a smooth, ovoid, or lobulated endobronchial mass with occasional punctuate calcifications and variable contrast enhancement. Lymphoma of the trachea is rare, usually related to mucosa-associated lymphoid tissue. The CT appearance is indistinguishable from other neoplasms.

6.2.2 Secondary Tracheobronchial Malignancy

Direct invasion of the central airways by neoplasm of the thyroid, oesophagus, lung, and larynx is much more common that haematogenous metastases. CT shows the primary neoplasm and its extension by contiguity within the main airways (endoluminal mass, destruction of cartilage, and tracheobronchial-oesophageal fistula).

Many cancers have the potential to metastasize to the trachea and bronchi. Endotracheal or endobronchial metastases appear as endotracheal nodules or eccentric thickening of the airway wall or soft tissue attenuation with contrast enhancement.

6.2.3 Benign Tracheobronchial Neoplasms

Benign tracheal neoplasms are rare. On CT, they present as endoluminal masses confined within the tracheobronchial lumen without evidence of involvement of surrounding structures. Benign neoplasms are typically sharply marginated, round, and smaller than 2 cm in diameter. Histology mainly includes hamartomas, lipomas, leiomyomas, fibromas, chondromas, and schwannomas. Endobronchial hamartomas represent 30% of intrathoracic hamartomas. The presence of fat with or without calcification is diagnostic.

Respiratory papillomatosis (laryngotracheobronchial papillomatosis) is a neoplastic disease caused by human papillomavirus (HPV) infection transmitted from mother to child at birth or acquired from orogenital contact. Papillomas arise in the larynx and can involve trachea and proximal bronchi in up to 50% of cases. Involvement of the lungs is rare, occurring in fewer than 1% of patients, and manifests on imaging studies as multiple lung nodules and cavitary and cystic lesions in the parenchyma. Malignant transformation into squamous cell carcinoma is a rare but serious complication of respiratory papillomatosis.

6.3 Nonneoplastic Tracheobronchial Disorders (Tables 6.2, 6.3, and 6.4) [4, 5, 7]

6.3.1 Posttraumatic Stenosis

Posttraumatic strictures of the trachea are usually the result of ischemic injury from a cuffed endotracheal or tracheostomy tube or extrinsic neck trauma. The two principal sites of stenosis following intubation or tracheostomy tube are at the stroma or at the level of the endotracheal or tracheostomy tube balloon.

Postintubation stenosis extends for several centimetres and typically involves trachea above the level of the thoracic inlet. Posttracheostomy stenosis typically begins 1.0–1.5 cm distal to the inferior margin of the tracheostomy stoma and extends over 1.5–2.5 cm. These strictures typically have an hourglass configuration with thickened tracheal wall. Less commonly the tracheal or bronchial stenosis may present as a thin membrane or granulation tissue protruding into the airway lumen.

> **Key Point**
> - CT with multiplanar reformations clearly depicts the severity and length of the stricture.

6.3.2 Infections

A number of infections, both acute and more often chronic, may affect the trachea and proximal bronchi, resulting in both focal and diffuse airway disease. Subsequent fibrosis may result in localized airway narrowing. The most common causes of infectious tracheobronchitis are acute bacterial tracheitis in immunocompromised patients, tuberculosis, rhinoscleroma (*Klebsiella rhinoscleromatis*), and necrotizing invasive aspergillosis. On CT, the extent of irregular and circumferential tracheobronchial narrowing is readily apparent, and in some patients, an accompanying mediastinitis is evident, manifesting as infiltration of mediastinal fat. In the fibrotic or healed phase, the airway is narrowed but has a smooth and normal thickness wall. Occasionally, because of the presence of chronic fibrous or granulomatous cheilitis/mediastinitis, tuberculosis of the trachea and/or proximal bronchi may mimic airway malignancy on CT.

6.3.3 Granulomatosis with Polyangiitis (Wegener Granulomatosis)

Inflammatory lesions may be present with or without subglottic or bronchial stenosis, ulcerations, and pseudotumours. Radiologic manifestations include thickening of the subglottic and proximal trachea with a smooth symmetric or asymmetric narrowing over variable length. Tracheal rings can become thickened and calcified. Cartilaginous erosions and ulcerations also may be seen. Stenosis can develop in any main, lobar, or segmental bronchus. Developing nodular or polypoid lesions can protrude into the airway lumen.

6.3.4 Relapsing Polychondritis

Relapsing polychondritis is a rare systemic autoimmune disease that affects cartilage at various sites, including the ears, nose, joints, and tracheobronchial tree. Symmetric subglottic stenosis is the most frequent manifestation in the chest. As the disease progresses, the distal trachea and bronchi may be involved. CT scans show smooth thickening of the airway wall associated with diffuse narrowing. In the early stages of the disease, the posterior wall of the trachea is spared, but in advanced disease, circumferential wall thickening can occur. Tracheobronchomalacia can develop as a result of weakening of cartilage, resulting in considerable luminal collapse on expiration. Marked destruction of the cartilaginous rings with fibrosis may cause stenosis.

6.3.5 Amyloidosis

Deposition of amyloid in the trachea and bronchi may occur in association with systemic amyloidosis or as an isolated process. CT scans show focal or, more commonly, diffuse thickening of the airway wall and narrowing of the lumen. Calcification may be present. Narrowing of the proximal bronchi can lead to distal atelectasis, bronchiectasis, or both with or without obstructive pneumonia.

6.3.6 Tracheobronchopathia Osteochondroplastica (TO)

TO is a rare disorder characterized by the presence of multiple cartilaginous nodules and bony submucosal nodules on the luminal surface of the trachea and proximal airways. TO involves males more frequently than females, and most patients are older than 50 years. Histologically, the nodules contain heterotopic bone, cartilage, and calcified acellular protein matrix. Because it contains no cartilage, the posterior wall of the trachea is spared. On CT, tracheal cartilages are thickened and show irregular calcifications. The nodules may protrude from the anterior and lateral walls into the lumen; they usually show foci of calcification.

6.3.7 Sabre-Sheath Trachea

Characterized by narrowing of the transverse diameter and increase of the sagittal diameter of the intrathoracic trachea, this deformity is almost always associated with COPD. The pathogenesis is unclear but likely results from altered mechanics from intrathoracic pressure changes associated with COPD. On radiographs and CT, the internal transverse diameter of the trachea is decreased to half or less than the corresponding sagittal diameter. The trachea usually shows a smooth inner margin but occasionally has a nodular contour. Calcification of the tracheal cartilage is common.

6.3.8 Tracheobronchomegaly (Mounier-Kuhn Syndrome)

This abnormality is characterized by abnormal dilation of the trachea and main bronchi and recurrent lower respiratory tract infection. The aetiology is not fully understood, but many patients have congenitally atrophic smooth muscle and elastin fibres. Mounier-Kuhn syndrome is often associated with tracheal diverticulosis and bronchiectasis. The subglottic trachea typically has a normal diameter, but the tracheal diameter expands toward the carina, often involving the central bronchi, as well. Atrophic mucosa prolapses between cartilage rings and gives the trachea a characteristically corrugated appearance. Corrugations may become exaggerated to form sacculations or diverticula. On CT a tracheal diameter of greater than 3 cm (measured 2 cm above the aortic arch) and diameter of 2.4 cm and 2.3 cm for the right and left bronchi, respectively, are diagnosing criteria. Additional findings include tracheal scalloping or diverticula (especially along the posterior membranous tracheal wall).

6.3.9 Tracheobronchomalacia and Excessive Dynamic Airway Collapse [8, 9, 10]

Tracheobronchomalacia (TBM) and excessive dynamic airway collapse (EDAC) may be responsible for expiratory central airway collapse (ECAC) which is an accepted term to describe the narrowing of central airway during expiration. TBM is characterized as a weakened or destroyed cartilage in the central airways resulting in expiratory airflow limitation. EDAC is characterized by excessive bulging of the posterior membrane inside the central airway lumen during expiration without cartilage collapse.

At CT, the diagnosis of EDAC is based on the narrowing of the lumen diameter by more than 70% on expiration compared with that on inspiration. The 50% reduction in airway cross-sectional area during forced expiration is inadequate to define abnormal collapse. No threshold of end-expiration collapse reliably predicts EDAC. Therefore dynamic expiratory imaging should be considered when there is high clinical suspicion for ECAC. In addition, dynamic expiratory multislice CT may offer feasible alternative to bronchoscopy in patients with suspected TBM or EDAC by showing complete relapse or collapse greater than 80% of airway lumen.

6.3.10 Broncholithiasis

Broncholithiasis is a rare condition characterized by erosion into or distortion of a bronchus from an adjacent calcified lymph node. The underlying abnormality is usually granulomatous lymphadenitis caused by *Mycobacterium tuberculosis* or fungi such as *Histoplasma capsulatum*. A few cases associated with silicosis have been reported. Calcified material in the bronchial lumen or bronchial distortion results in airway obstruction. This leads to collapse, obstructive pneumonitis, mucoid impaction, or bronchiectasis. Occasionally, patients will expectorate calcific fragments (lithoptysis). Broncholithiasis is recognized on CT by the presence of a calcified endobronchial or peribronchial lymph node, associated with bronchopulmonary complication related to obstruction in the absence of an associated soft tissue mass.

6.4 Tracheobronchial Fistula, Dehiscence, and Diverticula (Table 6.5) [2, 11]

Peripheral bronchopleural fistulas are most commonly caused by necrotizing pneumonia or secondary to trauma. Nodobronchial and nodobronchoesophageal fistulas are characterized by the presence of gas in cavitated hilar or mediastinal lymph nodes adjacent to the airways and are usually caused by tuberculosis. Occasionally, congenital tracheal diverticula and tracheobronchoesophageal fistulas may not present until adulthood, especially the H-type.

Malignant neoplasia, particularly oesophageal, is the most common cause of tracheoesophageal fistula in adults. Infection and trauma are the most frequent nonmalignant causes.

MDCT has a high degree of sensitivity and specificity for depicting bronchial dehiscence occurring after lung transplantation. Bronchial dehiscence is seen as a bronchial wall defect at the anastomosis associated with extraluminal gas collections.

The cardiac bronchus is an uncommon airway anomaly characterized by a supernumerary bronchus arising from the inferomedial aspect of the mid bronchus intermedius. The cardiac bronchus typically is a blind-ending pouch but

Table 6.5 Tracheobronchial dehiscence, fistulas, and diverticula

- Tracheal or bronchial rupture
- Bronchial dehiscence occurring after lung transplantation
- Tracheal diverticula (tracheocele)
- Paratracheal cyst
- Accessory cardiac bronchus
- Multiple tracheobronchial diverticula
- Nodobronchial and nodobronchoesophageal fistulas
- Tracheoesophageal fistulas
- Bronchopleural fistulas

occasionally supplies a very small number of pulmonary lobules. Most cardiac bronchi are clinically silent and thus are incidentally detected on chest CT. However, they may serve as a reservoir for retained secretions leading to chronic inflammation and hypervascularity, leading to recurrent episodes of infection or haemoptysis.

In smokers, bronchial diverticula or outpouchings may be seen as small airway collections in the wall of the main and lobar bronchi particularly well displayed on coronal reformations with minimal intensity projection. They express the fusion of multidepressions and dilations of the bronchial gland ducts forming a diverticulum, which herniates between and through the smooth muscle cellular bundles.

Paratracheal cysts are characterized by one or several cystic cavities present along the cervicothoracic part of the trachea. These cysts communicate with the tracheal lumen through a small wall defect visible on thin CT slices and located in the posterolateral angle of the trachea. The great majority is located on the right side.

6.5 Bronchiectasis [12, 13]

This chronic condition characterized by local, irreversible dilation of bronchi, usually associated with inflammation, remains an important cause of haemoptysis and chronic sputum production.

Pathologically, bronchiectasis is classified into three subtypes, reflecting increasing severity of disease: cylindrical, characterized by relatively uniform airway dilatation; varicose, characterized by nonuniform and somewhat serpentine dilation; and cystic. As bronchiectasis progresses, the lung parenchyma distal to the affected airway increasingly collapses.

The CT findings of bronchial dilation include lack of tapering of bronchial lumina (the cardinal sign of bronchiectasis), internal diameter of bronchi greater than that of the adjacent pulmonary artery (signet ring sign), bronchi visible within 1 cm of the costal pleura or abutting the mediastinal pleura, and mucus-filled dilated bronchi. With varicose bronchiectasis, the bronchial lumen assumes a beaded configuration. Cystic bronchiectasis appears as a string of cysts caused by sectioning irregular dilated bronchi along their lengths, or a cluster of cysts, caused by multiple dilated bronchi lying adjacent to each other. Cluster of cysts are most commonly associated with an atelectatic lobe. Fluid levels, caused by retained secretions, may be present in the dependent portion of the dilated bronchi. Accumulation of secretions within bronchiectatic airways is typically recognizable as lobulated V- or Y-shaped structures (finger in glove sign). CT may show a completely collapsed lobe containing bronchiectatic airways. Subtle degrees of volume loss may present in lobes in relatively early disease.

Table 6.6 Specific causes of disseminated bronchiectasis

- Acute, chronic, or recurrent infections
- Genetic abnormalities
  - Cystic fibrosis
  - Dyskinetic (immotile) cilia syndrome
  - Young syndrome
  - Williams-Campbell syndrome
  - Mounier-Kuhn syndrome (tracheobronchomegaly)
  - Immunodeficiency syndromes
  - Yellow nail syndrome
  - Alpha-1-antitrypsin deficiency
- Noninfectious inflammatory diseases
  - Allergic bronchopulmonary aspergillosis
  - Asthma
  - Systemic diseases (rheumatoid arthritis, Sjögren syndrome, systemic lupus erythematosus, inflammatory bowel disease)
  - Post-transplantation bronchiolitis obliterans syndrome

Associated CT findings of bronchiolitis are present in about 70% of patients with bronchiectasis. These abnormalities are very common in patients with severe bronchiectasis and can even precede the development of bronchiectasis. The obstructive defect on pulmonary function testing in patients with bronchiectasis is the consequence of an obstructive involvement of the small airways (constrictive). The extent and severity of bronchiectasis and bronchial wall thickening correlate with airflow obstruction [14]. In patients with bronchiectasis, bronchial wall thickening and the extent of decreased lung attenuation are the strongest determinants of airflow obstruction. In addition, bronchial wall thickening on baseline CT correlates with functional deterioration overtime [15].

MDCT with thin collimation is the optimal imaging test to assess the presence and extent of bronchiectasis. Several studies have shown that multiplanar reformations increase the detection rate of bronchiectasis, readers' confidence as to the distribution of bronchiectasis, and agreement among observers as to the diagnosis of bronchiectasis.

The reliability of CT for distinguishing among the causes of bronchiectasis is somewhat controversial. An underlying cause for bronchiectasis is found in fewer than half of patients, and CT features alone do not usually allow confident distinction between idiopathic bronchiectasis and known causes of bronchiectasis (Table 6.6).

6.6 Small Airway Diseases [2, 16]

Although normal bronchioles are below the resolution of thin-section CT, they can become detectable when inflammation of the airway wall and accompanying exudate develop. Some bronchiolar changes are too small to be visible directly but result in indirect signs on CT.

6.6.1 Small Centrilobular Nodular and Branching Linear Opacities (Tree-in-Bud)

Tree-in-bud opacities are defined as small centrilobular nodular and branching linear opacities, usually V- or Y-shaped, reflecting abnormally dilated bronchioles with thickened walls and mucus or exudate filling lumens. Associated peribronchiolar inflammation is often present, contributing to the CT appearance. Tree-in-bud opacities are characteristic of acute or chronic infectious bronchiolitis. They also occur in diffuse panbronchiolitis and aspiration.

6.6.2 Poorly Defined Centrilobular Nodules

Poorly defined centrilobular nodules reflect the presence of peribronchiolar inflammation in the absence of airway filling. When the distribution of nodules is diffuse and homogeneous, the pattern is suggestive of bronchiolar or vascular diseases. Bronchiolar disease associated with poorly defined centrilobular nodules includes respiratory bronchiolitis, hypersensitivity pneumonitis, and follicular bronchiolitis.

6.6.3 Decreased Lung Attenuation and Mosaic Perfusion

Areas of decreased lung attenuation associated with decreased vessel calibre on CT reflect bronchiolar obstruction and associated reflex vasoconstriction. In acute bronchiolar obstruction, decreased perfusion represents a physiologic reflex of hypoxic vasoconstriction, whereas irreversible vascular remodelling occurs with chronic bronchiolar obstruction. The areas of decreased lung attenuation related to hypoperfusion can be patchy or widespread. They are poorly defined or sharply demarcated giving a geographical outline, representing a collection of affected pulmonary lobules. Redistribution of blood flow to the normally ventilated areas causes localized increased attenuation. The patchwork of abnormal areas of low attenuation and normal lung or less diseased areas results in mosaic attenuation on CT, also termed mosaic perfusion. Expiratory CT accentuates the pattern of mosaic attenuation where areas of air trapping remain low in attenuation, whereas normal lung increases in attenuation. Usually the regional heterogeneity of lung attenuation is apparent at full inspiration.

> **Key Point**
> - MiniP is helpful in detecting mosaic attenuation.

However, with more extensive air trapping, the lack of regional homogeneity of lung attenuation can be challenging to detect on inspiratory scans, and, as a result, mosaic attenuation becomes visible only on expiratory scans. In patients with particularly severe and widespread involvement of the small airways, the patchy distribution of hypoattenuation and mosaic pattern is lost. Inspiratory scans show an apparent uniformity of decreased attenuation in the lungs and scans obtained at end expiration may appear similar to inspiration scan. In these patients, the most striking features are paucity of pulmonary vessels and lack of change of the cross-sectional area of lung between inspiration and expiration. Mosaic attenuation may be seen in patients who have constrictive bronchiolitis, bronchiolitis associated with hypersensitivity pneumonitis, asthma, and COPD.

6.6.4 Expiratory Air Trapping

Lobular areas of air trapping may be readily apparent on expiratory CT but are occult on inspiratory CT. Foci of lobular air trapping are usually well-demarcated reflecting the geometry of individual or joined lobules. Lobular areas of air trapping may be present on expiratory CT scans of normal individuals, especially in the medial and posterior basal and apical portions of the superior segments of the lower lobes. However, when lobular air trapping is present in the nondependent portions of the lung or the overall extent is equal or greater than one segment, air trapping should be considered as abnormal. Expiratory air trapping occurs in smokers and in patients with asthma, constrictive bronchiolitis, and bronchiolitis associated with hypersensitivity pneumonitis and sarcoidosis.

6.7 Constrictive (Obliterative) Bronchiolitis [2, 16]

Constrictive bronchiolitis, characterized by submucosal circumferential fibrosis along the central axis of terminal bronchioles, is the result of a variety of causes and, rarely, is idiopathic (Table 6.7).

The main thin-section CT findings usually consist of areas of decreased lung attenuation associated with vessels of decreased calibre on inspiratory scans and air trapping on expiratory scans. Bronchial wall thickening and bronchiectasis, both central and peripheral, are also commonly present.

The areas of decreased lung attenuation and perfusion may be confined to or predominant in one lung, particularly in Swyer-James or MacLeod syndrome, that is a variant form of postinfectious constrictive bronchiolitis in which the constrictive bronchiolar lesions affect predominantly one lung.

Table 6.7 Causes of and association with obliterative (constrictive) bronchiolitis

- Postinfection
  - Childhood viral infection (adenovirus, respiratory syncytial virus, influenza, parainfluenza)
  - Adulthood and childhood (*Mycoplasma pneumoniae*, *Pneumocystis jiroveci* in AIDS patients, endobronchial spread of tuberculosis, bacterial bronchiolar infection)
- Post-inhalation (toxic fumes and gases)
- Diffuse aspiration bronchiolitis (chronic occult aspiration in the elderly, patients with dysphagia)
- Connective tissue disorders (rheumatoid arthritis, Sjögren syndrome)
- Allograft recipients (bone marrow transplant, heart-lung, or lung transplant)
- Drugs (penicillamine, lomustine)
- Ulcerative colitis
- Other conditions
  - Bronchiectasis
  - Cystic fibrosis
  - Hypersensitivity pneumonitis
  - Diffuse idiopathic pulmonary neuroendocrine cell hyperplasia (DIPNECH)
  - Excessive *Sauropus androgynus* (katuk, sweet leaf, or star gooseberry) ingestion
- Idiopathic

6.8 Asthma [17]

The main clinical indication for imaging patients with asthma is to identify diseases that may mimic asthma clinically, particularly hypersensitivity pneumonitis, constrictive bronchiolitis, and tracheal or carinal obstruction by neoplastic or nonneoplastic tracheal disorders. CT of patients with asthma can be normal or shows bronchial abnormalities. Mucoid impaction and linear bands, reflecting subsegmental or segmental atelectasis, are reversible on follow-up. Bronchial wall thickening is commonly present and has been shown to correlate with clinical severity and duration of asthma and the degree of airflow obstruction. It also correlates with pathologic measures of remodelling from bronchial biopsies [18]. Bronchiectasis may also be present, and its extent is associated with an increased severity of asthma.

In patients with persistent moderate asthma, mosaic attenuation reflects remodelling in the small airways. The extent of expiratory air trapping does not change after inhalation of salbutamol. This allows to exclude the hypothesis of bronchoconstriction to explain gas trapping in these patients and to reinforce the role of airway remodelling. In contrast, in patients with mild or moderate uncontrolled asthma, therapy with inhaled corticosteroids reduces the degree of air trapping on CT, suggesting that CT can be used as a surrogate marker for assessing disease control.

6.9 Airway Disease in COPD [19]

Airway disease phenotypes of COPD include abnormalities of the small and large airways. Poorly defined centrilobular nodules primarily in the upper lobes reflect inflammatory changes in and around the bronchioles (respiratory bronchiolitis), which are reversible after smoking cessation and steroids. Mosaic attenuation and expiratory air trapping reflect remodelling of the small airways (obstructive bronchiolitis).

Bronchial wall thickening is frequently present. Bronchial wall thickness is one of the strongest determinants of FEV1 in patients with COPD. The measures of airway thickness are also associated with chronic bronchitis with bronchodilator responsiveness and with a paradoxical response to bronchodilators. In addition, CT studies have consistently showed reduced airway lumen dimensions and fewer peripheral airways in COPD.

Moderate tubular bronchiectasis can occur, particularly in the lower lobes, as a result of injury to cartilage. Bronchiectasis is often associated with more severe COPD exacerbations, lower airway bacterial colonization, and increased sputum inflammatory markers [20]. However, the presence of bilateral varicose and cystic bronchiectasis in patients with panlobular emphysema should raise the diagnosis of alpha-1-antitrypsin deficiency.

6.10 Concluding Remarks

Volumetric thin-collimation CT acquisition at full inspiration and expiration has tremendously improved the accuracy of imaging in the detection and characterization of airway disease. Both proximal and distal airway disease may be identified and correctly assessed in terms of extent and severity.

CT and endoscopy play complementary roles in the assessment of tracheobronchial lesions, including neoplasms, inflammation, and infection.

CT remains the imaging technique of reference in the diagnosis and extent assessment of bronchiectasis. It has gained much interest from the respiratory physicians in the assessment of obstructive lung disease, including COPD, chronic asthma, and constrictive bronchiolitis.

Take-Home Messages

- Volumetric thin-collimation CT with multiplanar reformations along the long axis and strictly perpendicular to the central axis of the airways has improved detection, characterization, and extent assessment of any tracheal or bronchial lesion.
- MIP images are helpful to detect foci of inflammatory or infectious lesions in terminal bronchioles.
- Expiratory CT scan and minIP are helpful to detect gas trapping due to obstruction of the bronchiolar lumens.
- Dynamic expiratory CT images may offer feasible alternative to bronchoscopy in patients with suspected tracheobronchomalacia or expiratory dynamic airway collapse by showing complete relapse or collapse greater than 80% of airway lumen.

References

1. Beigelman-Aubry C, Brillet PY, Grenier PA. MDCT of the airways: technique and normal results. Radiol Clin N Am. 2009;47:185–201.
2. Grenier PA, Beigelman-Aubry C, Fetita C, et al. New frontiers in CT imaging of airway disease. Eur Radiol. 2002;12:1022–44.
3. Ferretti GR, Bithigoffer C, Righini CA, et al. Imaging of tumors of the trachea and central bronchi. Radiol Clin N Am. 2009;47:227–41.
4. Chung JH, Kanne JP, Gilman MD. CT of diffuse tracheal diseases. AJR Am J Roentgenol. 2011;196:W240–8.
5. Kang EY. Large airway diseases. J Thorac Imaging. 2011;26:249–62.
6. Ngo AV, Walker CM, Chung JH, et al. Tumors and tumorlike conditions of the large airways. AJR Am J Roentgenol. 2013;201:301–13.
7. Grenier PA, Beigelman-Aubry C, Brillet PY. Nonneoplastic tracheal and bronchial stenoses. Radiol Clin N Am. 2009;47:243–60.
8. Murgu S, Colt H. Tracheobronchomalacia and excessive dynamic airway collapse. Clin Chest Med. 2013;34:527–55.
9. Lee EY, Litmanovich D, Boiselle PM. Multidetector CT evaluation of tracheobronchomalacia. Radiol Clin N Am. 2009;47:261–9.
10. Ridge CA, O'donnell CR, Lee EY, Majid A, et al. Tracheobronchomalacia: current concepts and controversies. J Thorac Imaging. 2011;26:278–89.
11. Sverzellati N, Ingegnoli A, Calabrò E, et al. Bronchial diverticula in smokers on thin-section CT. Eur Radiol. 2010;20:88–94.
12. Javidan-Nejad C, Bhalla S. Bronchiectasis. Radiol Clin N Am. 2009;47:289–306.
13. Feldman C. Bronchiectasis: new approaches to diagnosis and management. Clin Chest Med. 2011;32:535–46.
14. Roberts HR, Wells AU, Milne DG, et al. Airflow obstruction in bronchiectasis: correlation between computed tomography features and pulmonary function tests. Thorax. 2000;55:198–204.
15. Sheehan RE, Wells AU, Copley SJ, et al. A comparison of serial computed tomography and functional change in bronchiectasis. Eur Respir J. 2002;20:581–7.
16. Pipavath SN, Stern EJ. Imaging of small airway disease (SAD). Radiol Clin N Am. 2009;47:307–16.
17. Kauczor HU, Wielpütz MO, Owsijewitsch M, et al. Computed tomographic imaging of the airways in COPD and asthma. J Thorac Imaging. 2011;26:290–300.
18. Aysola RS, Hoffman EA, Gierada D, et al. Airway remodeling measured by multidetector CT is increased in severe asthma and correlates with pathology. Chest. 2008;134:1183–91.
19. Ley-Zaporozhan J, Kauczor HU. Imaging of airways: chronic obstructive pulmonary disease. Radiol Clin N Am. 2009;47:331–42.
20. Martínez-García MÁ, Soler-Cataluña JJ, Donat Sanz Y, et al. Factors associated with bronchiectasis in patients with COPD. Chest. 2011;140:1130–7.

7

Imaging of Pulmonary Infection

Tomás Franquet and Johnathan H. Chung

Learning Objectives

- To know the variable imaging findings of pulmonary infections.
- To understand the limitations of imaging in the diagnosis of pulmonary infections.
- To appreciate the importance of additional clinical information in the diagnosis of respiratory infections.

Respiratory infections are the commonest illnesses occurring in humans, and pneumonia is the leading cause of death due to infectious disease. Pneumonia is an acute infection of the pulmonary parenchyma that is associated with at least some symptoms of acute infection, accompanied by the presence of an acute infiltrate on a chest radiograph. The number of immunocompromised patients has increased in the last three decades because of three main phenomena: the AIDS epidemic, advances in cancer chemotherapy, and expanding solid organ and hematopoietic stem cell transplantation. The spectrum of organisms known to cause respiratory infections is broad and constantly increasing as new pathogens are identified and an increasing number of patients have decreased immunity due to disease or medications.

Epidemiologically, pneumonia can be classified into community-acquired pneumonia (CAP), hospital-acquired pneumonia (HAP), ventilator-associated pneumonia (VAP), and healthcare-associated pneumonia (HCAP) [1, 2].

T. Franquet (✉)
Department of Radiology, Hospital de Sant Pau. Universidad Autonoma de Barcelona, Barcelona, Spain
e-mail: Tfranquet@santpau.cat

J. H. Chung
Department of Radiology, The University of Chicago Medicine, Chicago, IL, USA

7.1 Community-Acquired Pneumonia (CAP)

Community acquired pneumonia refers to an acute infection of the lung in patients who did not meet any of the criteria for HCAP, presenting select clinical features (e.g., cough, fever, sputum production, and pleuritic chest pain) and accompanied by an acute infiltrate on a chest radiograph. Pulmonary opacities are usually evident on the radiograph within 12 h of the onset of symptoms [3]. Although the imaging findings do not allow a specific etiologic diagnosis, CAP diagnosis and disease management most frequently involve chest radiography, and other imaging modalities are not usually required [4].

The spectrum of causative organisms of CAP includes gram-positive bacteria such as *Streptococcus pneumoniae* (pneumococcus), *Haemophilus influenzae*, and *Staphylococcus aureus*, as well as atypical organisms such as *Mycoplasma pneumoniae*, *Chlamydia pneumoniae*, or *Legionella pneumophila* and viral agents such as influenza A virus and respiratory syncytial viruses [5]. However, many community-acquired pneumonias are still commonly caused by *S. pneumoniae* and are lobar in appearance.

7.1.1 Radiographic Patterns of CAP

The radiographic patterns of CAP are often related to the causative agent. Infection of the lower respiratory tract, acquired by way of the airways and confined to the lung parenchyma and airways, typically presents radiologically as one of three patterns: (a) focal nonsegmental or lobar pneumonia, (b) multifocal bronchopneumonia or lobular pneumonia, and (c) focal or diffuse "interstitial" pneumonia.

7.2 Hospital-Acquired Pneumonia (HAP)

Hospital-acquired pneumonia (HAP) may be defined as one occurring after admission to the hospital, which was neither present nor in a period of incubation at the time of admission. Hospital-acquired pneumonia (nosocomial) is the leading cause of death from hospital-acquired infections and an important public health problem. It occurs most commonly among intensive care unit (ICU) patients requiring mechanical ventilation.

7.3 Ventilator-Associated Pneumonia (VAP)

Microorganisms responsible for VAP may differ according to the population of patients in the ICU, the durations of hospital and ICU stays, and the specific diagnostic method(s) used. The spectrum of causative pathogens of VAP in humans is *Staphylococcus aureus*, *Pseudomonas aeruginosa*, and Enterobacteriaceae [6].

Chest radiograph is most helpful when it is normal and rules out pneumonia. However, pulmonary opacities were detected by computed tomography (CT) scan in 26% of cases with a normal portable chest X-ray. When infiltrates are present, the particular pattern is of limited value for differentiating among cardiogenic pulmonary edema, noncardiogenic, pulmonary edema, hemorrhage, atelectasis, and pneumonia.

7.4 Healthcare-Associated Pneumonia (HCAP)

When pneumonia is associated with healthcare risk factors such as prior hospitalization, dialysis, residing in a nursing home, and immunocompromised state, it is now classified as a healthcare-associated pneumonia (HCAP). The number of individuals receiving healthcare outside the hospital setting, including home wound care or infusion therapy, dialysis, nursing homes, and similar settings, is constantly increasing [7].

Key Points

- Pneumonia is the leading cause of death due to infectious disease.
- A variety of organisms that may present with similar clinical symptoms result in similar radiographic manifestations.
- The radiographic manifestations of a given organism may be variable depending on the immunologic status of the patient.

7.5 Clinical Utility and Limitations of Chest Radiography and CT

A clinical diagnosis of pneumonia can usually be readily established on the basis of signs, symptoms, and chest radiographs, although distinguishing pneumonia from conditions such as left heart failure, pulmonary embolism, and aspiration pneumonia may sometimes be difficult.

Differentiation of etiologies based solely on the radiograph is not reliable, yet the pattern of abnormalities should be very useful in formulating a differential diagnosis of the nature of disease [8].

7.5.1 Chest Radiography

Chest radiographs are of limited value in predicting the causative pathogen but are of good use to determine the extent of pneumonia and to detect complications (i.e., cavitation, abscess formation, pneumothorax, pleural effusion), to detect additional or alternative diagnoses, and, in some cases, to guide invasive diagnostic procedures.

The most common radiographic manifestations of respiratory infection are foci of consolidation, ground-glass opacities, or reticulonodular opacities. Other less common radiographic findings include hilar and mediastinal lymphadenopathy, pleural effusion, cavitation, and chest wall invasion [8, 9].

7.5.2 Computed Tomography

Computed tomography, particularly high-resolution CT (HRCT), has been shown to be more sensitive than the radiograph in the detection of subtle abnormalities and may show findings suggestive of pneumonia up to 5 days earlier than chest radiographs. CT is recommended in patients with clinical suspicion of infection and normal or nonspecific radiographic findings, in the assessment of suspected complications of pneumonia or suspicion of an underlying lesion such as pulmonary carcinoma.

7.6 Patterns of Pulmonary Infection

Pneumonias are usually divided according to their chest imaging appearance into lobar pneumonia, bronchopneumonia, and interstitial pneumonia.

In lobar pneumonia the inflammatory exudate begins in the distal airspaces adjacent to the visceral pleura and then spreads via collateral air drift routes (pores of Kohn) to produce uniform homogeneous opacification of partial or complete segments of the lung and occasionally an entire lobe.

As the airways are not primarily involved and remain patent, there is little to no volume loss, and air bronchograms are common. Some pneumonias present as spherical- or nodular-shaped consolidations.

Bronchopneumonia (lobular pneumonia) is characterized histologically by peribronchiolar inflammation manifesting radiologically as patchy airspace nodules with poorly defined margins. Radiologically a bronchopneumonia is characterized by large heterogeneous, scattered opacities which only later, with worsening of disease, become more homogeneous. An air bronchogram is usually absent. The most common causative organisms of bronchopneumonia are *S. aureus*, *H. influenzae*, *P. aeruginosa*, and anaerobic bacteria [8].

Characteristic manifestations of bronchopneumonia on HRCT include centrilobular ill-defined nodules and branching linear opacities, airspace nodules, and multifocal lobular areas of consolidation [10].

The term atypical pneumonia (interstitial pneumonia) was initially applied to the clinical and radiographic appearance of lung infection not behaving or looking like that caused by *S. pneumoniae* [11]. Today, when new diagnostic techniques such as direct antigen detection, polymerase chain reaction, and serology (ELISA) have moved beyond the initial diagnostic methods, a debate with regard to the appropriate use of the term "atypical pneumonia" is open [12].

Radiographically focal or diffuse small heterogeneous opacities are seen uniformly distributed in the involved lung. Frequently these opacities are described as reticular or reticulonodular. The usual causes of interstitial pneumonia are viral and mycoplasma infections [9].

7.7 Aerobic Bacteria

7.7.1 Gram-Positive Cocci

7.7.1.1 Streptococcus Pneumoniae

Streptococcus pneumoniae, a gram-positive coccus, is the most common bacterial cause of CAP among patients who require hospitalization. Risk factors for the development of pneumococcal pneumonia include the extremes of age, chronic heart or lung disease, immunosuppression, alcoholism, institutionalization, and prior splenectomy. The characteristic clinical presentation is abrupt in onset, with fever, chills, cough, and pleuritic chest pain. The typical radiographic appearance of acute pneumococcal pneumonia consists of a homogeneous consolidation that crosses segmental boundaries (nonsegmental) but involves only one lobe (lobar pneumonia) (Fig. 7.1). Occasionally, infection is manifested as a spherical focus of consolidation that simulates a mass (round pneumonia). Complications, such as cavitation and pneumatocele formation, are rare. Pleural effusion is common and is seen in up to half of patients.

7.7.1.2 Staphylococcus aureus

Pneumonia caused by *S. aureus* usually follows aspiration of organisms from the upper respiratory tract. Risk factors for the development of staphylococcal pneumonia include underlying pulmonary disease (e.g., COPD, carcinoma), chronic illnesses (e.g., diabetes mellitus, renal failure), or viral infection. The clinical presentation of staphylococcal pneumonia is changing and of particular importance is the dramatic increase of the incidence of methicillin-resistant *Staphylococcus aureus* (MRSA) infections in recent years. Increasingly, previously healthy young people without traditional risk factors for *S. aureus* disease are presenting with severe necrotizing infection and high mortality.

Fever, cough, and purulent sputum are prominent symptoms in cases of post-aspirative staphylococcal pneumonia. Severe pneumonia caused by community-associated methicillin-resistant *Staphylococcus aureus* (MRSA) carrying genes for Panton-Valentine leukocidin has been described in immunocompetent young adults.

The characteristic pattern of presentation is as a bronchopneumonia (lobular pneumonia) that is bilateral in 40% of patients. The radiographic manifestations usually consist of bilateral patchy areas of consolidation. Air bronchograms are uncommon. Other features are cavitation, pneumatoceles, pleural effusions, and spontaneous pneumothorax (Fig. 7.2). Pneumatoceles are seen especially in children [13].

7.7.2 Gram-Positive Bacilli

7.7.2.1 Actinomycosis

Thoracic actinomycosis is a chronic suppurative pulmonary or endobronchial infection caused by *Actinomyces* species, most frequently *Actinomyces israelii* considered to be a gram-positive branching filamentous bacterium. Pulmonary infection is characterized pathologically by bronchopneumonia with focal or multifocal abscess formation. Actinomycosis has the ability to spread across fascial planes to contiguous tissues without regard to normal anatomic barriers. On CT, parenchymal actinomycosis is characterized by airspace consolidation with cavitation or central areas of low attenuation and adjacent pleural thickening. Endobronchial actinomycosis can be associated with a foreign body (direct aspiration of a foreign body contaminated with *Actinomyces* organisms) or a broncholith (secondary colonization of a preexisting endobronchial broncholith by aspirated *Actinomyces* organisms).

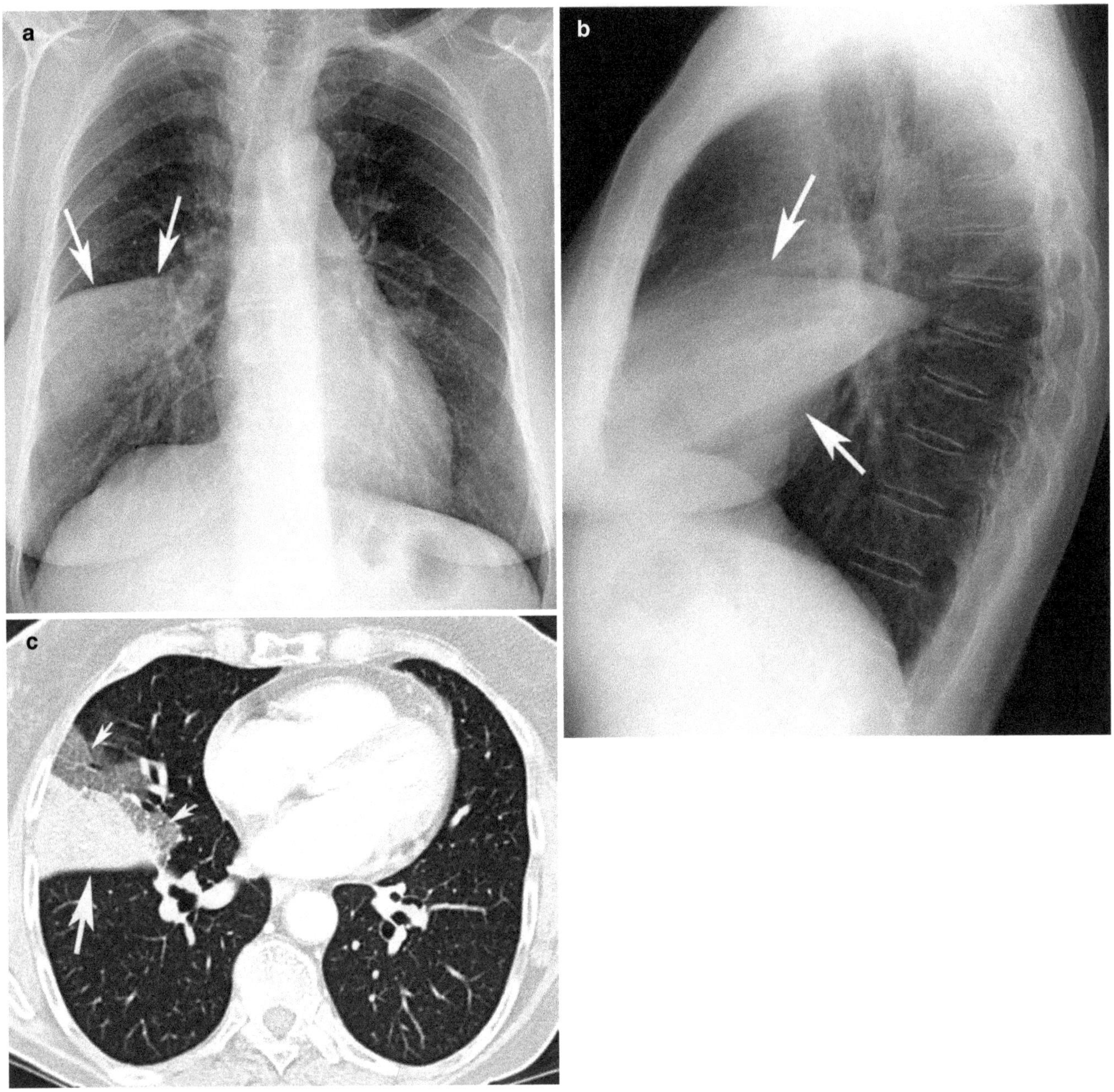

Fig. 7.1 (**a**, **b**, **c**) Lobar pneumonia. (**a**) Posteroanterior and lateral (**b**) chest radiographs in this patient with fever and cough demonstrate lateral segment right middle lobe consolidation (arrows). (**c**) Axial contrast-enhanced CT image shows a mixed opacity of consolidation (arrow) and ground-glass opacity (small arrows) consistent with lobar pneumonia

7.7.2.2 Nocardia Species

Nocardia is a genus of filamentous gram-positive, weakly acid fast, aerobic bacteria that affects both immunosuppressed and immunocompetent patients. *Nocardia asteroides* is responsible of 80% of infections by this organism in man. Pulmonary nocardiosis can be an acute, subacute, or chronic disease. Nocardiosis usually begins with a focus of pulmonary infection and may disseminate through hematogenous spread to other organs, most commonly to the CNS. Imaging findings are variable and consist of unifocal or multifocal consolidation and single or multiple pulmonary nodules [14]. *Nocardia asteroides* infection may complicate alveolar proteinosis.

7.7.3 Gram-Negative Bacilli

Gram-negative pneumonias are chiefly caused by *Klebsiella pneumoniae*, *Enterobacter* sp., *Serratia marcescens*, *Escherichia coli*, *Proteus* sp., and *Pseudomonas aeruginosa*. Patients affected are invariably debilitated by a chronic medical or pulmonary disease. The lower lobes

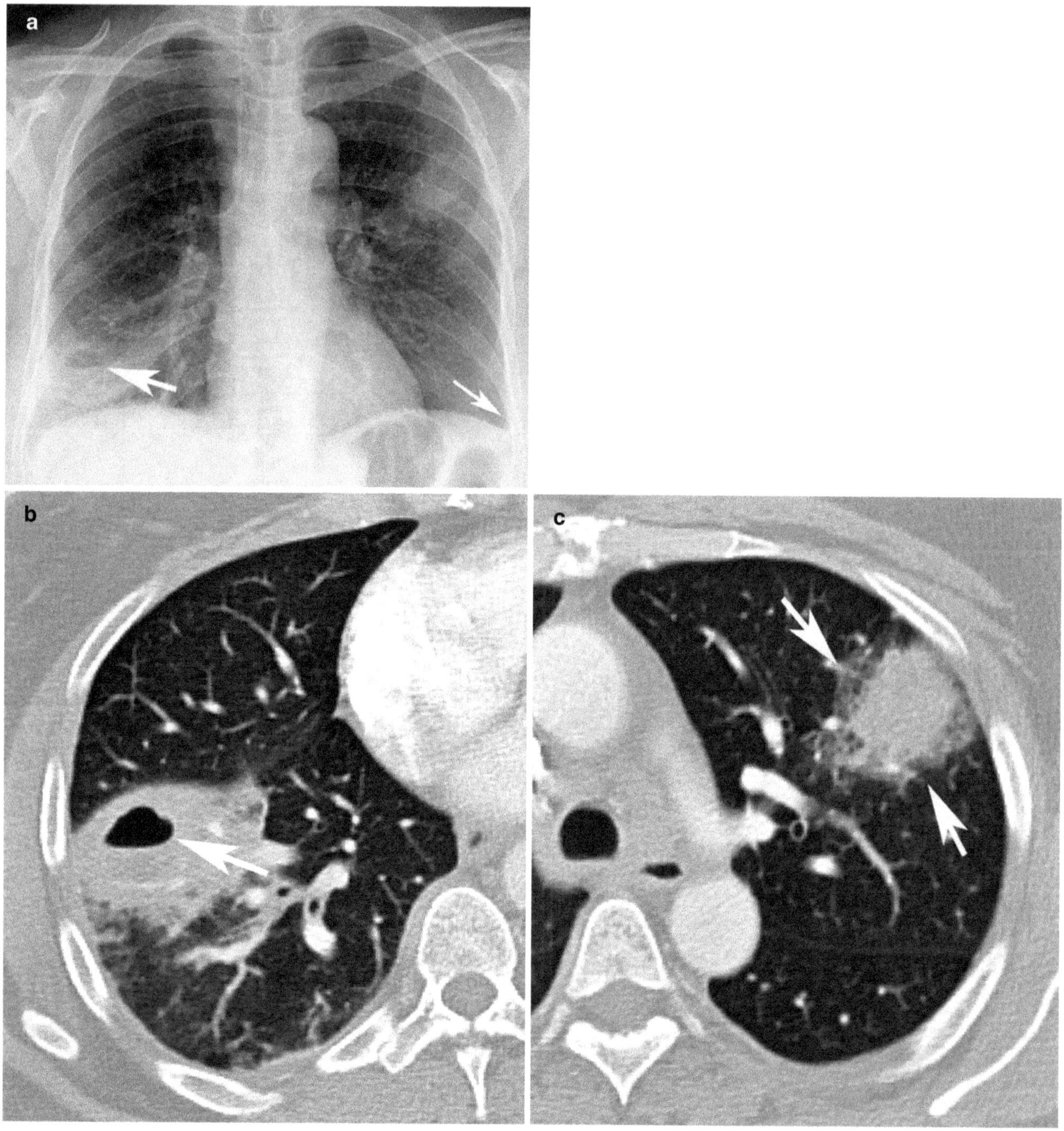

Fig. 7.2 (**a, b, c**) *Staphylococcus aureus* pneumonia: (**a**) Posteroanterior chest radiograph demonstrates a dominant right basilar and left upper lung mass-like opacities with cavitation in the right basilar opacity (arrow). Small left pleural effusion is also seen (small arrow). (**b, c**) Axial contrast-enhanced CT shows a cavitary mass within the right lower lobe (arrow) and a mass in the left upper lobe demonstrating surrounding ground-glass opacity (halo sign) (arrows)

tend to be affected, and the radiographic pattern is similar to that seen with *S. aureus* infections in adults.

7.7.3.1 Klebsiella

Klebsiella pneumoniae is among the most common gram-negative bacteria accounting for 0.5–5.0% of all cases of pneumonia. These features are bulging fissures, sharp margins of the advancing border of the pneumonic infiltrate and early abscess formation. CT findings consist of ground-glass attenuation, consolidation, and intralobular reticular opacity, often associated with pleural effusion. Complications of *Klebsiella pneumonia* include abscess formation, parapneumonic effusion, and empyema.

7.7.3.2 Escherichia coli

Escherichia coli accounts for 4% of cases of CAP and 5–20% of cases of HAP or HCAP. It occurs most commonly in debilitated patients. The typical history is one of abrupt onset of fever, chills, dyspnea, pleuritic pain, and productive cough in a patient with preexisting chronic disease.

The radiographic manifestations usually are those of bronchopneumonia; rarely a pattern of lobar pneumonia may be seen.

7.7.3.3 *Pseudomonas aeruginosa*

Pseudomonas aeruginosa is a gram-negative bacillus that is the most common cause of nosocomial pulmonary infection. It causes confluent bronchopneumonia that is often extensive and frequently cavitates (Fig. 7.3). The radiologic manifestations are nonspecific and consist most commonly of patchy areas of consolidation and widespread poorly defined nodular opacities [9].

7.7.3.4 Chlamydia

Chlamydia pneumoniae is the most commonly occurring gram-negative intracellular bacterial pathogen. It is frequently involved in respiratory tract infections and has also been implicated in the pathogenesis of asthma in both adults and children. Symptoms include sore throat, headache, and a nonproductive cough that can persist for months if treatment is not initiated early.

Chest radiographs tend to show less extensive abnormalities than are seen with other causes of pneumonia. On CT, *C. pneumoniae* pneumonia demonstrates a wide spectrum of

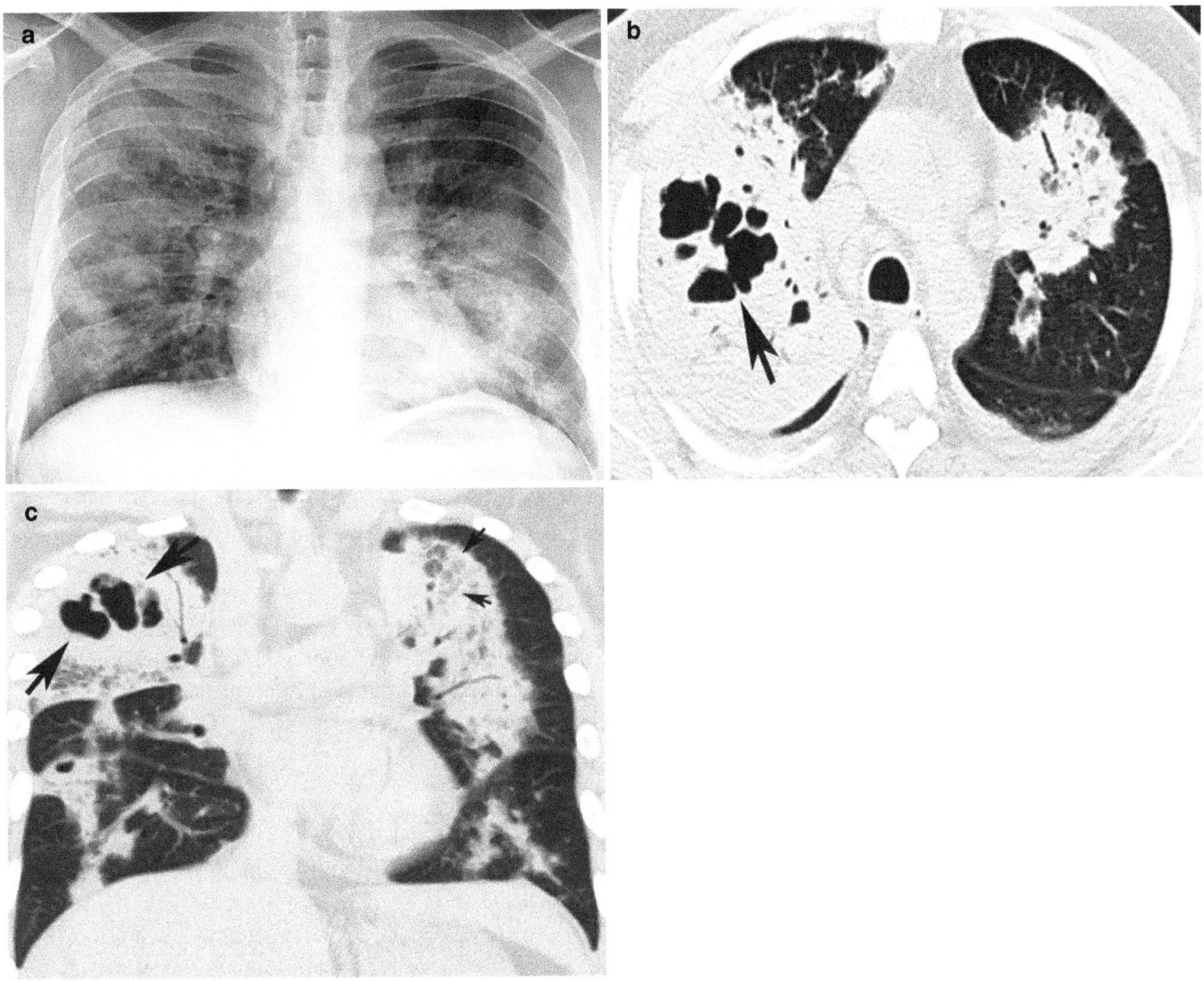

Fig. 7.3 (**a**, **b**, **c**) Pseudomonas aeruginosa pneumonia: (**a**) Posteroanterior chest radiograph demonstrates multifocal lung consolidation bilaterally consistent with bronchopneumonia. (**b**) Axial and (**c**) coronal CT images demonstrate bilateral multifocal lung consolidations; cavitary necrosis is observed within the right upper lobe consolidation (arrows); mild superimposed ground-glass opacity is also present (small arrows)

findings that are similar to those of *S. pneumoniae* pneumonia and *M. pneumoniae*. Cavitation and hilar or mediastinal adenopathy are uncommon.

7.7.3.5 Rickettsial Pneumonia

The most common rickettsia lung infection is sporadic or epidemic Q-fever pneumonia caused by *Coxiella burnetii*, an intracellular, gram-negative bacterium.

Infection is acquired by inhalation from farm livestock or their products and occasionally from domestic animals. Imaging findings consist of multilobar airspace consolidation, solitary or multiple nodules surrounded by a halo of "ground-glass" opacity and vessel connection, and necrotizing pneumonia.

7.7.3.6 *Francisella tularensis*

Tularemia is an acute, febrile, bacterial zoonosis caused by the aerobic gram-negative bacillus *Francisella tularensis*. It is endemic in parts of Europe, Asia, and North America. Primary pneumonic tularemia occurs in rural settings. Humans become infected after introduction of the bacillus by inhalation, intradermal injection, or oral ingestion. Chest radiographic findings are scattered multifocal consolidations, hilar adenopathy, and pleural effusion.

7.7.4 *Gram-Negative Coccobacilli*

7.7.4.1 *Haemophilus influenza*

Haemophilus influenzae is a pleomorphic, gram-negative coccobacillus that accounts for 5–20% of CAP in patients in whom an organism can be identified successfully. Factors that predispose to Haemophilus pneumonia include COPD, malignancy, HIV infection, and alcoholism. The typical radiographic appearance of *Haemophilus influenza* pneumonia consists of multilobar involvement with lobar or segmental consolidation and pleural effusion.

7.7.4.2 *Legionella* Species

Legionella is a pathogenic gram-negative bacterium with at least 50 species. It is one of the most common causes of severe community-acquired pneumonia in immunocompetent hosts. Human infection may occur when Legionella contaminates water systems, such as air conditioners and condensers. Risk factors for the development of *L. pneumophila* pneumonia include immunosuppression, posttransplantation, cigarette smoking, renal disease, and exposure to contaminated drinking water. Patients with *Legionella* pneumonia usually present with fever, cough, initially dry and later productive, malaise, myalgia, confusion, headaches, and diarrhea. Thirty percent of patients develop pleuritic chest pain.

Imaging findings include peripheral airspace consolidation similar to that seen in acute *S. pneumoniae* pneumonia. In many cases, the area of consolidation rapidly progresses to occupy all or a large portion of a lobe (lobar pneumonia) or to involve contiguous lobes or to become bilateral. Cavitation is uncommon in immunocompetent patients, and pleural effusion may occur in 35–63% of cases.

7.7.5 Gram-Negative Cocci

7.7.5.1 *Moraxella catarrhalis*

Moraxella catarrhalis (formerly known as *Branhamella catarrhalis*) has emerged as a significant bacterial pathogen of humans over the past two decades. It is an intracellular gram-negative coccus now recognized as one of the common respiratory pathogens [15]. *M. catarrhalis* causes otitis media and sinusitis in children and mild pneumonia and acute exacerbation in older patients with COPD. It is currently considered the third most common cause of community-acquired bacterial pneumonia (after *S. pneumoniae* and *H. influenzae*). The majority of patients with pneumonia (80–90%) have underlying chronic pulmonary disease. Chest radiographs show bronchopneumonia or lobar pneumonia that usually involves a single lobe.

7.8 Miscellaneous Infections

7.8.1 *Mycoplasma pneumoniae*

M. pneumoniae is one of the most common causes of community-acquired pneumonia. It accounts for up to 37% of CAP in persons treated as outpatients. Patients with COPD appear to be more severely affected with *M. pneumoniae* than normal hosts.

The radiographic findings in *M. pneumoniae* are variable and in some cases closely resemble those seen in viral infections of the lower respiratory tract. Chest radiograph shows fine linear opacities followed by segmental airspace consolidation [16].

Key Points

- A "tree-in-bud" pattern is a characteristic CT manifestation of infectious bronchiolitis.
- Focal areas of consolidation secondary to infection in immunocompromised patients are most commonly due to bacterial pneumonia.
- Interstitial and/or mixed interstitial and airspace opacities in CAP are typically due to viruses or *M. pneumoniae*.

7.9 Mycobacteria

7.9.1 *Mycobacterium Tuberculosis*

Mycobacterium tuberculosis accounts for more than 95% of pulmonary mycobacterial infections. Other mycobacterial species, *M. kansasii* and *M. avium–intracellulare* complex (MAC), account for the remainder.

Factors that contribute to the large number of cases seen worldwide are human immunodeficiency virus (HIV) infection, inner city poverty, homelessness, and immigration from areas with high rates of infection. Other predisposing conditions are diabetes mellitus, alcoholism, silicosis, and malignancy.

7.9.1.1 *Primary tuberculosis*

This form is seen in infants and children. With improved control of tuberculosis in western societies, however, more people reach adulthood without exposure, and primary patterns of disease are being seen with increasing frequency in adulthood and represents about 23–34% of all adult cases of tuberculosis.

Although primary tuberculosis typically presents with radiographic manifestations, chest radiograph may be normal in 15% of cases. Lymphadenopathy is the most common manifestation of primary tuberculosis in children and occurs with or without pneumonia. In adults hilar or mediastinal lymphadenopathy is less common declining to about 50% of cases in the older population. Pleural effusion occurs in children, who usually have parenchymal or nodal disease, or in teenagers and young adults, when it is frequently isolated.

7.9.1.2 *Postprimary tuberculosis*

Most cases are due to reactivation of quiescent lesions, but occasionally a new infection from an exogenous source occurs. Pathologically, the ability of the host to respond immunologically results in a greater inflammatory reaction and caseous necrosis.

The radiological manifestations may overlap with those of primary tuberculosis, but the absence of lymphadenopathy, more frequent cavitation, and a predilection for the upper lobes are more typical of postprimary tuberculosis. A Rasmussen aneurysm is a rare life-threatening complication of cavitary tuberculosis caused by granulomatous weakening of a pulmonary arterial wall.

Endobronchial spread can occur with or without cavitary disease and is similar to that seen with primary tuberculosis leading to the appearance of the typical images of "tree-in-bud" [17, 18].

After antituberculous treatment healing results in scar formation. The fibrosis produces well-defined, upper lobe nodular and linear opacities, often with evidence of severe volume loss and pleural thickening. Residual thin-walled cavities may be present in both active and inactive disease.

Although classically a manifestation of primary disease, miliary tuberculosis is now more commonly seen as a postprimary process in older patients. Multiple small (1–2 mm) discrete nodules are scattered evenly throughout both lungs.

A tuberculoma may occur in the setting of primary or postprimary tuberculosis and represents localized parenchymal disease that alternately activates and heals. It usually calcifies and frequently remains stable for years [19].

7.9.1.3 *Pulmonary Nontuberculous Mycobacteria (NTMB)*

As mentioned above, 1–3% of pulmonary mycobacterial infections are caused by agents other than *M. tuberculosis*: usually *M. avium–intracellulare* complex (*MAC*) and less commonly *M. kansasii*. Patients are often predisposed by reason of underlying debilitating disease, immune compromise, chronic airflow obstruction, previous pulmonary tuberculosis, or silicosis and following lung transplantation [20]. Clinically, MAC may be an indolent process with symptoms of cough, with or without sputum production.

More commonly, MAC presents with a radiological pattern that does not resemble that of postprimary tuberculosis. It consists of multiple nodules, with or without small ring opacities, showing no specific lobar predilection and bronchiectasis particularly in the lingula and right middle lobe. The most typical form of pulmonary nontuberculous mycobacteria (NTMB) infection is frequently associated to elderly men with underlying lung disease and to elderly white women without underlying lung disease (Lady Windermere syndrome). Radiological findings consist of mild to moderate cylindrical bronchiectasis and multiple 1–3 mm diameter centrilobular nodules.

7.10 Fungal Infections

Fungi involved in pulmonary infections are either pathogenic fungi, which can infect any host, or saprophytic fungi, which infect only immunocompromised hosts. Pathogenic fungi include coccidioidomycosis, blastomycosis, and histoplasmosis. Saprophytes include Pneumocystis, Candidiasis, Mucormycosis, and Aspergillosis. Pulmonary fungal infections may be difficult to diagnose, and a definitive diagnosis of pulmonary fungal infections is made by isolating the fungus from tissue specimen.

7.10.1 Aspergillus Infection

Aspergillosis is a fungal disease caused by *Aspergillus* species, usually *A. fumigatus* that can take different forms depending on an individual's immune response to the organism. Classically, pulmonary aspergillosis has been categorized into saprophytic, allergic, and invasive forms [21, 22].

Aspergillus mycetomas are saprophytic growths which colonize a preexisting cavity in the lung (e.g., from sarcoidosis or tuberculosis). Most cavities and thus mycetomas are in the upper lobes or superior segments of the lower lobes.

Allergic bronchopulmonary aspergillosis (ABPA) describes a hypersensitivity reaction which occurs in the major airways. It is associated with elevated serum IgE, positive serum precipitins, and skin reactivity to *Aspergillus*. The radiographic appearances consist of nonsegmental areas of opacity most common in the upper lobes, lobar collapse, branching thick tubular opacities due to bronchi distended with mucus and fungus, and occasionally pulmonary cavitation. The mucus plugs in ABPA are usually hypodense, but in up to 20% of patients, the mucus can be hyperdense on CT (Fig. 7.4).

Angioinvasive aspergillosis is seen in immunocompromised hosts with severe neutropenia. This form is characterized by invasion and occlusion of small-to-medium pulmonary arteries, developing necrotic hemorrhagic nodules or infarcts. The most common pattern seen in CT consists of multiples nodules surrounded by a halo of ground-glass attenuation (halo sign) or pleural-based wedge-shaped areas of consolidation [21].

7.10.2 Candidiasis

Candida species has been increasingly recognized as an important source of fungal pneumonia in immunocompromised patients, particularly in those with underlying malignancy (acute leukemia and lymphoma), intravenous drug abuse, and acquired immune deficiency syndrome

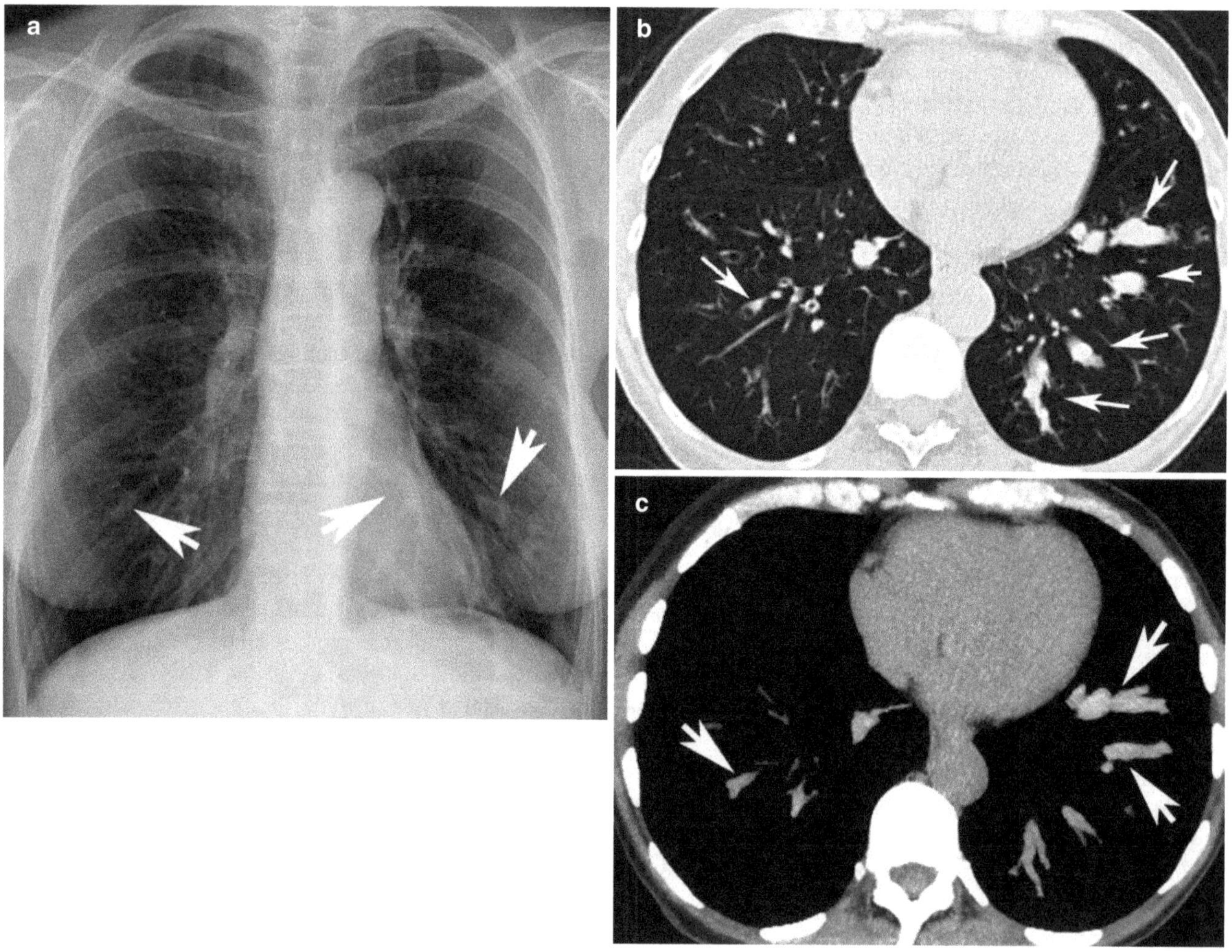

Fig. 7.4 (**a**, **b**, **c**) Allergic bronchopulmonary aspergillosis: (**a**) Posteroanterior chest radiograph demonstrates basilar branching opacities suggestive of mucus-filled bronchiectasis (arrows). (**b**) Axial CT image confirms the presence of left basilar bronchiectasis, mucus-filled airways (arrows). (**c**) Hyperdensity of mucus-filled airways on axial MIP image (arrows) from chest CT is diagnostic of allergic bronchopulmonary aspergillosis

(AIDS), and following bone marrow transplantation. The most common thin-section CT findings of pulmonary candidiasis consist of multiple bilateral nodular opacities often associated with areas of consolidation and ground-glass opacity [23].

7.10.3 *Pneumocystis jiroveci*

Pneumocystis jiroveci a unique opportunistic fungal pathogen that causes pneumonia in immunocompromised individuals such as patients with AIDS, patients with organ transplants, and patients with hematologic or solid organ malignancies who are undergoing chemotherapy. In 90% of patients with *Pneumocystis jiroveci*, pneumonia chest radiographs show diffuse bilateral infiltrates in a perihilar distribution (Fig. 7.5). The most common high-resolution CT finding in *Pneumocystis jiroveci* pneumonia is diffuse ground-glass opacity [24].

7.10.4 Mucormycosis

Mucormycosis is an opportunistic fungal infection of the order Mucorales, characterized by broad, nonseptated hyphae that randomly branch at right angles.

The most common radiographic findings consist of lobar or multilobar areas of consolidation and solitary or multiple pulmonary nodules and masses with associated cavitation or an air-crescent sign [25].

7.11 Viral Pneumonias

Viruses can result in several pathologic forms of lower respiratory tract infection including tracheobronchitis, bronchiolitis, and pneumonia. Viral infections predispose to secondary bacterial pneumonia. Organizing pneumonia, a nonspecific reparative reaction, may result from a variety of causes or underlying pathologic processes including viral infections [26].

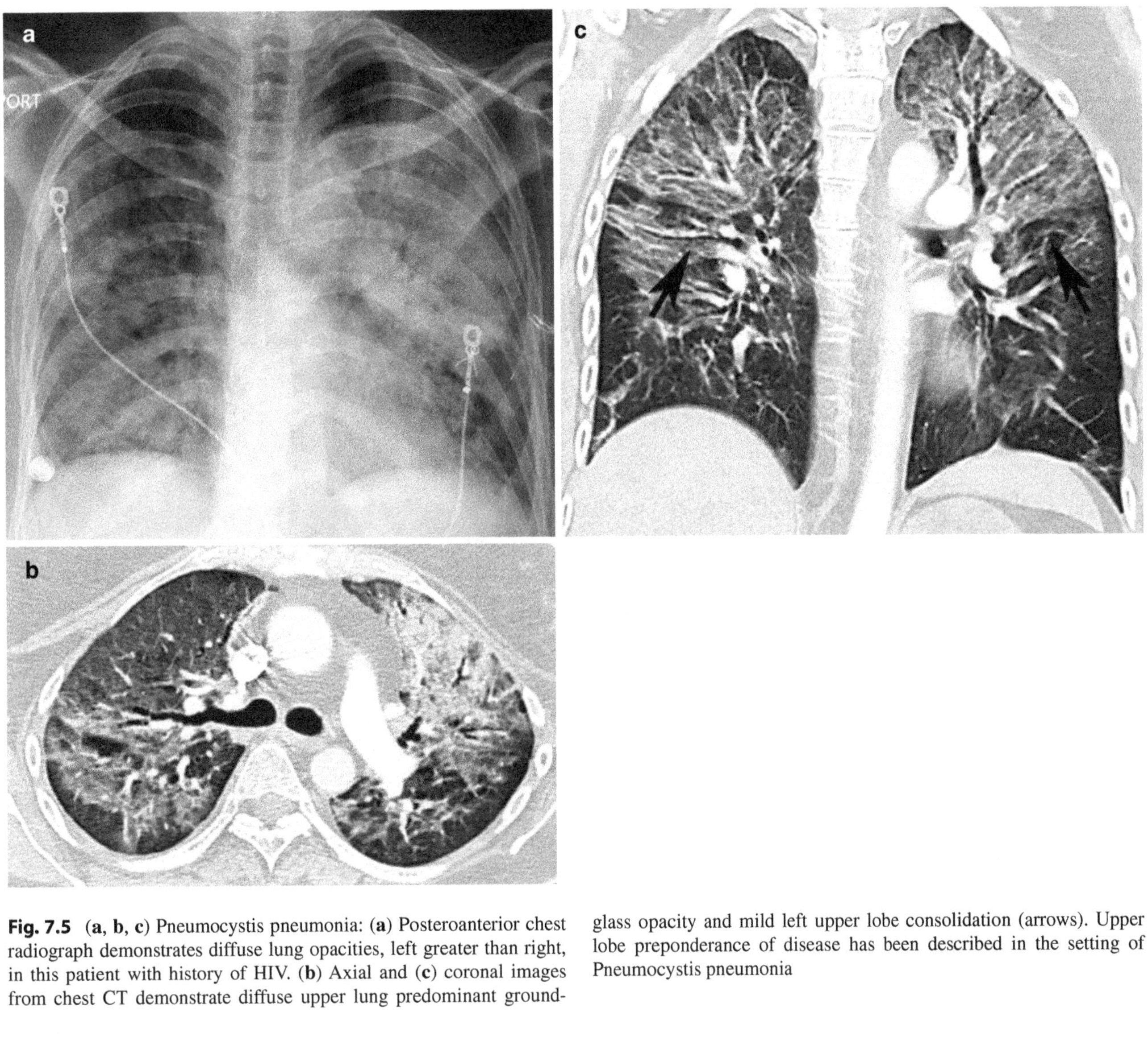

Fig. 7.5 (**a**, **b**, **c**) Pneumocystis pneumonia: (**a**) Posteroanterior chest radiograph demonstrates diffuse lung opacities, left greater than right, in this patient with history of HIV. (**b**) Axial and (**c**) coronal images from chest CT demonstrate diffuse upper lung predominant ground-glass opacity and mild left upper lobe consolidation (arrows). Upper lobe preponderance of disease has been described in the setting of Pneumocystis pneumonia

7.11.1 Influenza a

Influenza type A is the most important of the respiratory viruses with respect to the morbidity and mortality in the general population. In recent years, both influenza and parainfluenza viruses have been recognized as a significant cause of respiratory illness in immunocompromised patients, including solid organ transplant recipients. The predominant high-resolution CT findings are ground-glass opacities, consolidation, centrilobular nodules, and branching linear opacities.

7.11.2 Adenovirus

Adenovirus accounts for 5–10% of acute respiratory infections in infants and children but for less than 1% of respiratory illnesses in adults. Swyer-James-MacLeod syndrome is considered to be a post-infectious bronchiolitis obliterans (BO) secondary to adenovirus infection in childhood.

7.11.3 Respiratory Syncytial Virus (RSV)

Respiratory syncytial virus (RSV) is the most frequent viral cause of lower respiratory tract infection in infants. The major risk factors for severe RSV disease in children are prematurity (< 36 weeks gestation), congenital heart disease, chronic lung disease, immunocompromised status, and multiple congenital abnormalities. CT findings consist of small centrilobular nodules, airspace consolidation, ground-glass opacities, bronchial wall thickening, and "tree-in-bud" opacities (Fig. 7.6).

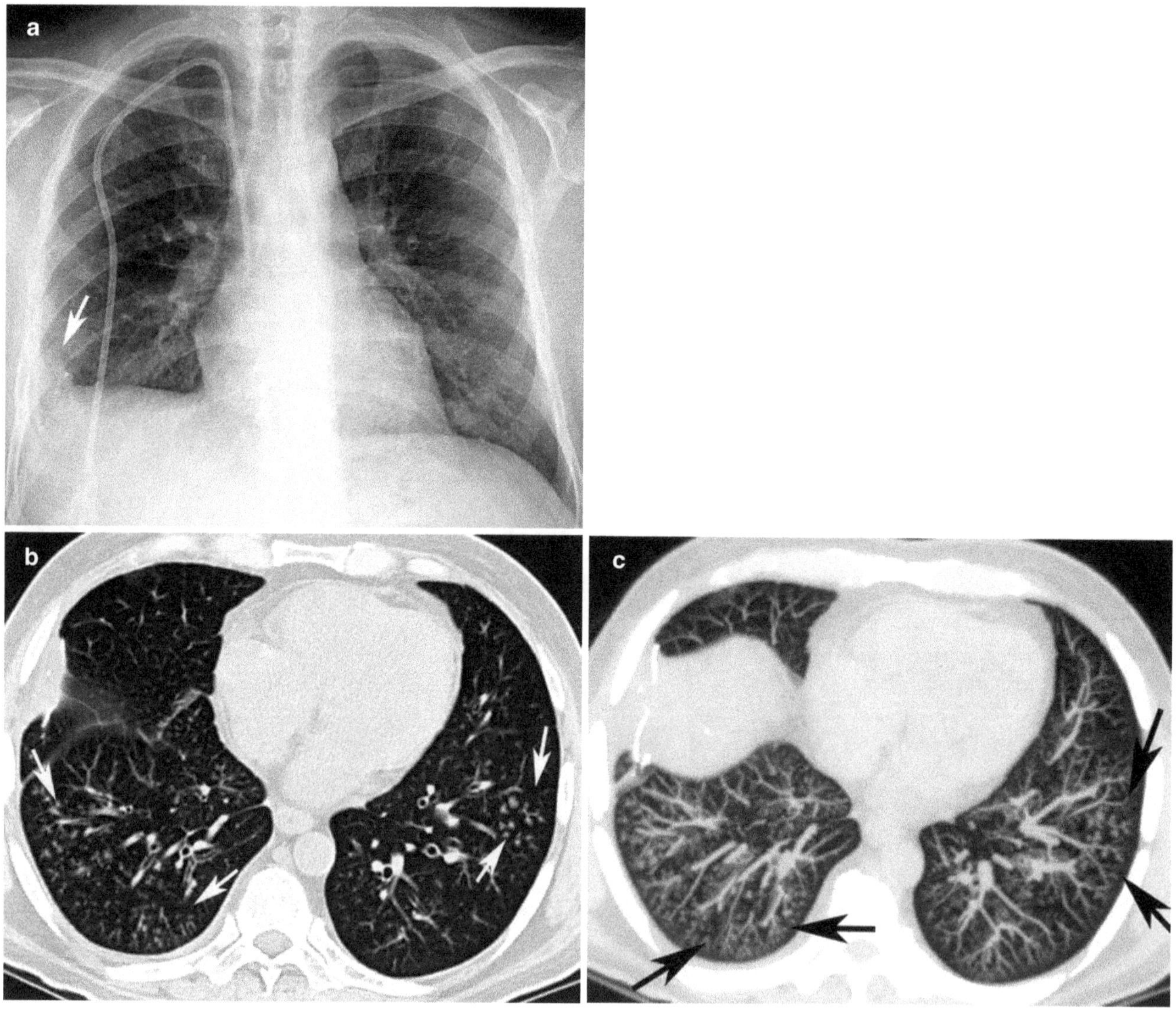

Fig. 7.6 (**a**, **b**, **c**) Respiratory syncytial virus pneumonia: (**a**) Posteroanterior chest radiograph demonstrates subtle basilar nodularity and mild right basilar pleuroparenchymal scarring (arrow). (**b**) Axial CT image and (**c**) MIP images from chest CT demonstrate tree-in-bud opacities in the lower lobes (arrows)

7.11.4 Epstein-Barr Virus (EBV)

Primary infection with EBV occurs early in life and presents as infectious mononucleosis with the typical triad of fever, pharyngitis, and lymphadenopathy, often accompanied by splenomegaly. Mild, asymptomatic pneumonitis occurs in about 5–10% of cases of infectious mononucleosis. The CT manifestations of EBV pneumonia are similar to those of other viral pneumonias. The findings usually consist of lobar consolidation, diffuse and focal parenchymal haziness, irregular reticular opacities, and multiple miliary nodules or small nodules with associated areas of ground-glass attenuation ("halo").

7.11.5 Varicella Virus

Varicella is a common contagious infection in childhood with increasing incidence in adults. Clinically presents in two forms: varicella (chickenpox) representing a primary disseminated disease in uninfected individuals and zoster (shingles) representing reactivation of latent virus (unilateral dermatomal skin eruption).

Pneumonia, although rare, is the most serious complication affecting adults with chickenpox. The thin-section CT appearances in varicella pneumonia reflect the multicentric hemorrhage and necrosis centered on airways. Common findings include numerous nodular opacities measuring 5–10 mm in diameter, some with a surrounding halo of ground-glass opacity, patchy ground-glass opacities, and coalescence of nodules.

7.11.6 *Cytomegalovirus (CMV)*

Cytomegalovirus pneumonia is a major cause of morbidity and mortality following hematopoietic stem cell (HSCT) and solid organ transplantation and in patients with AIDS in whom CD4 cells are decreased to fewer than 100 cells/mm^3. This complication characteristically occurs during the post-engraftment period (30–100 days after transplantation) with a median time onset of 50–60 days posttransplantation.

CT features of CMV pneumonia consist of lobar consolidation, diffuse and focal ground-glass opacities, irregular reticular opacities, and multiple miliary nodules or small nodules with associated areas of ground-glass attenuation ("halo").

7.12 New Emerging Viruses

7.12.1 Severe Acute Respiratory Distress Syndrome (SARS)

Severe acute respiratory distress syndrome (SARS) caused by SARS-associated coronavirus (SARS-CoV) is a systemic infection that clinically manifests as progressive pneumonia. Severe acute respiratory distress syndrome was first detected in the Guangdong Province of China in late 2002, with major outbreaks in Hong Kong, Guangdong, Singapore, and Toronto and Vancouver, Canada. Over 8000 people were affected, with a mortality rate of 10%. The typical clinical presentation consists of an incubation period of 2–10 days, early systemic symptoms followed within 2–7 days by dry cough or shortness of breath, the development of radiographically confirmed pneumonia by day 7–10, and lymphocytopenia in many cases. Histologically, acute diffuse alveolar damage with airspace edema is the most prominent feature. The imaging features consist of unilateral or bilateral ground-glass opacities, focal unilateral or bilateral areas of consolidation, or a mixture of both [27, 28].

7.12.2 Middle East Respiratory Syndrome (MERS)

MERS is a viral disease caused by a coronavirus (MERS-CoV), with most of the infections believed to have originated in Saudi Arabia and the Middle East. Most patients develop a severe acute respiratory illness. CT may depict ground-glass opacities, consolidation, interlobular thickening, and pleural effusion. During the subsequent weeks, other findings may be present, such as centrilobular nodules, a "crazy-paving" pattern, obliterative bronchiolitis, peribronchial air trapping, and organizing pneumonia [29].

7.12.3 Swine Influenza (H1N1)

In the spring of 2009, an outbreak of severe pneumonia was reported in conjunction with the concurrent isolation of a novel swine-origin influenza A (H1N1) virus, widely known as swine flu, in Mexico. On June 11, 2009, the World Health Organization declared the first pandemic of the twenty-first century caused by swine-origin influenza virus A (H1N1). The predominant CT findings are unilateral or bilateral ground-glass opacities with or without associated focal or multifocal areas of consolidation. On CT, the ground-glass opacities and areas of consolidation have a predominant peribronchovascular and subpleural distribution, resembling organizing pneumonia [30].

Key Points

- Primary TB occurs most commonly in children.
- The most typical form of pulmonary NTMB infection is frequently associated to elderly non-smoking white women without underlying lung disease (Lady Windermere syndrome).
- With respect to the morbidity and mortality, influenza type A is the most important of the respiratory viruses in the general population.

References

1. Burnham JP, Kollef MHCAP, HCAP HAP. VAP: the diachronic linguistics of pneumonia. Chest. 2017;152(5):909–10.
2. Musher DM, Thorner AR. Community-acquired pneumonia. N Engl J Med. 2015;372(3):294.
3. Hagaman JT, Rouan GW, Shipley RT, Panos RJ. Admission chest radiograph lacks sensitivity in the diagnosis of community-acquired pneumonia. Am J Med Sci. 2009;337(4):236–40.
4. Rider AC, Frazee BW. Community-acquired pneumonia. Emerg Med Clin North Am. 2018;36(4):665–83.
5. Ishiguro T, Yoshii Y, Kanauchi T, et al. Re-evaluation of the etiology and clinical and radiological features of community-acquired lobar pneumonia in adults. J Infect Chemother. 2018;
6. Chastre J, Fagon JY. Ventilator-associated pneumonia. Am J Respir Crit Care Med. 2002;165(7):867–903.
7. Micek ST, Reichley RM, Kollef MH. Health care-associated pneumonia (HCAP): empiric antibiotics targeting methicillin-resistant Staphylococcus aureus (MRSA) and Pseudomonas aeruginosa predict optimal outcome. Medicine (Baltimore). 2011;90(6):390–5.
8. Ketai L, Jordan K, Busby KH. Imaging infection. Clin Chest Med. 2015;36(2):197–217.. viii
9. Franquet T. Imaging of community-acquired pneumonia. J Thorac Imaging. 2018;33(5):282–94.
10. Tanaka N, Matsumoto T, Kuramitsu T, et al. High resolution CT findings in community-acquired pneumonia. J Comput Assist Tomogr. 1996;20(4):600–8.
11. Basarab M, Macrae MB, Curtis CM. Atypical pneumonia. Curr Opin Pulm Med. 2014;20(3):247–51.
12. Murdoch DR, Chambers ST. Atypical pneumonia--time to breathe new life into a useful term? Lancet Infect Dis. 2009;9(8):512–9.
13. Vilar J, Domingo ML, Soto C, Cogollos J. Radiology of bacterial pneumonia. Eur J Radiol. 2004;51(2):102–13.
14. Kanne JP, Yandow DR, Mohammed TL, Meyer CA. CT findings of pulmonary nocardiosis. AJR Am J Roentgenol. 2011;197(2):W266–72.
15. Verduin CM, Hol C, Fleer A, van Dijk H, van Belkum A. Moraxella catarrhalis: from emerging to established pathogen. Clin Microbiol Rev. 2002;15(1):125–44.
16. Reittner P, Muller NL, Heyneman L, et al. Mycoplasma pneumoniae pneumonia: radiographic and high-resolution CT features in 28 patients. AJR Am J Roentgenol. 2000;174(1):37–41.
17. Im JG, Itoh H, Han MC. CT of pulmonary tuberculosis. Semin Ultrasound CT MR. 1995;16(5):420–34.
18. Rossi SE, Franquet T, Volpacchio M, Gimenez A, Aguilar G. Tree-in-bud pattern at thin-section CT of the lungs: radiologic-pathologic overview. Radiographics. 2005;25(3):789–801.
19. Burrill J, Williams CJ, Bain G, Conder G, Hine AL, Misra RR. Tuberculosis: a radiologic review. Radiographics. 2007;27(5):1255–73.
20. Kendall BA, Winthrop KL. Update on the epidemiology of pulmonary nontuberculous mycobacterial infections. Semin Respir Crit Care Med. 2013;34(1):87–94.
21. Franquet T, Muller NL, Gimenez A, Guembe P, de La Torre J, Bague S. Spectrum of pulmonary aspergillosis: histologic, clinical, and radiologic findings. Radiographics. 2001;21(4):825–37.
22. Gefter WB. The spectrum of pulmonary aspergillosis. J Thorac Imaging. 1992;7(4):56–74.
23. Franquet T, Muller NL, Lee KS, Oikonomou A, Flint JD. Pulmonary candidiasis after hematopoietic stem cell transplantation: thin-section CT findings. Radiology. 2005;236(1):332–7.
24. Kanne JP, Yandow DR, Meyer CA. Pneumocystis jiroveci pneumonia: high-resolution CT findings in patients with and without HIV infection. AJR Am J Roentgenol. 2012;198(6):W555–61.
25. Hammer MM, Madan R, Hatabu H. Pulmonary Mucormycosis: radiologic features at presentation and over time. AJR Am J Roentgenol. 2018;210(4):742–7.
26. Franquet T. Imaging of pulmonary viral pneumonia. Radiology. 2011;260(1):18–39.
27. Wong KT, Antonio GE, Hui DS, et al. Thin-section CT of severe acute respiratory syndrome: evaluation of 73 patients exposed to or with the disease. Radiology. 2003;228(2):395–400.
28. Muller NL, FitzGerald JM. Severe acute respiratory syndrome (SARS). Thorax. 2003;58(11):919.
29. Das KM, Lee EY, Langer RD, Larsson SG. Middle East respiratory syndrome coronavirus: what does a radiologist need to know? AJR Am J Roentgenol. 2016;206(6):1193–201.
30. Ajlan AM, Khashoggi K, Nicolaou S, Muller NL. CT utilization in the prospective diagnosis of a case of swine-origin influenza A (H1N1) viral infection. J Radiol Case Rep. 2010;4(3):24–30.

8

Current Concepts in the Diagnosis and Staging of Lung Cancer

Brett W. Carter and Jeremy J. Erasmus

Learning Objectives

- Understand the role of imaging in diagnosing and staging lung cancer.
- Describe the tumor (T), lymph node (N), and metastasis (M) descriptors and stage groups outlined in the eighth edition of the TNM staging system (TNM-8).
- Employ TNM-8 to properly characterize and stage lung cancers with multiple sites of pulmonary involvement, including those with multiple tumor nodules, ground-glass lesions, and consolidation.

8.1 Introduction

Lung cancer is a major cause of cancer-related mortality worldwide and is the leading cause of cancer-related mortality in the United States in both men and women, accounting for more deaths than colorectal, breast, prostate, and pancreatic cancers combined [1, 2]. Lung cancer is staged using a typical tumor (T), node (N), and metastasis (M) scheme. The seventh edition of the tumor-node-metastasis (TNM) staging system for lung cancer (TNM-7) included key changes to the T and M descriptors and the recommendation that both small cell lung carcinoma and bronchopulmonary carcinoid tumors be staged with this system [3]. Updated revisions to the TNM staging system, in the form of the eighth edition (TNM-8), have been accepted by the Union for International Cancer Control (UICC) and the American Joint Committee on Cancer (AJCC) based on proposals from the International Association for the Study of Lung Cancer [4]. TNM-8 features additional changes to the T and M descriptors, modifications, and additions to the overall stage groups, new recommendations for the staging of patients with multiple sites of pulmonary involvement, and recommendations for lesion measurement. In this manuscript, we discuss the role of imaging in the diagnosis of lung cancer and the key features of TNM-8 with which radiologists must be familiar.

B. W. Carter (✉) · J. J. Erasmus
Department of Diagnostic Radiology, The University of Texas MD Anderson Cancer Center, Houston, TX, USA
e-mail: bcarter2@mdanderson.org; jerasmus@mdanderson.org

8.2 Diagnosis of Lung Cancer

8.2.1 Clinical Symptoms

Most patients diagnosed with lung cancer manifest in the fifth and sixth decades of life [5]. Approximately three-fourths of patients demonstrate clinical symptoms at the time of presentation, the most common of which include cough (50–75%), hemoptysis (25–50%), dyspnea (25%), and chest pain (20%). Nonspecific symptoms related to systemic manifestations of the malignancy such as anorexia, weight loss, or fatigue may be present. Clinical symptoms also depend on the local effects of the primary tumor, the presence of regional or distant metastases, and the coexistence of paraneoplastic syndromes. While patients with solitary, peripherally located tumors tend to be asymptomatic, those with central endobronchial tumors may demonstrate fever, dyspnea, hemoptysis, and cough. Symptoms related to invasion of the mediastinum and associated vital structures include chest pain, vocal cord paralysis and hoarseness, facial and upper truncal edema, headaches, neck vein distention and enlarged collateral chest wall vessels (as seen in superior vena cava obstruction), and dysphagia (as seen in esophageal involvement). Lung cancers may produce symptoms via the release of bioactive substances or hormones or result in immune-mediated neural tissue destruction caused by antibody or cell-mediated immune responses. Such paraneoplastic syndromes occur in 10–20% of lung cancer patients, the most common of which are related to the release of antidiuretic and adrenocorticotropin hormones, which can result in hyponatremia and serum hypo-osmolarity and in Cushing's syndrome (central obesity, hypertension, glucose intolerance, plethora, hirsutism), respectively [5].

8.2.2 Imaging Evaluation of Pulmonary Nodules

Once a solitary pulmonary nodule is identified, it may be further evaluated with cross-sectional imaging techniques such as computed tomography (CT) and/or positron emission tomography (PET)/CT. Key features that should be assessed include morphology, density, growth, and metabolic activity.

8.2.2.1 Morphology and Density

Pulmonary nodules may be described as solid or subsolid, the latter of which includes part-solid (combination of solid and ground-glass components) and nonsolid (pure ground-glass) nodules. Updated guidelines for the evaluation of solid and subsolid pulmonary nodules have been published by the Fleischner Society but are beyond the scope of this manuscript. Continuous improvement in CT technology has enabled the widespread utilization of thin collimation imaging and improved the detection and characterization of subsolid pulmonary nodules [6]. In general, subsolid nodules that persist on CT have a higher incidence of malignancy than solid nodules, as 63% of part-solid nodules are malignant as compared to 18% for ground-glass opacities and 7% for solid nodules [6]. For subsolid nodules, the likelihood of malignancy varies according to the size of the soft tissue component on CT. The frequency of lobulation, spiculation, and pseudocavitation (small focal lucencies) has also been reported to be significantly higher in malignant part-solid nodules. The "classic" morphology of a lung cancer has often been described as irregular or "spiculated"; however, it is important to recognize that benign lesions may occasionally demonstrate this appearance. Similarly, although many benign pulmonary nodules have a smooth margin, malignant lesions, including lung cancer, can have a similar manifestation.

The presence of intralesional fat (defined as Hounsfield Units of −40 to −120 on CT) almost always represents a benign hamartoma or, less commonly, lipoid pneumonia. Pulmonary metastases may contain fat in the setting of a primary soft tissue tumor that contains fat such as a liposarcoma, although this is rare. Different patterns of calcification may be identified within pulmonary nodules, some of which are typically benign and others of which tend to be malignant. For instance, central, popcorn, and laminated patterns of calcification tend to be benign and may be seen in the setting of granulomatous disease or hamartomas. Eccentric and stippled patterns of calcification are more concerning for malignant lesions.

8.2.2.2 Growth

The stability of nodules can be assessed by comparison to any chest radiographs or CT examinations performed in the past. In general, solid pulmonary nodules that have been stable for >2 years are considered benign and may represent granulomas, hamartomas, or intrapulmonary lymph nodes. The determination of stability for subsolid nodules, including part-solid and nonsolid (pure ground-glass) nodules is more complex, as such lesions can remain stable for a long period of time (>2 years) due to slow growth rates.

Lung cancers typically double in volume (defined as an increase of 26% in diameter) between 30 and 400 days (with an average of 240 days). Extremely rapid doubling times are more likely to reflect a benign etiology. For example, volume doubling times <20–30 days are suggestive of an infectious or inflammatory etiology but can occur with lymphoma or rapidly growing metastases. Small lung cancers may demonstrate long volume doubling times. For instance, in a screening study analyzing the growth rates of small lung cancers on CT, the doubling time ranged from 52 to 1733 days (mean of 452 days), and 20% of these malignancies had a volumetric doubling time >2 years [7]. These lesions were typically well-differentiated adenocarcinomas. For subsolid nodules, an increase in overall size, density, and/or an associated solid component should raise the suspicion for malignancy [8].

8.2.2.3 Metabolic Activity

PET/CT using the radiopharmaceutical [^{18}F]-fluoro-2-deoxy-D-glucose (FDG), a D-glucose analog labeled with fluorine-18, compliments conventional radiologic assessment of lung nodules. The reported sensitivity and specificity for detecting malignant pulmonary lesions are 97% and 78%, respectively. Thus, when solid nodules measuring 1 cm or greater in diameter demonstrate little to no FDG uptake, the likelihood of malignancy is generally considered to be low. One of the limitations of PET/CT is that the spatial resolution of PET scanners is in the range of 6 mm; therefore, smaller lesions may not appear FDG-avid even when cancer cells are present. Other limitations include false-positive studies with benign lesions, such as infection, inflammation, and granulomatous disease, and false-negative examinations due to indolent neoplasms such as bronchopulmonary carcinoid and lesions in the adenocarcinoma spectrum (adenocarcinoma in situ and minimally invasive adenocarcinoma), small foci of metastasis, and non-enlarged lymph nodes (those measuring <10 mm).

Key Point

- In the evaluation of pulmonary nodules for potential malignancy, the most important features to consider include morphology, density, growth over time, and metabolic activity on FDG PET/CT.

8.3 Patient Evaluation and the Role of Imaging

Once a diagnosis of lung cancer has been made, a variety of imaging techniques are available to further evaluate patients. For non-small cell lung cancer, the National Comprehensive Cancer Network (NCCN) recommends that the initial patient evaluation include (1) pathology review, (2) history and physical examination, (3) CT of the chest and upper abdomen with intravenous contrast (including coverage of the adrenal glands), (4) laboratory studies (typically complete blood count, platelets, and chemistry profile), and (5) smoking cessation counseling [9]. Additional imaging examinations including FDG PET/CT and magnetic resonance (MR) imaging may be used depending on the clinical stage and have specific advantages and disadvantages.

8.3.1 Computed Tomography

CT with intravenous contrast is the imaging modality of choice for evaluating most patients with lung cancer, as the modality accurately demonstrates the location and size of the primary lesion, the extent of local disease, and the relationship of the tumor to intrathoracic structures. Additionally, it can be used to determine the presence of intrathoracic and extrathoracic lymph node metastases, which are typically considered abnormal when they measure >1 cm in short-axis diameter. However, the strictly anatomic information provided by limits its effectiveness in this regard. For instance, in one study, 44% of metastatic nodes measured <1 cm, and 77% of patients without lymph node metastases had nodes measuring >1 cm [10].

8.3.2 FDG PET/CT

FDG PET/CT is more accurate than CT or stand-alone PET in determining the tumor classification, with integrated PET/CT correctly predicting the tumor stage in 86% of cases compared to 68% with CT and 46% with PET [11]. Additionally, FDG PET/CT can distinguish between tumor and associated post-obstructive atelectasis/pneumonitis, with the former typically demonstrating greater FDG uptake [12]. As FDG PET/CT combines the anatomic information of CT and the functional information of PET, it is more accurate than CT in detecting lymph node metastases. Early studies demonstrated a pooled average sensitivity, specificity, positive predictive value, negative predictive value, and accuracy of PET/CT of, respectively, 73%, 91%, 71%, 90%, and 86%, compared to 74%, 73%, 52%, 88%, and 73% of CT alone and 83%, 81%, 71%, 89%, and 82% of PET alone [13]. FDG PET/CT is superior to both CT and PET in identifying distant metastatic disease, particularly soft tissue and pleural metastases, and is better than nuclear medicine bone scintigraphy as the imaging modality of choice for detecting osseous metastases [13].

8.3.3 MR Imaging

MR imaging is typically not routinely performed in the evaluation of patients with lung cancer; however, it has been shown to be superior to CT and FDG PET/CT for identifying invasion of the mediastinum and chest wall and evaluating the heart, pericardium, and vascular structures [14, 15]. Characteristic MR imaging features of chest wall invasion include (1) infiltration or disruption of the normal extrapleural fat plane on T1-weighted imaging, (2) hyperintensity of the parietal pleura on T2-weighted imaging, (3) rib destruction on short tau inversion recovery (STIR) sequences, and (4) fixation of the tumor to the chest wall during breathing on cine MR imaging. MR imaging is better than CT in differentiating between the primary neoplasm and post-obstructive atelectasis/pneumonitis, the former of which typically usually shows higher signal on T2-weighted imaging than the central tumor [14]. MR imaging is the best imaging modality for identifying brain and liver metastases and can be used to diagnose adrenal metastases; specifically, chemical shift techniques can be used to differentiate adrenal metastases from adenomas, with reported sensitivity and specificity of 100% and 81%, respectively.

Key Point
- Once a diagnosis of lung cancer has been made, most patients are further assessed with contrast-enhanced CT. Additional imaging modalities such as FDG PET/CT and MR imaging may be obtained depending on the suspected clinical stage and/or further evaluation of specific findings.

8.4 Lung Cancer Staging

8.4.1 Rationale and Methodology for TNM-8

A significant limitation of the International Association for the Study of Lung Cancer (IASLC) Staging Project that informed TNM-7 was the retrospective nature of the database. An international group led by the IASLC collected new lung cancer cases with retrospective and prospective clinical information for the creation of a large database that would ultimately inform TNM-8 [4, 16]. The database included data on 94,708 cases diagnosed between 1999 and 2010 gathered from 35 sources in 16 countries, 4667 of which were submitted through an online electronic data capture system stored at Cancer Research and Biostatistics in Seattle, Washington. Of these cases, 17,552 were excluded due to unknown or different histologic type and incomplete stage information. Thus, 77,156 patients (70,967 with non-small cell lung cancer and 6189 with small cell lung cancer) with clinical and pathologic staging information were available for analysis.

8.4.2 Modifications to TNM-8

8.4.2.1 T Classification

The tumor (T) classification assigns specific descriptors to characterize the primary lung cancer [17] (Table 8.1). When evaluating tumors, the key imaging features to consider include lesion size (typically measured in long-axis diameter), the presence or absence of local invasion, and the presence or absence of tumor nodules. Analysis of the new lung cancer staging database evaluated the impact of these features on patient survival, and several significant changes are introduced in TNM-8.

8.4.2.2 Tumor Size

The overall size of the primary lung cancer is one of the most important considerations in T descriptor determination, and significant differences in survival between lung cancers of various sizes have influenced additional changes introduced in TNM-8. Analysis of the new lung cancer staging database revealed separation of T1 lesions from T2 lesions based on a size threshold of 3 cm and progressively worse survival for each cut point of 1 cm. Thus, T1 lung cancers are divided into three groups at 1 cm thresholds: T1a tumors measuring 1 cm or less, T1b nodules measuring greater than 1 cm and less than or equal to 2 cm, and T1c lesions measuring greater than 2 cm and less than or equal to 3 cm. Similarly, T2 lung cancers are divided into two groups: T2a lesions measuring greater than 3 cm and less than or equal to 4 cm and T2b tumors measuring greater than 4 cm and less than or equal to 5 cm. Finally, T3 lesions measure greater than 5 cm and less than or equal to 7 cm, and T4 tumors measure greater than 7 cm in TNM-8.

8.4.2.3 Involvement of Main Bronchi

A lung cancer invading a main bronchus 2 cm or more from the carina was classified as T2, whereas involvement of the more proximal aspect of a main bronchus was classified as a

Table 8.1 TNM Descriptors for TNM-8

T descriptor	Definition
TX	Tumor cannot be assessed or tumor proven by the presence of malignant cells in sputum or bronchial washings but not visualized by imaging or bronchoscopy
T0	No evidence of the primary tumor
Tis	Carcinoma in situ
T1	Tumor ≤3 cm in greatest dimension, surrounded by lung or visceral pleura, without bronchoscopic evidence of invasion more proximal than the lobar bronchus
T1a	Tumor ≤1 cm in greatest dimension
T1b	Tumor >1 cm but ≤2 cm in greatest dimension
T1c	Tumor >2 cm but ≤3 cm in greatest dimension
T2	Tumor >3 cm but ≤5 cm or tumor with any of the following features: Involvement of a main bronchus regardless of distance from carina, invasion of the visceral pleura, associated with partial or complete lung atelectasis/pneumonitis
T2a	Tumor >3 cm but ≤4 cm in greatest dimension
T2b	Tumor >4 cm but ≤5 cm in greatest dimension
T3	Tumor >5 cm or one that directly invades any of the following structures: Parietal pleura, chest wall (including superior sulcus tumors), phrenic nerve, parietal pericardium, or separate tumor nodule(s) in the same lobe
T4	Tumor measuring >7 cm that invades any of the following structures: Mediastinum, diaphragm, heart, great vessels, trachea, recurrent laryngeal nerve, esophagus, vertebral body, carina, or separate tumor nodule(s) in a different lobe of the same lung
N descriptor	Definition
NX	Lymph nodes cannot be assessed
N0	No regional lymph nodes
N1	Ipsilateral peribronchial and/or ipsilateral hilar lymph nodes and intrapulmonary nodes, including involvement by direct extension
N2	Ipsilateral mediastinal and/or subcarinal lymph node(s)
N3	Contralateral mediastinal, contralateral hilar, ipsilateral or contralateral scalene, or supraclavicular lymph node(s)
M descriptor	Definition
M0	No metastasis
M1	Metastasis
M1a	Separate tumor nodule(s) in contralateral lung; malignant pleural effusion or pleural thickening/nodules/masses; malignant pericardial effusion or pericardial thickening/nodules/masses
M1b	Single distant (extrathoracic) metastasis in single organ
M1c	Multiple distant (extrathoracic) metastases in single or multiple organs

Adapted from [25]

T3 lesion in TNM-7. Analysis of the new lung cancer staging database revealed that lung cancers invading a main bronchus less than 2 cm from the carina, but without direct invasion of the carina, were associated with better survival compared to lung cancers with other characteristic T3 features. Thus, in TNM-8, lung cancers involving a main bronchus, regardless of the distance from the carina, are grouped together as T2 tumors.

8.4.2.4 Atelectasis or Pneumonitis of the Lung

A lung cancer resulting in partial atelectasis or pneumonitis, defined as involving less than an entire lung, was classified as T2 in TNM-7, whereas atelectasis or pneumonitis of an entire lung was classified as a T3 lesion. Analysis of the new lung cancer staging database revealed that patients with complete atelectasis or pneumonitis of a lung had better survival than those with other characteristics T3 features. Thus, partial and complete forms of lung atelectasis and pneumonitis are grouped together as T2 lesions in TNM-8 (Fig. 8.1).

8.4.2.5 Diaphragmatic Invasion

In TNM-7, invasion of the diaphragm was included in T3. Analysis of the new database demonstrated that the 5-year survival of patients with this feature was worse than that of patients with other T3 lung cancers but similar to that of patients with T4 tumors. Therefore, diaphragmatic invasion has been reclassified as T4 in TNM-8 (Fig. 8.2).

8.4.2.6 Involvement of the Mediastinal Pleura

In TNM-7, involvement of the mediastinal pleura was classified as T3. Analysis of the new database showed that lung cancers with this feature were associated with a better prognosis than other T3 lesions; however, only a small number of cases were available. It was also noted that mediastinal pleura invasion was rarely used in clinical staging reports as it can be difficult to accurately determine. Therefore, invasion of the mediastinal pleura has been eliminated from the T classification in TNM-8.

Key Point

- The most important features to consider in the classification of tumors include lesion size, location, and local extension. Modifications to the T classification have been made on the basis of 1 cm increments in tumor size; grouping of lung cancers that result in partial or complete lung atelectasis or pneumonitis; grouping of tumors with involvement of a main bronchus irrespective of distance from the carina; reassignment of diaphragmatic invasion in terms of T classification; and elimination of mediastinal pleural invasion.

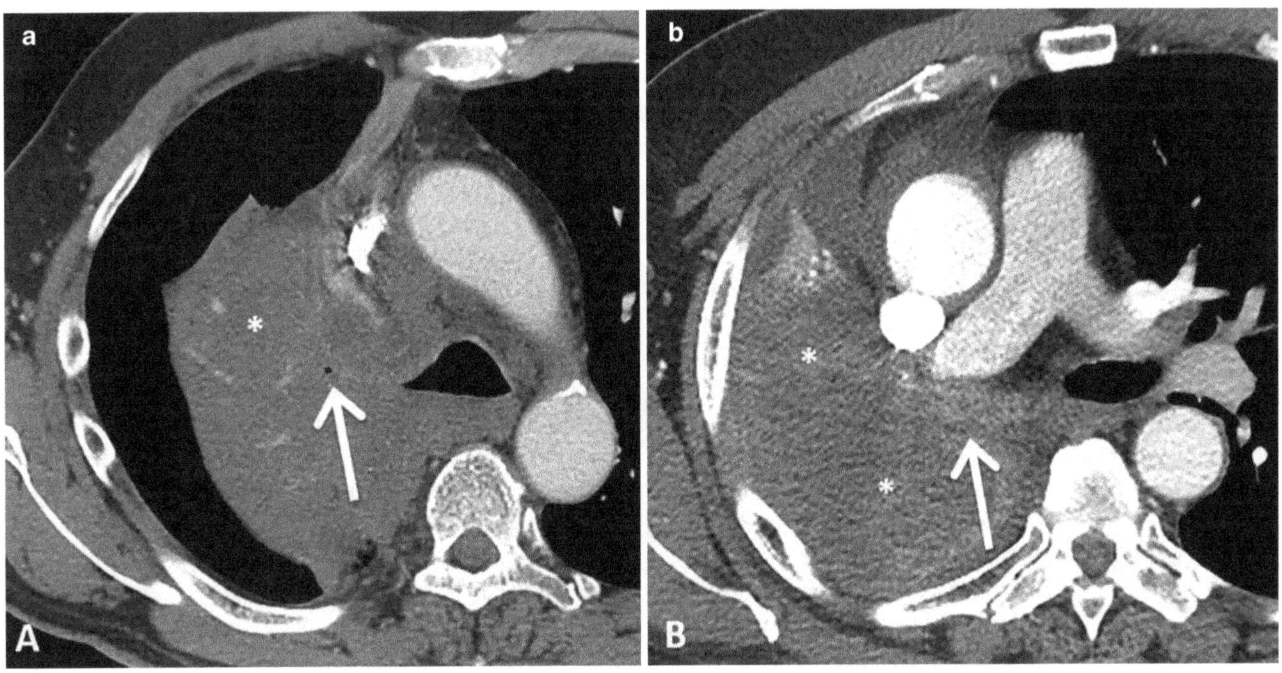

Fig. 8.1 Atelectasis/pneumonitis. (**a**) Contrast-enhanced axial CT of a 63-year-old man with non-small cell lung cancer demonstrates occlusion of the right upper lobe bronchus (arrow) and complete atelectasis of the right upper lobe (*) due to a right perihilar mass. (**b**) Contrast-enhanced axial CT of a 55-year-old man with non-small cell lung cancer demonstrates complete occlusion of the right main bronchus (arrow) and complete atelectasis of the right lung (*) due to a large right perihilar mass. In TNM-8, partial and complete lung atelectasis/pneumonitis are grouped together as a T2 descriptor

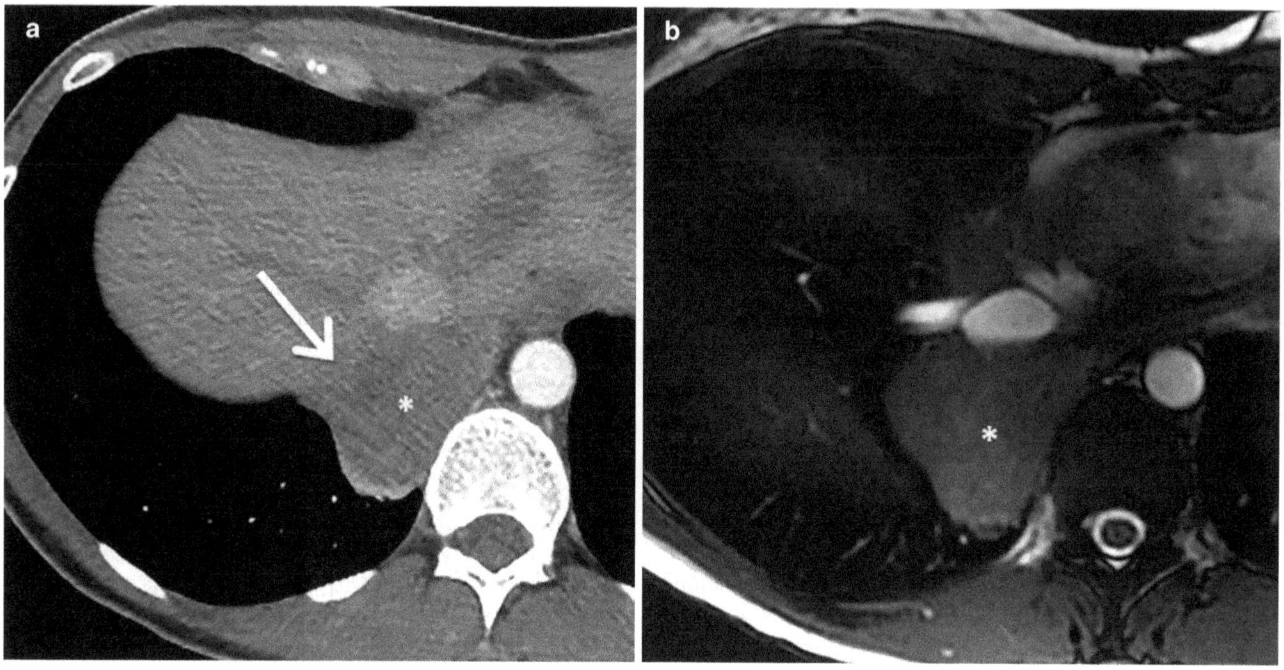

Fig. 8.2 Diaphragmatic invasion. (**a**) Axial contrast-enhanced axial CT of a 61-year-old man with non-small cell lung cancer shows a mass (*) in the right lower lobe inseparable from the right hemidiaphragm (arrow). (**b**) Axial cine T2-weighted MR confirmed invasion of the right hemidiaphragm. Because the 5-year survival of patients with diaphragmatic invasion is similar to that of patients with other T4 tumors, diaphragmatic invasion has been reclassified from T3 to T4 in TNM-8

8.4.2.7 Lymph Node (N) Classification

The lymph node (N) classification assigns specific descriptors that are related to the presence or absence of intrathoracic lymph node disease (Table 8.1). In contrast to primary lung cancers, for which the long-axis diameter is measured and reported, lymph nodes are typically measured in short-axis diameter. IASLC recommends use of a standardized lymph node map that assigns nodes into specific supraclavicular, upper, aorticopulmonary, subcarinal, lower, hilar/interlobar, and peripheral zones [18]. The analysis of the new database revealed that the current N classification provides consistent separation of prognostically distinct groups. Thus, the lymph node descriptors are unchanged for TNM-8 [19]. N0 is defined as the absence of lymph node disease. N1 is characterized by ipsilateral peripheral or hilar lymph nodes, N2 includes ipsilateral mediastinal including subcarinal lymph nodes, and N3 involves ipsilateral or contralateral supraclavicular lymph node or contralateral mediastinal, hilar/interlobar, or intrapulmonary lymph nodes.

The potential prognostic impact of the number of lymph node stations involved and skip metastases was also evaluated. To assess the former, pathologic staging (pN) was divided into several groups, in which the letter "a" denoted single lymph node station involvement and the letter "b" represented multiple lymph node station involvement within an N category. Therefore, single (pN1a) and multiple (pN1b) pN1 stations and single (pN2a) and multiple (pN2b) pN2 stations were delineated. No significant difference was seen between the pN1b and pN2a groups, although survival differences between the pN1a and pN1b groups and between the pN2a and pN2b groups were significant. To assess the skip metastases, pN2a was divided into several components, in which a designation ending in "1" indicated the presence of skip metastases and a designation ending in "2" indicated the absence of skip metastases. Thus, single pN2 with skip (no pN1 involvement, pN2a1) and single pN2 without skip (pN1 and pN2 involvement, pN2a2) categories were recognized. Although the survival of patients with pN2a1 was better than those with pN1b, this difference was not significant. Although significant differences in survival were present between the pN2a1 and pN2a2 groups and between the pN2a2 and pN2b groups, no significant difference was present between the pN1b and pN2a1 groups.

For the purposes of clinical staging, IASLC recommends that radiologists document the number of lymph node stations involved and classify the N category using descriptors such as N1a (single lymph node station), N1b (multiple lymph node stations), N2a (single lymph node station), and N2b (multiple lymph node stations). The presence or absence of skip metastasis (pN2a1 or pN2a2) should be noted when such information is available.

Key Point

- The current nomenclature for lymph node classification is maintained in TNM-8 due to consistent separation of prognostically distinct groups, which is primarily based on lymph node location. In general, ipsilateral hilar (N1) lymph nodes are considered resectable, ipsilateral mediastinal or subcarinal lymph nodes (N2) may be resectable (usually after induction chemotherapy), and contralateral mediastinal lymph nodes and scalene or supraclavicular adenopathy (N3) are generally considered unresectable.

8.4.2.8 Metastasis (M) Classification

The metastasis (M) classification assigns specific descriptors reflecting the absence (M0) or presence (M1) of intrathoracic or extrathoracic metastatic disease (Table 8.1). The M classification for TNM-7 included M1a and M1b components for intrathoracic and extrathoracic metastatic disease, respectively. Analysis of the new lung cancer staging database revealed that patients with a single metastasis in one extrathoracic organ (median survival of 11.4 months) had similar survival to that of patients with M1a (median survival of 11.5 months) but better survival compared to patients with multiple metastases in one or more extrathoracic organs (median survival of 6.3 months) [20]. Therefore, M1 is divided into M1a, M1b, and M1c components based on survival differences. M1a, or intrathoracic metastatic disease, describes pleural or pericardial spread of disease and tumor nodules in the contralateral lung (Fig. 8.3). M1b and M1c describe extrathoracic metastatic disease, the former of which includes a single metastasis involving a single distant (extrathoracic) organ and the latter of which includes multiple metastases in one or more distant (extrathoracic) organs (Fig. 8.4). Overall, the most common sites of metastatic disease include the brain, liver, adrenal glands, and bone.

It is recommended that radiologists document the following features on imaging studies performed for the purposes of clinical staging: (1) the number and location of metastatic lesions, (2) the diameter of individual metastases, and (3) the number and location of organs affected.

Key Point

- The M1 descriptor is subdivided into M1a (intrathoracic metastatic disease, including pleural or pericardial spread, cardiac metastasis, and contralateral tumor nodule), M1b (extrathoracic metastatic disease, with one lesion in one distant organ), and M1c (extrathoracic metastatic disease, with more than one lesion in one or more distant organs) based on the location and number of metastases.

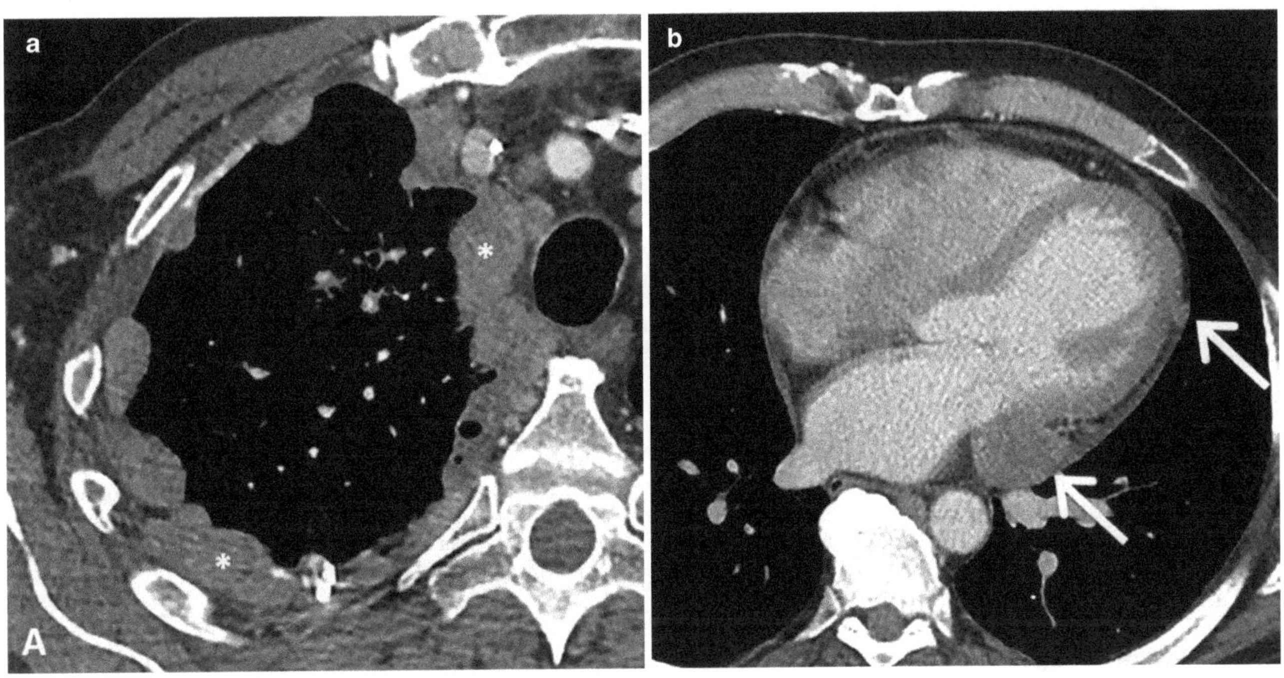

Fig. 8.3 Intrathoracic metastases. (**a**) Contrast-enhanced axial CT of a 66-year-old man with non-small cell lung cancer demonstrates extensive pleural thickening and nodularity (*) in the right hemithorax compatible with metastatic disease. (**b**) Contrast-enhanced axial CT of a 57-year-old woman with non-small cell lung cancer shows several nodules (arrows) involving the pericardium and a small amount of pericardial fluid, compatible with metastatic disease. M1a is used to describe pleural or pericardial spread of disease and tumor nodules in the contralateral lung

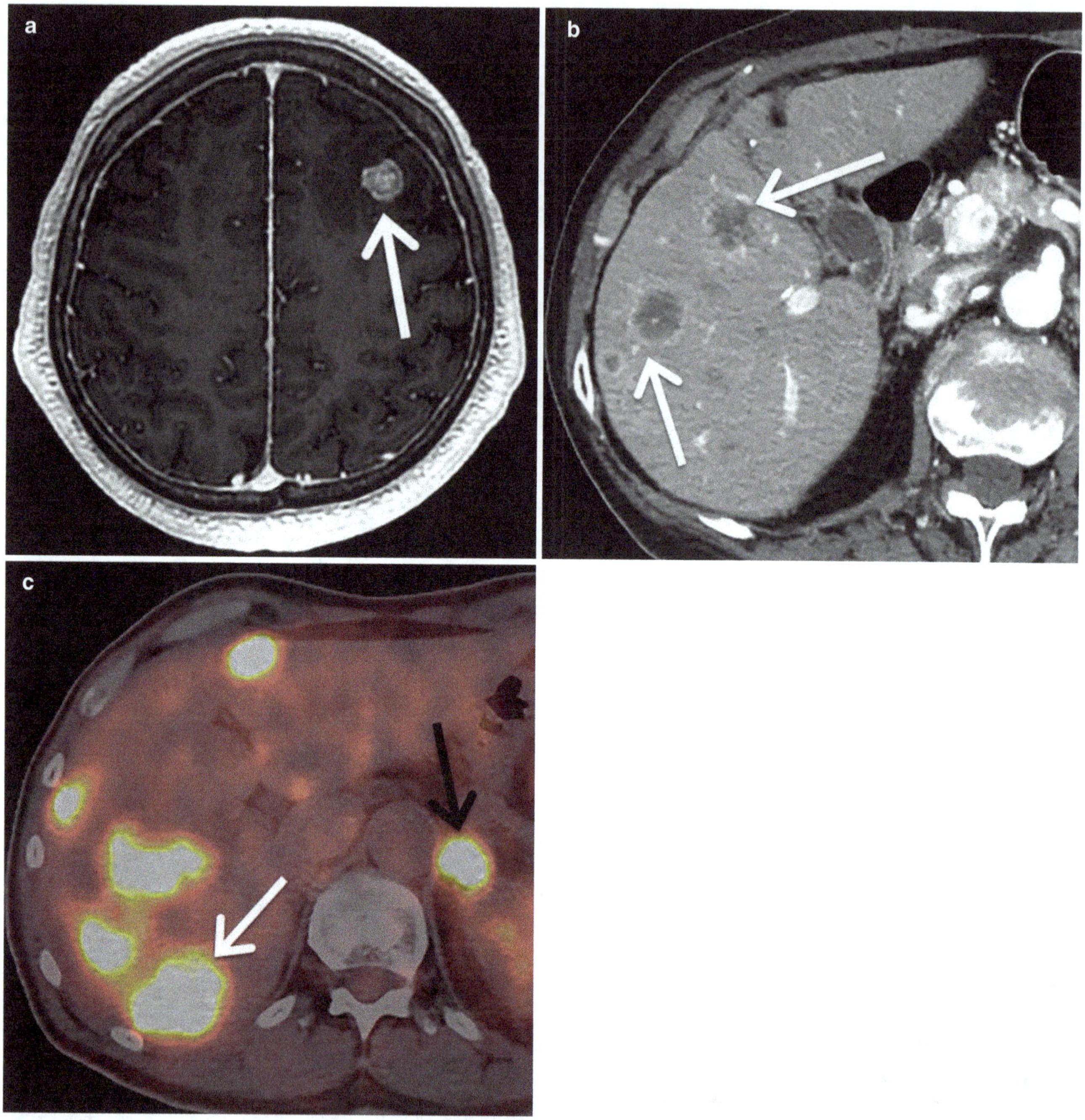

Fig. 8.4 Distant (extrathoracic) metastases. (**a**) Axial contrast-enhanced T1-weighted MR image of a 53-year-old man with non-small cell lung cancer demonstrates an enhancing metastasis (arrow) with surrounding edema in the left middle frontal gyrus. (**b**) Contrast-enhanced axial CT of a 64-year-old man with non-small cell lung cancer demonstrates numerous heterogeneously hypodense masses in the liver (arrows), consistent with metastases. C. Fused axial FDG PET/CT of a 71-year-old man with non-small cell lung cancer demonstrates hepatic (white arrow) and left adrenal (black arrow) metastases. TNM-8 recognizes differences in survival based on both the location and number of metastases; thus, distant metastatic disease is designated as M1b (solitary metastasis in a single distant organ) and M1c (multiple metastases in one or more distant organs)

8.4.3 Stage Groups

Due to changes to the T and M descriptors in TNM-8, the stage groups in TNM-7 have been modified, and new groups have been added [21] (Table 8.2). For example, in response to the separation of T1 lesions into T1a, T1b, and T1c components based on 1 cm increments, three new associated stages have been created and designated as IA1, IA2, and IA3, respectively. In another instance, to describe cases of locally advanced tumors (including T3 and T4

Table 8.2 Stage Groups for TNM-8

Stage	Tumor	Node	Metastasis
Occult carcinoma	TX	N0	M0
Stage 0	Tis	N0	M0
Stage IA1	T1a (mi)	N0	M0
	T1a	N0	M0
Stage IA2	T1b	N0	M0
Stage IA3	T1c	N0	M0
Stage IB	T2a	N0	M0
Stage IIA	T2b	N0	M0
Stage IIB	T1a-c	N1	M0
	T2a	N1	M0
	T2b	N1	M0
Stage IIIA	T1a-c	N2	M0
	T2a-b	N2	M0
	T3	N1	M0
	T4	N0	M0
	T4	N1	M0
Stage IIIB	T1a-c	N3	M0
	T2a-b	N3	M0
	T3	N2	M0
	T4	N2	M0
Stage IIIC	T3	N3	M0
	T4	N3	M0
Stage IVA	Any T	Any N	M1a
	Any T	Any N	M1b
Stage IVB	Any T	Any N	M1c

mi minimally invasive
Adapted from [25]

lesions) with N3 but no evidence of metastatic disease, a new stage designated as stage IIIC has been created for TNM-8. Intrathoracic metastatic disease, including pleural, pericardial, and cardiac spread, as well as tumor nodules in the contralateral lung, remains classified as stage IVA. A single metastasis to a single distant organ (M1b) is considered stage IVA, whereas multiple distant metastases in one or more distant organs (M1c) are classified as stage IVB.

8.4.4 Lung Cancers with Multiple Sites of Pulmonary Involvement

Multiple distinct patterns of lung cancer manifesting with several sites of pulmonary involvement have been described, including multiple primary lung cancers, lung cancers with one or more tumor nodules, multiple ground-glass lesions, and consolidation [22]. Recommendations for the staging of tumors resulting in these patterns is included for the first time in TNM-8 and are based on review of the literature and expert opinion provided by IASLC.

8.4.4.1 Multiple Primary Lung Cancers

When a lung cancer is identified on an imaging examination and there are multiple additional lung lesions, the radiologist must consider data from several sources when attempting to determine whether such lesions represent multiple primary lung cancers. IASLC recommends that the decision to classify two (or more) lung lesions as synchronous primary lung cancers or two foci of a single lung cancer should be based on multidisciplinary evaluation that incorporates clinical, relevant findings on prior and current imaging and histopathologic findings obtained at image-guided or surgical biopsy or surgical resection [22, 23]. If two (or more) lung lesions are determined to represent separate primary lung cancers, then each separate malignancy should be staged using TNM-8.

8.4.4.2 Lung Cancer with One or More Tumor Nodules

When a lung cancer is identified on an imaging examination with one or more nodules, these other lesions may or may not be of the same histologic subtype as the primary lesion. Tumor nodules related to the primary malignancy should be suspected when one or more solid lung nodule is identified along with a dominant lung lesion resulting in the "classic" lung cancer appearance, such as a spiculated nodule or mass. Analysis of the new lung cancer staging database revealed a progressive decrease in survival with increasing distance between a primary lung cancer and associated tumor nodule. Thus, patient survival is better when lung cancers have tumor nodules in the same lobe as the primary tumor (T3) compared with those lesions with nodules in a different ipsilateral lobe (T4) or the contralateral lung (M1a) [22, 24] (Fig. 8.5).

8.4.4.3 Multiple Ground-glass Lesions

In general, lung cancers appearing as multiple lesions with ground-glass or lepidic features are almost always adenocarcinoma, tend to affect women and nonsmokers, and are associated with excellent patient outcomes and infrequent recurrences [22, 25]. Compared to other types of lung cancer, subsolid adenocarcinomas tend to have a lower likelihood of resulting in lymph node spread or metastasis, have a greater propensity for developing additional subsolid lung cancers, and are more likely to behave in an indolent manner [25].

IASLC recommends that the term multifocal adenocarcinoma be used to describe lung lesions if a malignant subsolid nodule is present (suspected at clinical staging or histopathologically proven) and if other ground-glass lesions are present [25]. This definition also includes cases in which a subsolid lesion with a 50% or greater solid (invasive) component appears to have arisen from a ground-glass nodule and other ground-glass opacities are present. The term multifocal lung adenocarcinoma should not be applied to patients with multiple ground-glass nodules likely representing benign lesions or preneoplastic/preinvasive lesions such as atypical adenomatous hyperplasia.

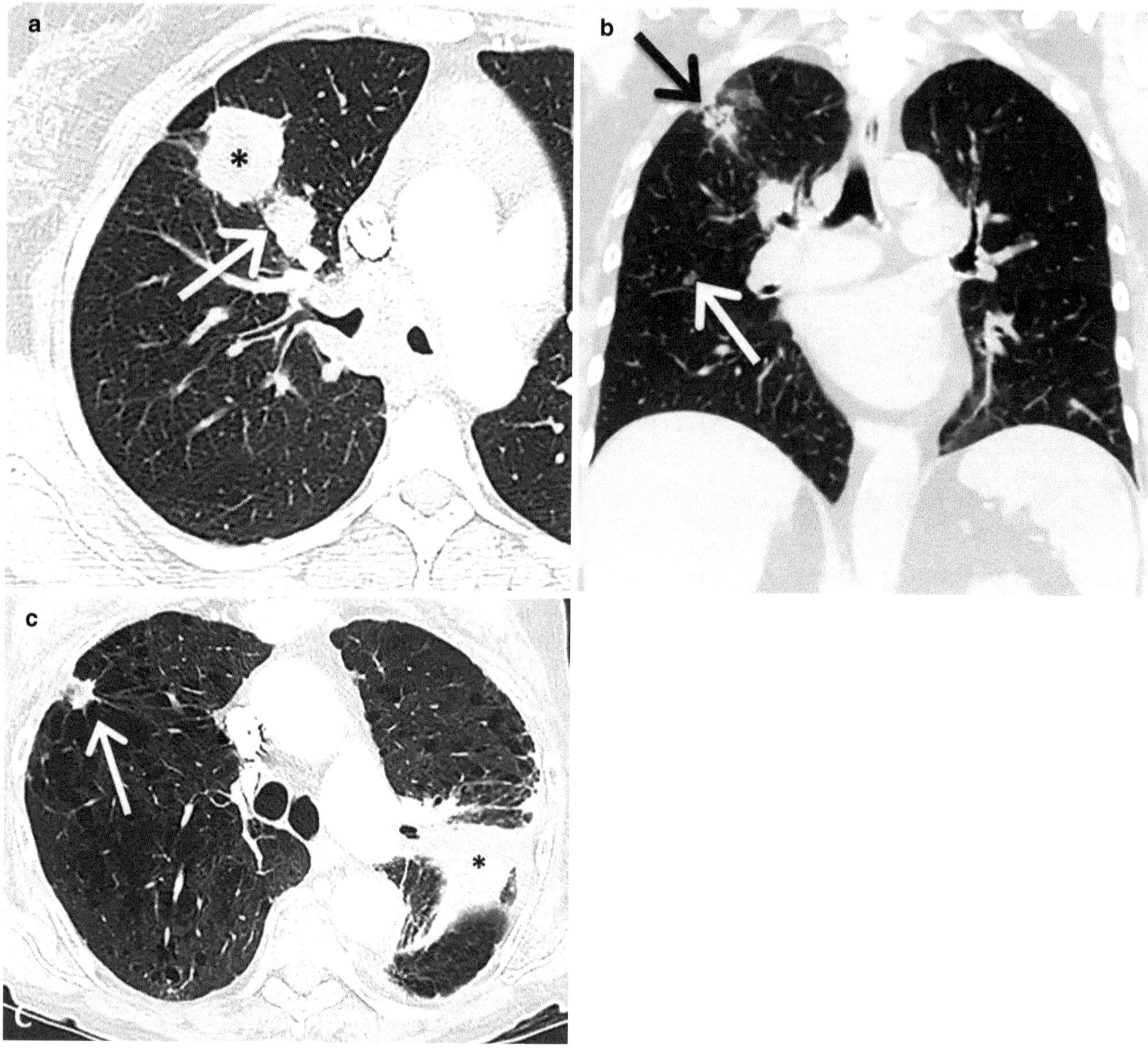

Fig. 8.5 Lung cancers with separate tumor nodules. (**a**) Contrast-enhanced axial CT of a 39-year-old woman with non-small cell lung cancer demonstrates the tumor in the right upper lobe (*) and a separate tumor nodule (arrow) in the adjacent lung. These findings are designated as T3. (**b**) Contrast-enhanced coronal CT of a 72-year-old woman with non-small cell lung cancer demonstrates the tumor in the right upper lobe (*) and a separate tumor nodule in the middle lobe (arrow). These findings are classified as T4. (**c**) Contrast-enhanced axial CT of a 63-year-old man with non-small cell lung cancer demonstrates the tumor in the left lung (*) and a separate tumor nodule in the right upper lobe (arrow). Biopsy of the right upper lobe nodule confirmed malignancy, and these findings are designated as M1a

For the purposes of staging, IASLC recommends that the T classification be determined by the lesion with the highest-level T descriptor and the number of lesions (#)—or simply "(m)" for multiple—indicated in parentheses (Fig. 8.6). Lesion size is determined by the largest diameter of the solid component measured on CT or the largest diameter of the invasive component at pathologic examination. Adenocarcinoma in situ and minimally invasive adenocarcinoma should be classified as Tis and T1a(mi), respectively [26]. It is recommended that the T(#/m) multifocal classification should be used regardless of whether these lesions are suspected on the basis of imaging or if there is histopathologic proof and regardless of whether the lesions are in the same lobe or in different lobes of the same or different lung. Once the T classification has been determined, the N and M descriptors apply to all of the tumor foci collectively.

8.4.4.4 Consolidation

The dominant manifestation of some lung cancers may appear as diffuse consolidation or a "pneumonic type" of adenocarcinoma, most of which are invasive mucinous adenocarcinomas [27–29]. These lesions manifest as a

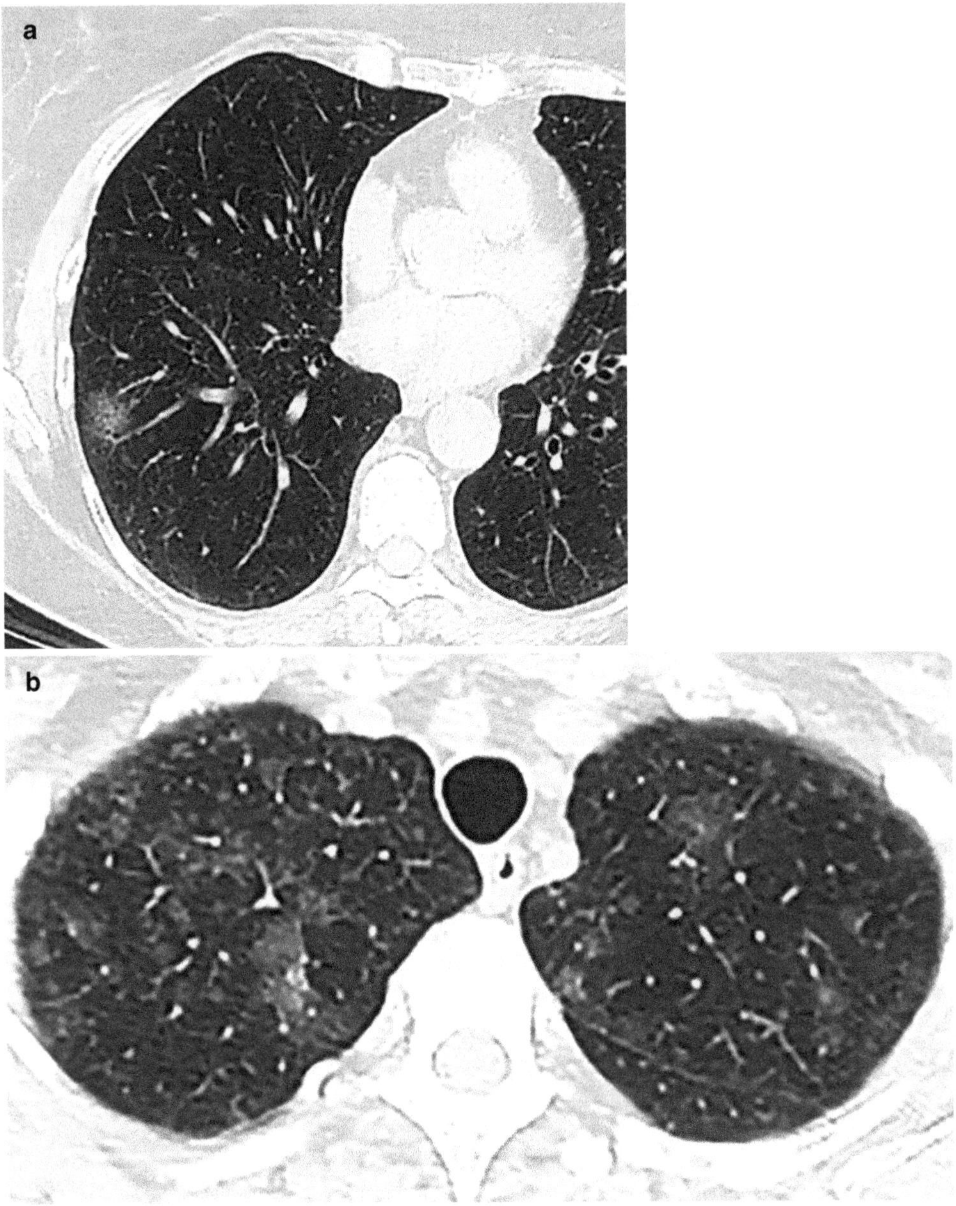

Fig. 8.6 Multiple ground-glass lesions (multifocal adenocarcinoma). (**a**) Unenhanced axial CT of a 58-year-old woman with multifocal lung adenocarcinoma demonstrates several ground-glass nodules in the right lung, the largest of which measures 1.6 cm. (**b**) Unenhanced axial CT of a 64-year-old woman with multifocal lung adenocarcinoma shows numerous ground-glass nodules bilaterally, the largest of which measures 4.5 cm. In the setting of multiple ground-glass lesions, the IASLC recommends the utilization of the dominant lesion for T descriptor purposes. In the first case, the nodule is classified as a T1b lesion, and the overall descriptor can be listed as either T1b (# of lesions) or T1b (m). In the second case, the nodule is classified as a T2b lesion, and the overall descriptor can be listed as either T2b (# of lesions) or T2b (m)

consolidative pattern on CT without evidence of an obstructed bronchus and may only involve a specific region (such as a segment or lobe), multiple regions (appearing confluent or separate), or the lung in a diffuse manner. Lymph node involvement and metastatic disease are uncommon at presentation, even in the setting of extensive lung disease [30–32]. Progression is typically slow; however, the overall survival is worse compared with that of patients with multifocal ground-glass lesions.

For the purposes of staging, IASLC recommends that, when the lung cancer involves a single area, the T classification is determined by the size of the lesion. When multiple sites of involvement are present, the disease is characterized as T3 if confined to one lobe, T4 if different lobes of the same lung are affected, and M1a if both lungs are involved (Fig. 8.7). When disease is present within both lungs, the T classification is based on the appropriate T category for the lung with the greatest extent of tumor involvement. For a lesion that is confined to a single lobe but is difficult to measure reliably, the T3 descriptor should be used. Lesions in which there is extension of tumor into an adjacent lobe or a discrete separate area of involvement of an adjacent lobe is identified should be classified as T4. Once the T classification has been determined, the N and M descriptors apply to all of the tumor foci collectively. This algorithm should also be used to stage lung cancers presenting with a miliary pattern of disease, characterized by numerous small pulmonary nodules in the lungs. Miliary disease is often difficult to measure, and a single lobe should be classified as T3 without regard to size.

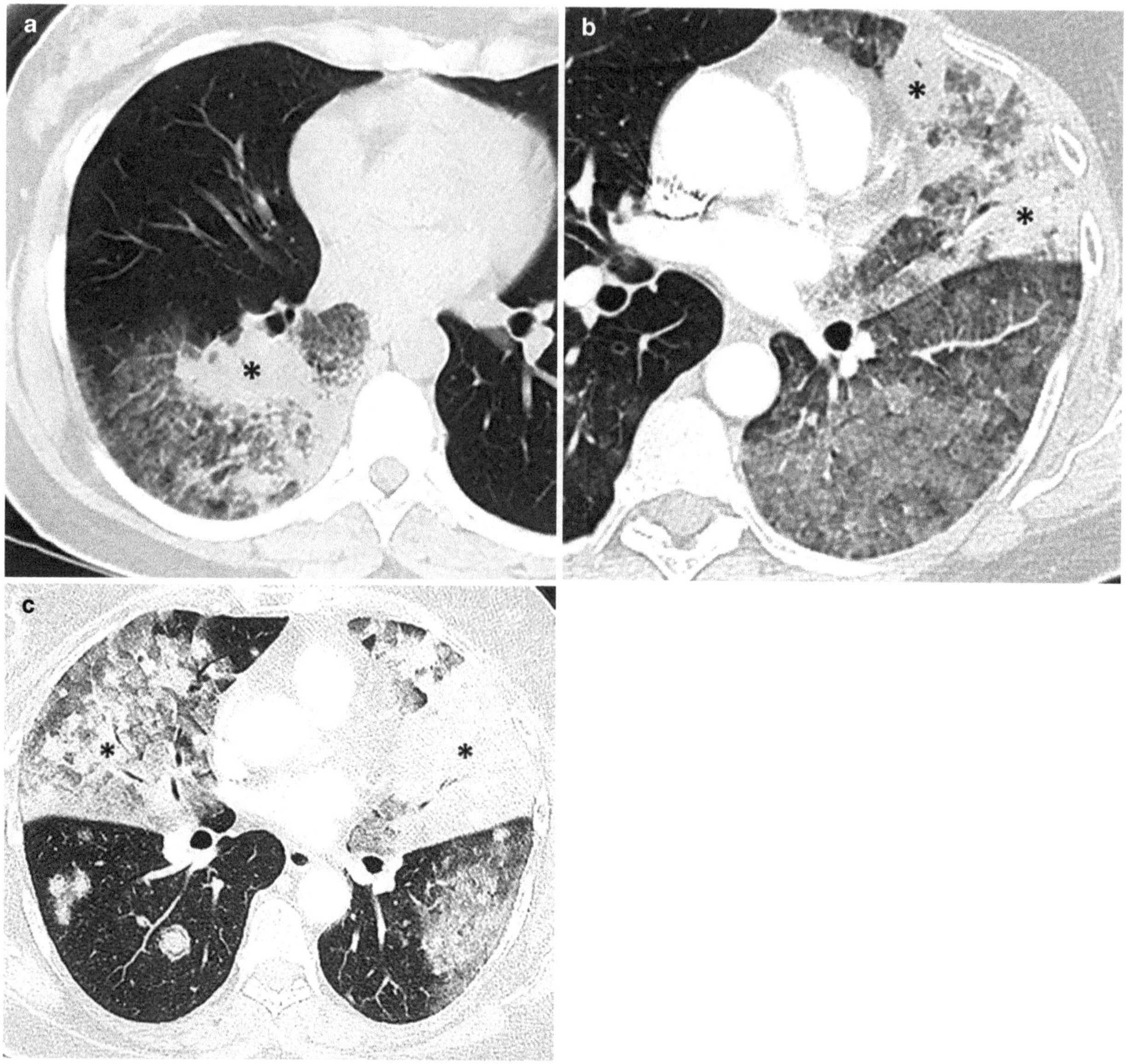

Fig. 8.7 Lung cancer manifesting as consolidation. (**a**) Unenhanced axial CT of a 69-year-old woman with non-small cell lung cancer demonstrates consolidation isolated to the right lower lobe (*) with surrounding ground-glass opacity. As this lesion is limited to the right lower lobe, it is designated as T3. (**b**) Contrast-enhanced axial CT of a 49-year-old woman with multifocal adenocarcinoma demonstrates multifocal consolidation (*) in the left upper lobe and extensive ground-glass opacities in the left lung. As these lesions are present in both lobes of the left lung, the designation is T4. (**c**) Contrast-enhanced axial CT of a 53-year-old woman with multifocal adenocarcinoma shows consolidation and extensive ground-glass opacities in the lungs bilaterally. As consolidation is present in both lungs, the designation is M1a

Key Point

- A subcommittee of the IASLC staging and prognostic factors committee identified four distinct patterns of disease in cases of lung cancer characterized by multiple sites of pulmonary involvement, including multiple primary lung cancers, lung cancers with separate tumor nodules, multiple ground-glass lesions, and consolidation. Specific criteria have been outlined in order to categorize and stage lesions with these patterns of disease.

8.4.5 Tumor Measurement

For the purposes of initial clinical staging on cross-sectional imaging, lung cancers should be measured and reported in centimeters with millimeter increments. Solid and nonsolid lesions should be measured on the image showing the greatest tumor dimension, regardless of plane (axial, sagittal, or coronal), whereas part-solid lesions should be measured on the image showing the largest average tumor diameter and the greatest diameter of the solid component of the lesion. For the purpose of determining the T classification, the

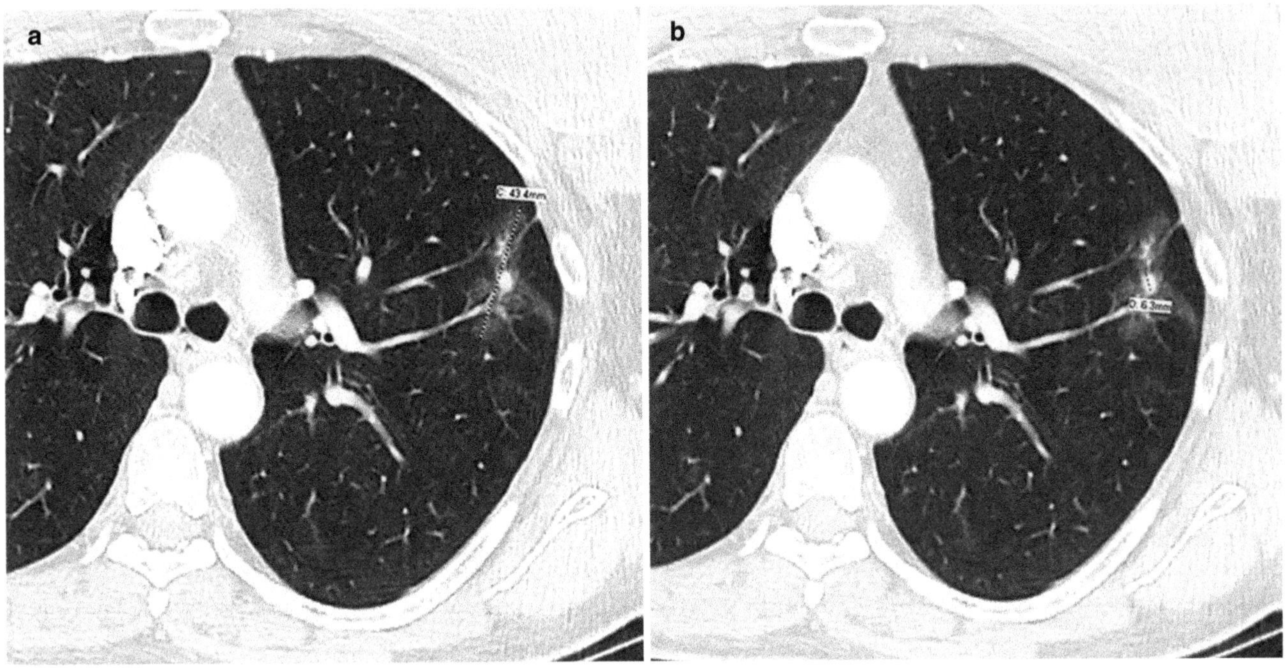

Fig. 8.8 Measurement of part-solid tumors. (**a**) and (**b**) Contrast-enhanced axial CT of a 57-year-old woman demonstrates a part-solid nodule in the left upper lobe with measurement of the entire lesion (A) and just the solid component (B). For the purpose of evaluating part-solid lesions, IASLC recommends that the image showing the largest average tumor diameter and the greatest diameter of the solid component of the lesion be used. For determining the T descriptor, the longest diameter of the solid component should be used for part-solid lesions

longest diameter should be used for solid and nonsolid lesions, and the longest diameter of the solid component should be used for part-solid lesions [17, 26] (Fig. 8.8).

Regarding optimal CT scan technique, thin-section images (specifically, 1 mm sections if possible for small lesions measuring 10 mm or less) help reduce the variability in measurement and allow visualization of specific tumor features such as density, shape, and margin due to enhanced spatial resolution [33–36]. It is recommended that lung or intermediate window settings should be used to detect and measure the solid components of subsolid lesions and that the long-axis measurement of the largest solid component should be identified.

8.4.6 Small Cell Lung Cancer

IASLC first recommended that SCLC should be evaluated with the TNM staging system at the release of TNM-7. A separate staging system developed by the Veterans Administration Lung Study Group that divides SCLC into two subgroups, limited-stage SCLC and extensive-stage SCLC, based on the extent of disease and the ability to treat in a single radiation portal, is still often used in current clinical practice. Limited-stage SCLC is confined to one hemithorax and can be treated in a single radiation portal, and extensive-stage SCLC, which includes all other cases. The TNM staging system has been shown to better differentiate stage-specific survival compared with the Veterans Administration Lung Study Group system [37, 38]. Analysis of the new database confirmed the prognostic value of TNM staging in patients with SCLC, and the IASLC recommends its use for staging of patients with SCLC. Radiologists should record the following information regarding SCLC: (a) the number of extrathoracic metastatic sites, (b) the number of organs involved, (c) the diameter of individual metastatic sites, (d) the types of examinations and studies used for staging, and (e) whether patients with brain metastases are symptomatic or asymptomatic [39].

8.5 Concluding Remarks

The revised TNM staging system, TNM-8, includes important modifications to the T and M classifications, changes and additions to stage groups, and the introduction of new recommendations regarding the staging of lung cancers with multiple pulmonary sites of involvement and guidelines for tumor measurement. Understanding TNM-8 will allow radiologists to accurately stage patients with lung cancer and optimize patient management.

Take-Home Messages

- Lung cancer is a major cause of cancer mortality, and accurate staging is crucial to the formulation of effective treatment strategies.
- Revisions to the eighth edition of the tumor-node-metastasis (TNM) staging system are based on significant differences in patient survival.
- TNM-8 features changes to the T and M descriptors, modifications and additions to the overall stage groups, new recommendations for the staging of patients with multiple sites of pulmonary involvement, and recommendations for lesion measurement.

References

1. Centers for Disease Control and Prevention. National Center for Health Statistics. CDC WONDER On-line Database, compiled from Compressed Mortality File 1999-2012 Series 20 No. 2R, 2014.
2. American Cancer Society. Cancer facts and figures, 2017. Accessed 30 Jan 2017.
3. Goldstraw P, Crowley J, Chansky K, et al. The IASLC lung cancer staging project: proposals for the revision of the TNM stage groupings in the forthcoming (seventh) edition of the TNM classification of malignant Tumours. J Thorac Oncol. 2007;2:706–14.
4. Carter BW, Lichtenberger JP 3rd, Benveniste MK, de Groot PM, Wu CC, Erasmus JJ, Truong MT. Revisions to the TNM staging of lung cancer: rationale, significance, and clinical application. Radiographics 2018;38(2):374-391.
5. Ost DE, Yeung SC, Tanoue LT, Gould MK. Clinical and organizational factors in the initial evaluation of patients with lung cancer: diagnosis and management of lung cancer, 3rd ed: American College of Chest Physicians evidence-based clinical practice guidelines. Chest. 2013;143(5 Suppl):e121S–41S.
6. Henschke CI, Yankelevitz DF, Mirtcheva R, et al. CT screening for lung cancer: frequency and significance of part-solid and nonsolid nodules. AJR. Am J Roentgenol. 2002;178(5):1053–7.
7. Hasegawa M, Sone S, Takashima S, et al. Growth rate of small lung cancers detected on mass CT screening. Br J Radiol. 2000;73(876):1252–9.
8. Kakinuma R, Ohmatsu H, Kaneko M, et al. Progression of focal pure ground-glass opacity detected by low-dose helical computed tomography screening for lung cancer. J Comput Assist Tomogr. 2004;28(1):17–23.
9. National Comprehensive Cancer Network. NCCN Clinical Practice Guidelines in Oncology (NCCN Guidelines®). Non-Small Cell Lung Cancer, 2018. Accessed 12 Sept 2018.
10. Prenzel KL, Mönig SP, Sinning JM, et al. Lymph node size and metastatic infiltration in non-small cell lung cancer. Chest. 2003;123(2):463–7.
11. Pauls S, Buck AK, Hohl K, et al. Improved non-invasive T-staging in non-small cell lung cancer by integrated 18F-FDG PET/CT. Nuklearmedizin. 2007;46(1):9–14.. quiz N1-2
12. Steinert HC. PET and PET-CT of lung cancer. Methods Mol Biol. 2011;727:33–51.
13. Chao F, Zhang H. PET/CT in the staging of the non-small-cell lung cancer. J Biomed Biotechnol. 2012;2012:783739.
14. Ohno Y, Koyama H, Dinkel J, Hintze C. Lung cancer. In: Kauczor HU, editor. MRI of the lung. Heidelberg, Springer; 2009: 179–216.
15. Ohno Y, Adachi S, Motoyama A, et al. Multiphase ECG triggered 3D contrast-enhanced MR angiography: utility for evaluation of hilar and mediastinal invasion of bronchogenic carcinoma. J Magn Reson Imaging. 2001;13:215–24.
16. Rami-Porta R, Bolejack V, Giroux DJ, et al. The IASLC lung cancer staging project: the new database to inform the eighth edition of the TNM classification of lung cancer. J Thorac Oncol. 2014;9(11):1618–24.
17. Rami-Porta R, Bolejack V, Crowley J, et al. The IASLC lung cancer staging project: proposals for the revisions of the T descriptors in the forthcoming eighth edition of the TNM classification for lung cancer. J Thorac Oncol. 2015;10:990–1003.
18. Rusch VW, Asamura H, Watanabe H, et al. The IASLC lung cancer staging project: a proposal for a new international lymph node map in the forthcoming seventh edition of the TNM classification for lung cancer. J Thorac Oncol. 2009;4(5):568–77.
19. Asamura H, Chansky K, Crowley J, et al. The International Association for the Study of Lung Cancer lung cancer staging project: proposals for the revision of the N descriptors in the forthcoming 8th edition of the TNM classification for lung cancer. J Thorac Oncol. 2015;10(12):1675–84.
20. Eberhardt WEE, Mitchell A, Crowley J, et al. The IASLC lung cancer staging project: proposals for the revision of the M descriptors in the forthcoming (8th) edition of the TNM classification of lung cancer. J Thorac Oncol. 2015;10:1515–122.
21. Goldstraw P, Chansky K, Crowley J, et al. The IASLC lung cancer staging project: proposals for revision of the TNM stage groupings in the forthcoming (eighth) edition of the TNM classification for lung cancer. J Thorac Oncol. 2016;11(1):39–51.
22. Detterbeck FC, Nicholson AG, Franklin WA, et al. The IASLC lung cancer staging project: summary of proposals for revisions of the classification of lung cancers with multiple pulmonary sites of involvement in the forthcoming eighth edition of the TNM classification. J Thorac Oncol. 2016;11(5):639–50.
23. Detterbeck FC, Franklin WA, Nicholson AG, et al. The IASLC lung cancer staging project: background data and proposed criteria to distinguish separate primary lung cancers from metastatic foci in patients with two lung tumors in the forthcoming eighth edition of the TNM classification for lung cancer. J Thorac Oncol. 2016;11(5):651–65.
24. Detterbeck FC, Bolejack V, Arenberg DA, et al. The IASLC lung cancer staging project: background data and proposals for the classification of lung cancer with separate tumor nodules in the forthcoming eighth edition of the TNM classification for lung cancer. J Thorac Oncol. 2016;11(5):681–92.
25. Detterbeck FC, Marom EM, Arenberg DA, et al. The IASLC lung cancer staging project: background data and proposals for the application of TNM staging rules to lung cancer presenting as multiple nodules with ground glass or Lepidic features or a pneumonic type of involvement in the forthcoming eighth edition of the TNM classification. J Thorac Oncol. 2016;11(5):666–80.
26. Travis WD, Asamura H, Bankier AA, et al. The IASLC lung cancer staging project: proposals for coding T categories for subsolid nodules and assessment of tumor size in part-solid tumors in the forthcoming eighth edition of the TNM classification of lung cancer. J Thorac Oncol. 2016;11(8):1204–23.
27. Wislez M, Massiani M-A, Milleron B, et al. Clinical characteristics of pneumonic-type adenocarcinoma of the lung. Chest. 2003;123:1868–77.
28. Akira M, Atagi S, Kawahara M, Iuchi K, Johkoh T. High resolution CT findings of diffuse bronchioloalveolar carcinoma in 38 patients. Am J Roentgenol. 1999;173:1623–9.
29. Battafarano RJ, Meyers BF, Guthrie TJ, Cooper JD, Patterson GA. Surgical resection of multifocal non-small cell lung cancer is associated with prolonged survival. Ann Thorac Surg. 2002;74:988–94.

30. Barlesi F, Doddoli C, Gimenez C, et al. Bronchioloalveolar carcinoma: myths and realities in the surgical management. Eur J Cardiothorac Surg. 2003;24:159–64.
31. de Perrot M, Chernenko S, Waddell TK, et al. Role of lung transplantation in the treatment of bronchogenic carcinomas for patients with end-stage pulmonary disease. J Clin Oncol. 2004;22:4351–6.
32. Ahmad U, Wang Z, Bryant AS, et al. Outcomes for lung transplantation for lung cancer in the united network for organ sharing registry. Ann Thorac Surg. 2012;94:935–41.
33. Petrou M, Quint LE, Nan B, Baker LH. Pulmonary nodule volumetric measurement variability as a function of CT slice thickness and nodule morphology. AJR Am J Roentgenol. 2007;188:306–12.
34. Goo JM, Tongdee T, Tongdee R, Yeo K, Hildebolt CF, Bae KT. Volumetric measurement of synthetic lung nodules with multi-detector row CT: effect of various image reconstruction parameters and segmentation thresholds on measurement accuracy. Radiology. 2005;235:850–6.
35. Ravenel JG, Leue WM, Nietert PJ, Miller JV, Taylor KK, Silvestri GA. Pulmonary nodule volume: effects of reconstruction parameters on automated measurements—a phantom study. Radiology. 2008;247:400–8.
36. Wang Y, de Bock GH, van Klaveren RJ, et al. Volumetric measurement of pulmonary nodules at low-dose chest CT: effect of reconstruction setting on measurement variability. Eur Radiol. 2010;20:1180–7.
37. Ignatius Ou SH, Zell JA. The applicability of the proposed IASLC staging revisions to small cell lung cancer (SCLC) with comparison to the current UICC 6th TNM edition. J Thorac Oncol. 2009;4(3):300–10.
38. Kalemkerian GP, Akerley W, Bogner P, et al. Small cell lung cancer. J Natl Compr Cancer Netw. 2013;11(1):78–98.
39. Nicholson AG, Chansky K, Crowley J, et al. The International Association for the Study of Lung Cancer lung cancer staging project: proposals for the revision of the clinical and pathologic staging of small cell lung cancer in the forthcoming eighth edition of the TNM classification for lung cancer. J Thorac Oncol. 2016;11(3):300–11.

9

Diseases of the Chest Wall, Pleura, and Diaphragm

Aine M. Kelly and Thomas Frauenfelder

Learning Objectives
- To learn which imaging modalities to use in evaluating the chest wall, pleura, and diaphragm.
- To generate a differential diagnosis for diseases of the chest wall, pleura, and diaphragm.
- To distinguish extrapulmonary pathology from pulmonary pathology on imaging studies.
- To apply physics principles when assessing fluid and air in the pleural space.
- To become familiar with the imaging appearances in diaphragmatic trauma.

9.1 Introduction

When imaging the chest wall, pleura, and diaphragm, chest radiography is helpful in problem-solving, whereas in the mediastinum, CT is much more useful. With extrapulmonary lesions arising in the superior sulcus (apical) region, or chest wall masses, magnetic resonance imaging (MRI) is excellent because of its tissue characterization abilities.

In general, normal variants, unlike disease, are reasonably symmetric and often bilateral, and thus a side-by-side comparison can be made. The soft tissues, fat, and musculature should be fairly symmetric. When assessing for skeletal abnormalities, which are frequently challenging to see, it is critical to examine the individual bones carefully, one by one. To help differentiate an extrapulmonary (chest wall, pleural, or diaphragmatic) lesion from a pulmonary parenchymal lesion, assessing the angle the mass makes with the lung edge (obtuse angle for extra-parenchymal masses and acute angles for pulmonary masses) may be helpful. With extrapulmonary masses, it can be difficult to determine if it is arising from the chest wall or pleura, as their shapes may be similar, but the presence of bone destruction suggests an extrapleural origin.

A. M. Kelly (✉)
Department of Radiology, University of Michigan, Ann Arbor, MI, USA
e-mail: ainekell@med.umich.edu

T. Frauenfelder
Institute of diagnostic and interventional Radiology, University Hospital Zurich, Zurich, Switzerland
e-mail: Thomas.frauenfelder@usz.ch

9.2 Chest Wall Disease

The chest wall should normally be symmetric with the most common causes of apparent asymmetry being patient rotation or thoracic kyphoscoliosis. The more lucent side is that to which the patient is rotated toward (e.g., in a right anterior oblique (RAO)/left posterior oblique (LPO) position, the left side becomes more lucent). Chest radiography is useful to detect subcutaneous emphysema and calcification and to evaluate skeletal disease.

Key Point
- Normal variants tend to be symmetric.

9.3 Hyperlucent or Hyperopaque Hemithorax

Asymmetry in the opacity (hyperlucency or hyper-opacity) of the hemithoraces has many causes, and a reliable approach (once rotation has been excluded) is to start from the outside (skin) and work inward (through subcutaneous tissues, muscles, bones, pleura, and pulmonary parenchyma), to reach the vasculature (pulmonary arteries). Tables 9.1 and 9.2 depict the most common causes of a hyperlucent or hyperopaque hemithorax.

Table 9.1 Causes of a hyperlucent hemithorax

Rotation to that side—patient positioning or thoracic kyphoscoliosis
Mastectomy or chest wall resection on the ipsilateral side
Poland syndrome—congenital
Stroke/polio—acquired disease
Subcutaneous emphysema (e.g., from trauma)
Pneumothorax
Emphysema
Hypoplastic lung
Pulmonary artery hypoplasia

Table 9.2 Causes of a hyperopaque hemithorax

Rotation away from that side—patient positioning or thoracic kyphoscoliosis
Chest wall mass on the ipsilateral side
Pleural effusion—large
Fibrothorax
Consolidation involving most of the ipsilateral lung
Mass—large, in ipsilateral lung
Pneumonectomy or lobectomy on the contralateral side

Key Point

- With unequal lucency of the hemithoraces, it is helpful to start by working one's way in from the outside (skin and subcutaneous tissues) to the inside (pulmonary vasculature) to evaluate the cause. Don't forget patient rotation and kyphoscoliosis!

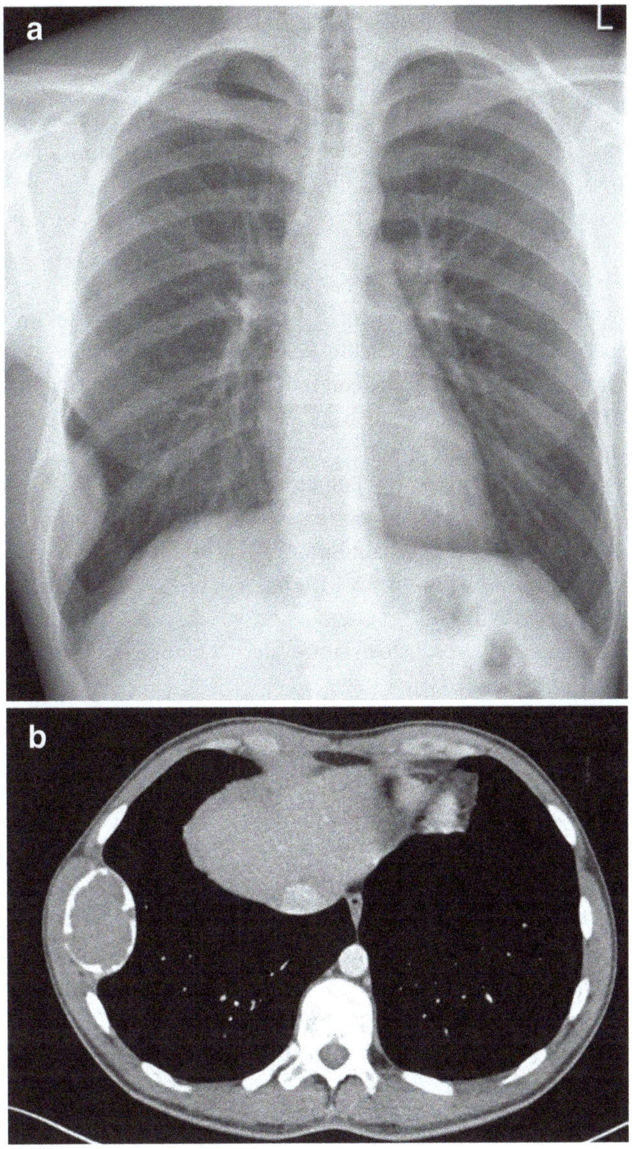

Fig. 9.1 (**a**, **b**). A 25-year-old male with a palpable hard mass in the right lateral chest wall. Frontal chest radiography (**a**) shows an expansile oval lesion of the right eighth rib laterally, with a hazy matrix. Axial CT demonstrates an expansile lesion of the lateral right rib with well-defined borders

9.4 Soft Tissue Masses

These need to be differentiated from asymmetries due to patient positioning, contralateral surgery (such as mastectomy), and contralateral atrophy (e.g., poliomyelitis or stroke). Lipomas are the most common benign primary tumor, and the patient can often provide a history of a stable or slowly enlarging soft mass. Other benign entities include hemangiomas, neurogenic lesions (neurofibromas, schwannomas), and fibromatosis. Neurofibromas arise from intercostal nerves or paraspinal ganglia which can be multiple in von Recklinghausen disease, neurofibromatosis type 1. The most common nonneoplastic tumor of the thoracic skeleton is fibrous dysplasia, accounting for 30% of chest wall benign bone tumors [1]. These slow-growing tumors arise in the posterolateral ribs and are usually asymptomatic until pathologic fractures or pressure symptoms occur. On imaging, fibrous dysplasia presents as an expansile lytic lesion with a "ground glass" or hazy or matrix (Fig. 9.1).

Chest wall malignancies are rare and can result from direct spread of or metastatic disease from adjacent tumors including primary bronchogenic neoplasms, mesothelioma, thymoma, and breast cancer. Plasmacytoma and multiple myeloma are the most common malignant neoplasms of the thoracic skeleton and can present as extrapulmonary masses with bone destruction, similar appearances to other metastases [2]. Well-defined bone lesions with a punched-out appearance are found, which can erode, expand, and destroy cortex, sometimes with surrounding bone reaction, the so-called soap bubble appearance. Other primary chest wall malignant bone tumors are rare and include chondrosarcoma, osteosarcoma, Ewing's sarcoma family of tumors, (evaluate for chondroid or osseous matrix here), multiple myeloma/plasmacytoma, fibrosarcoma, and malignant fibrohisticytoma in adults. Malignant soft tissue masses are a heterogenous group and include undifferentiated pleomorphic sarcoma, liposarcoma, angiosarcoma, and malignant peripheral nerve sheath tumor (which result from malignant transformation of a peripheral chest wall neurofibroma in neurofibromatosis 1 patients) [3–6].

SAPHO (synovitis, acne, pustulosis, hyperostosis, and osteitis) syndrome is a distinct clinical entity representing involvement of the musculoskeletal and dermatologic systems. SAPHO syndrome can mimic some of the more common disease entities such as infection, tumor, and other inflammatory arthropathies. Treatment is empirical, including nonsteroidal anti-inflammatory drugs (NSAIDs) as first-line agents, as well as corticosteroids, disease-modifying antirheumatic drugs, antibiotics, and biological agents. Imaging can be helpful by offering a detailed evaluation of the abnormalities [7]. Ossification of the costoclavicular ligament and hyperostosis at the sternal end of the first ribs are important early findings.

9.5 Inflammatory Disease of the Chest Wall

Chest wall involvement with bacterial infection typically involves ribs and sternum but is rare. Hematogenous or direct spread from a nearby infectious process can cause osteomyelitis with *Staphylococcus aureus* or *Pseudomonas aeruginosa* most commonly implicated. Soft tissue swelling and underlying rib destruction with periosteal reaction may be seen by radiography in chronic cases of osteomyelitis; however, cross-sectional imaging with CT and MRI is much more sensitive and specific. MRI is more sensitive than CT in detecting early osteomyelitis manifest as marrow hypointensity on T1 and bone marrow edema on T2 images. On the other hand, CT better depicts cortical destruction and periosteal reaction compared with MRI.

Chest wall involvement with tuberculosis (TB) is uncommon, with hematogenous spread or, very rarely, direct extension from the adjacent pleural space (empyema necessitans) or the underlying lung parenchyma. Chest wall involvement with TB manifests as soft tissue masses with calcification and rim enhancement, and osseous and cartilaginous destruction can be seen [8]. In immunocompromised patients, fungal infections of the chest wall and bones can occur with *Aspergillus* species accounting for 80–90% of cases [9]. Thoracic actinomycosis can also invade the chest wall, creating fistulous tracts and empyema necessitatis. In post-op patients, nocardia infection can also cause destructive chest wall masses.

9.6 Calcification

Soft tissue calcification may be metastatic or dystrophic. Metastatic calcification is found with elevated serum calcium with calcium hydroxyapatite crystals being deposited in multiple locations, including the lung, stomach, kidney, and vascular system [10]. Dystrophic calcification occurs in altered, necrotic, or dead tissues, in patients with normal serum calcium and phosphorus levels, for example, in connective tissue disorders, like dermatomyositis, where it can be deposited in the subcutaneous tissues, muscles, and fascial planes as calcification universalis.

9.6.1 Pectus Excavatum

In this congenital variant of chest wall development (incidence 1/400–1/1000), the sternum is depressed relative to the anterior ribs and often tilts rightward, with the mediastinal structures displaced leftward [9, 11]. Many cases are asymptomatic and cosmetic only, but if severe [9].

9.6.2 Injuries to the Thoracic Skeleton/Rib Fractures/Trauma

Fractures of the upper ribs and scapulae suggest severe trauma and should prompt a search for associated injury to the aorta, great vessels, and brachial plexus [12]. Fractures of the sternum and medial clavicle have higher risks of associated vascular or cardiac injury. Sternal fractures are extremely difficult to see on frontal chest radiographs but may be seen on the lateral view. CT is indicated if they are suspected. Nearly all sternal fractures will be visible on CT, and adjacent hematoma can be demonstrated. With sternal fractures, one should evaluate for associated cardiac or vascular injury. For suspected fractures of the lower ribs, abdominal radiographs are more helpful, as they are better penetrated. Fractures of the lower ribs may be associated with hepatic, splenic, or renal injury, and abdominal CT is indicated in these cases.

A flail chest (or flail segment) occurs when there are five or more consecutive rib fractures (or three or more ribs are fractured in two or more places). During the respiratory cycle, the flail segment moves paradoxically which can result in ventilatory compromise. Fractures of the thoracic spine account for 15–30% of all spinal fractures, with the most vulnerable segment being the thoracolumbar junction (T9 to T12) region. More than two thirds of thoracic spine fractures are demonstrated by radiography, with almost all visible at CT. CT has the added advantage of demonstrating displacement or retropulsion of bone fragments into the spinal canal and impingement upon the spinal cord.

Key Point

- Fractures of the sternum are extremely difficult to see on radiographs, and CT with contrast is indicated to evaluate for aortic and vascular injury, if sternal fracture is suspected.

9.7 Thalassaemia

With chronic hemolytic anemias (most commonly thalassaemia), hematopoietic tissues outside the bone marrow produce blood (extramedullary hematopoiesis). Normal marrow tissue expands outside the medulla through permeative erosions or by reactivation of previously dormant hematopoietic tissues [13]. Erythropoiesis is ineffective, leading to expansion of bone marrow space in the vertebral column, ribs, long bones, skull, and characteristically the facial bones (frontal bossing). Paravertebral and rib lesions are most often incidental but can occasionally cause cord compression due to mass effect on the spinal canal. On chest radiographs, thalassemia can manifest as bilateral lobulated paravertebral masses with rib expansion.

Key Point

- Chest radiography still plays a key role in the evaluation of the chest wall, particularly for calcification and air but also to assess the skeletal structures.

9.8 Pleural Disease

When assessing for pleural effusion or pneumothorax on radiography, one must keep in mind the patient's positioning (whether supine, semi upright, or upright), as air will rise upward and fluid will gravitate downward within the pleural space and influence the appearances. In critically ill supine patients, air will rise to lie in the anterior inferior costophrenic sulcus, leading to the deep sulcus sign with radiolucency inferior and laterally. The ipsilateral hemidiaphragm may also be more sharply delineated due to the air above it. Conversely, pleural fluid will layer posteriorly and can "cap" over the lung apex. On upright radiographs, intraperitoneal "free" gas will rise to the highest point, under the diaphragmatic domes, if sufficient time is allowed. Alternatively, ill patients can be rolled onto their side for decubitus views to diagnose pneumothorax or effusions. For suspected pneumothorax, the abnormal side should be put up to allow any air to rise, whereas to evaluate effusions, the side should down to get fluid to layer along the inner ribs.

9.9 Pleural Effusion

On upright radiographs, free-flowing pleural fluid displaces the lung away from the costophrenic sulci and blunts the angle, producing a fluid meniscus sign. With small pleural effusions, on upright lateral chest radiographs, one needs to check the posterior costophrenic sulcus (the lowest point) to look for dependent fluid. On the frontal view, view the lateral costophrenic angle or sulcus but bear in mind that subpulmonic pleural fluid can be present without blunting the lateral costophrenic angle. With a subpulmonic effusion, the ipsilateral "hemidiaphragm" will be of uniform attenuation, with a more lateral position of the apparent dome of the hemidiaphragm (with a gradual sloping medial aspect and a more sharply sloping lateral aspect). On supine radiographs, a fluid meniscus or interface (with lung or normal pleura) may not be seen if free-flowing pleural fluid layers posteriorly. With large pleural effusions, in supine patients, an apical pleural cap may be visualized as fluid layers around the apex of the lung.

If there are fibrinous adhesions or scars, pleural effusions may become loculated into localized components. Pleural fluid tracking into fissures can have a tapering cigar-shaped appearance. If pleural fluid in a fissure has a more rounded shape, it can look mass-like giving a "pseudotumor" appearance. Clues to its nature include the "mass" being homogenous in density, with a smooth outline, and having a different shape on two orthogonal projections. One can also review prior radiographs and see a decrease in size or resolution on follow-up.

When pleural effusions are large, they can deviate the mediastinal structures toward the opposite side. A rare but serious complication of large pleural effusions is diaphragmatic inversion. With diaphragmatic inversion, during respiration, the two hemidiaphragms move in opposite directions. This causes air to move over and back between the two lungs (pendulum respiration), resulting in increased dead space and significant respiratory compromise. Symptoms can be relieved with thoracocentesis which restores the affected hemidiaphragm to its normal position. It is easier to diagnose left hemidiaphragm inversion, as this causes mass effect upon the left upper quadrant, displacing the stomach air bubble inferiorly.

In hospitalized patients, pleural effusions are most commonly related to congestive cardiac failure or postsurgical. With congestive heart failure, the effusions are usually relatively symmetric bilaterally but occasionally more asymmetric (right larger than left) or unilateral. When effusions are unilateral or asymmetric with the left larger than the right in nonsurgical patients, other causes should be considered including pneumonia, infarction, neoplasm, trauma, and connective tissue disorders (especially systemic lupus erythematosus and rheumatoid arthritis). In acute pulmonary embolus (PE), small unilateral or bilateral hemorrhagic pleural effusions may be found.

Upper abdominal pathologies can cause sympathetic pleural effusions, usually unilateral. These include subdiaphragmatic abscess, pancreatitis, splenic trauma, and ascites. Clinical history will help, and thoracentesis can help distinguish some entities, for example, elevated amylase with pancreatitis. With ascites, due to hepatic failure, bilateral pleural effusions may develop from leak of fluid through diaphragmatic defects or with third spacing from hypoalbuminemia. With suspected right subdiaphragmatic fluid collections, ultrasound can be very helpful, but for suspected left upper quadrant abscess, CT is better.

Trauma, as the etiology of unilateral pleural effusion, may be apparent when there are multiple rib fractures but less obvious when due to vascular damage in the absence of fractures. Another less apparent cause might include incorrectly placed enteric tubes or vascular catheters. Accidental feeding tube placement into the lung may be uneventful as long as the malposition is detected before feeding is commenced. Malpositioned tubes in the pleural space are usually symptomatic due to complications including tension pneumothorax and empyema.

Key Point

- Patient positioning for radiography affects the appearances of pleural fluid with fluid layering dependently and posteriorly in the supine position, and if there is sufficient fluid, an apical pleural cap may be seen.

9.10 Empyema

Patients with pneumonia commonly have small sympathetic pleural effusions. Infection of the pleural space (empyema) can occur as a complication of pneumonia, with infections such as *Mycobacterium tuberculosis* and fungi, known for involving the pleural space. Differentiating empyema from lung abscess on chest radiographs can be performed by evaluating the shape of the collection on orthogonal views. A lung abscess tends to make acute angles with the adjacent chest wall, while empyemas will make a more obtuse angle. Furthermore, lung abscesses are round and of similar appearances and size on different projections in contrast to empyemas, which tend to be oval or linear on one projection and more spherical on the orthogonal projection. On contrast-enhanced CT, empyema will have a space-occupying effect, deviating nearby bronchi and vessels, while bronchi and vessels will appear to enter and be obliterated by the lung abscess. The empyema will tend to have smoother margins than lung abscess which will be more ill-defined due to surrounding consolidation. In empyema, the "split pleura sign" with separation of the thickened visceral and parietal pleura may also be seen.

The presence of infection in the pleural space cannot be confirmed with imaging alone, and clinical (and laboratory) information are needed to support the diagnosis of infection. Imaging's role is to localize the source of infection to the pleural space, with the cause of pleural effusion often suggested based on clinical information. Early on, an empyema may be difficult to differentiate from a loculated pleural effusion. In some cases, thoracentesis and analysis of pleural fluid will be needed for diagnosis. Thoracic wall ultrasound can be helpful to guide thoracentesis.

9.11 Pneumothorax

Air can enter the pleural space in up to 40% of patients with acute chest trauma as a result of lung, tracheobronchial, or esophageal injury, and pneumothorax may be seen. To detect pneumothorax, upright frontal radiography is indicated as air tends to rise within the pleural space. However, if upright radiography is not feasible, lateral decubitus radiography (with the side of suspected pneumothorax up) is an alternative option. Computed tomography can identify many small and moderate-sized pneumothoraces which may not be visible on supine radiography.

Pneumothorax is best diagnosed by visualization of the visceral pleura outlined by air in the pleural space. Lucency and absence of vessels are less reliable signs which can be seen with presence of focal emphysema or bullae. As is the case with pleural effusions, detection of pneumothorax becomes difficult in the supine position, with the nondependent portion of the pleural space being at the anterior inferior costophrenic recess. Look for the deep sulcus sign, with lucency over the lower lateral chest and a sharply defined ipsilateral hemidiaphragm. A "too easily seen" sharply defined hemidiaphragm or increased lucency over the lung bases should raise concern for basilar pneumothorax, even without seeing the pleural line. A further sign is the "deep sulcus sign" corresponding to a sharply demarcated lateral sulcus. Pneumothorax can track into the fissures with air in the minor fissure a reported sign of supine pneumothorax.

Tension pneumothorax is a medical emergency, due to compression of mediastinal structures resulting in decreased venous return to the heart and hemodynamic collapse. As intrapleural pressure increases, the ipsilateral hemidiaphragm is depressed, with deviation of the mediastinal structures contralaterally.

Pneumothorax is most often due to trauma or iatrogenic (with surgery or other interventions), but they can also occur secondary to ruptured blebs, and with interstitial lung diseases, where honeycomb change or cysts increase the risk of pneumothorax (e.g., in lymphangiomyomatosis or eosinophilic granuloma).

Other causes of pneumothorax, with an apparently normal CXR, include cavitary lesions in a subpleural location, for example, metastases or tuberculosis. Cavitary metastases include mostly squamous primary neoplasms and sarcomas. Increased intrathoracic pressure can potentially cause pneumothorax with an otherwise normal or nearly normal CXR, as can occur in asthma and pregnancy. Bronchial injury or bronchopleural fistula should be suspected when there is persistent or increasing pneumothorax with a functioning chest tube in place or the tube is on suction.

Pneumothorax ex vacuo is a complication of lobar collapse, with a sudden increase in negative intrapleural pressure surrounding the collapsed lobe [14]. This results in gas from the ambient tissues and blood being drawn into the pleural space with the seal between the visceral and parietal pleura of the adjacent lobe or lobes remaining intact. Once the bronchial obstruction is relieved and the collapsed lobe re-expands, the pneumothorax will resolve. It is critical to recognize this entity, as treatment is to relieve the bronchial obstruction rather than to insert a pleural drainage catheter.

Key Point

- In the supine position, a pleural edge may not be seen with pneumothorax, and the radiologist may have to rely on secondary signs including the deep sulcus sign or a hemidiaphragm that is too clearly defined.

9.12 Hemothorax

Hemothorax resulting from injury to large central pulmonary vessels, systemic thoracic veins or arteries, or lacerated viscera can be catastrophic with hemodynamic collapse, requiring urgent surgical intervention, whereas bleeding from low-pressure pulmonary vessels is usually self-limited. Like pleural effusion, hemothorax may be difficult to detect in the supine position, due to layering posteriorly. On supine radiographs, signs of hemothorax include an apical pleural cap, hazy increased opacity projected over the hemithorax, and confluent lateral pleural opacification. Whenever rib fractures are found, a hemothorax should always be considered, and CT is the most accurate way to detect tiny amounts of pleural fluid. A hemothorax can be suggested by CT, when the pleural fluid attenuation is >35 to 40 HU, and dependent layering of the higher attenuation hematocrit elements may be visible with enough blood in the pleural space. Consider a chylous pleural effusion when there is delayed or late appearance of pleural fluid that continues to slowly accumulate over days, particularly with penetrating injuries or following thoracic surgery, secondary to thoracic duct disruption.

9.13 Pleural Plaques or Thickening

With repeated asbestos exposure, bilateral pleural plaques occur commonly and sometimes visibly calcify. They are typically located at the hemidiaphragmatic domes and beside the posterolateral lower ribs [15]. When calcified plaques are viewed en face, they appear as irregularly shaped, poorly marginated opacities, sometimes with scalloped outlines giving a holly leaf-like appearance. A clue to the extrapulmonary origin of pleural plaques is that their long axis doesn't run parallel to that of the underlying pulmonary vasculature and bronchi.

Unilateral pleural plaques can be seen with asbestos exposure but also occur with previous hemothorax in trauma or following empyema. A small hemithorax with extensive pleural calcification (fibrothorax) may be seen after tuberculosis and untreated hemothorax. Non-calcified pleural plaques (and pleural implants) are often better demonstrated with CT rather than by radiography, in contrast to pleural effusion or pneumothorax.

9.14 Pleural Implants and Masses

While pleural masses may be seen with metastatic disease, pleural effusions more commonly occur. Many pleural implants are obscured on chest radiography (and even on CT) by surrounding pleural fluid. Some pleural masses, such as malignant thymoma, cause unilateral multifocal pleural implants without accompanying pleural fluid. On contrast-enhanced CT, the higher attenuation soft tissue implants may be visualized, suggesting the malignant nature of the effusion. Intravenous contrast enhancement (and narrow soft tissue window widths) help distinguish the solid elements from pleural fluid. Dependent layering of hematocrit components with chronic pleural hematoma may look similar to malignant effusion and implants on CT.

Benign mesothelioma (benign fibrous tumor of the pleura) is often a single pleural mass, which ranges in size from small to very large [16]. These masses may be pedunculated and change in position and appearances by twisting around their pedicle. Large benign fibrous tumors are generally distinguishable from malignant mesothelioma due to their focal nature, with malignant mesothelioma being typically more widespread. Benign mesotheliomas are generally recogniz-

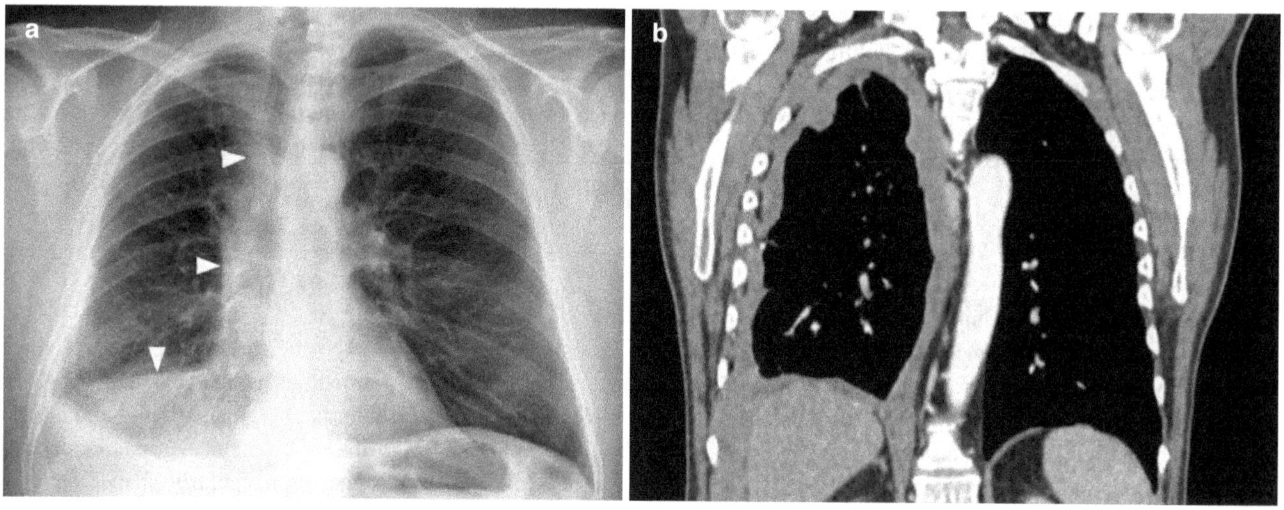

Fig. 9.2 (**a**, **b**): A 65-year-old man with progressive shortness of breath on exertion and a dry cough. Frontal chest radiography (**a**) demonstrates a smaller right hemithorax with circumferential pleural thickening, including the mediastinal or medial aspect (white arrowheads). Coronal contrast-enhanced CT (**b**) shows nodular pleural thickening over the hemidiaphragmatic and mediastinal aspects, with a decrease in volume of the right hemithorax

able as extra-parenchymal pleural lesions due to their shape, with a broad based ill-defined pleural base, making obtuse angles to the lung. Difficulty arises when they occur in the fissures, appearing rounded and more sharply defined, raising suspicion for malignancy. Multiplanar imaging with CT localizes the "mass" to the fissure, making benign fibrous tumor a more likely diagnosis. Clinical associations can sometimes help in distinguishing benign fibrous tumor, such as associated hypertrophic pulmonary osteoarthropathy, and sometimes hypoglycemia. Benign mesotheliomas undergo malignant degeneration in up to a third of cases, and therefore management includes imaging workup prior to excision.

Pleural metastases are much more common than primary pleural neoplasms. Many cancers metastasize to the pleura with those in close proximity most likely, including the lung and breast. When a pleural mass is found and there is primary neoplasm elsewhere, metastatic disease should still be considered even if the primary malignancy isn't one frequently associated with pleural spread.

Key Point

- Pleural implants are more commonly caused by metastatic disease, with the main primaries being the lung, breast, mesothelioma and thymoma locally, and ovarian cancer.

Malignant mesothelioma is the most common primary tumor associated with pleural effusion. Lobulated pleural masses occur along with effusions, often unilateral. Previous asbestos exposure (or bilateral calcified pleural plaques) is a helpful clue, but note that asbestos exposure is only documented in about half of malignant mesothelioma patients. Malignant mesothelioma can be differentiated from benign plaques by the involvement of the mediastinal pleura and the presence of pleural effusion. In some patients, a lack of mediastinal shift away from the affected side of and a decrease in volume in the presence of extensive pleural abnormality are clues to malignant mesothelioma [17, 18]. A differential to consider with circumferential nodular pleural masses often including the medial pleura are encountered is metastatic adenocarcinoma (Fig. 9.2).

Peritoneal metastases often occur with ovarian cancer, and malignant pleural effusions can occur when malignant seedlings pass through congenital hemidiaphragm defects. Massive malignant pleural effusions in ovarian cancer are known as Meigs syndrome.

Key Point

- Consider malignant mesothelioma or metastatic adenocarcinoma when lobulated pleural masses involving the mediastinal surface of the pleura are found.

9.15 Diaphragmatic Disease

On posteroanterior radiographs, the upper border of the right hemidiaphragm usually lies between the level of the fifth rib anteriorly and the anterior sixth–seventh rib interspace, typically a rib interspace higher than the left hemidiaphragm. On radiography, the diaphragm is inseparable from the abdominal structures below. On CT, the diaphragm is a thin soft-tissue attenuation linear structure which is thinner (and sometimes not clearly visible) toward the central tendon in contrast to the edges [19]. Muscle slips run obliquely along the inferior surface and may be asymmetric, with a mass-like appearance sometimes seen on cross section, especially in males, as they are more prominent. Prominent muscle slips with the muscle bulging upward on either side of the slips can give a scalloped appearance to the diaphragm, a normal variant. Multiplanar CT is useful to see the diaphragm due to the differences in attenuation of the diaphragm, adjacent intraperitoneal fat, nearby extrapulmonary fat, and aerated lung. Diaphragmatic defects (eventration) and hernias (Bochdalek posteriorly, Morgagni anteromedially) may be congenital or acquired (hiatus hernia, trauma, paresis, or paralysis). Predisposing conditions for all abdominal hernias include pregnancy, trauma, obesity, chronic constipation, and chronic cough.

9.16 Bochdalek Hernia

In adult patients, 90% of congenital diaphragmatic hernias found are Bochdalek hernias, more commonly left sided, possibly because of the protective effect of the liver on the right side [20]. Bochdalek hernias occur posterolaterally, through which intraperitoneal fat and, occasionally, solid organs such as kidneys or bowel loops pass through gaps between the costal and vertebral portions of the diaphragm [21]. Neonates and infants can present with respiratory compromise, with older children or adults sometimes presenting with acute or chronic gastrointestinal symptoms. Rarely, Bochdalek hernias can present as an acute abdomen due to complications of bowel incarceration, strangulation, perforation, or shock. With widespread CT imaging, most are discovered incidentally nowadays, as small defects, sometimes bilateral, particularly in patients with chronic obstructive airways disease. In these incidentally discovered Bochdalek hernias, no further action is needed. On CT imaging, discontinuity of the diaphragm posteriorly or posteromedially is usually easily seen with protrusion of peritoneal or retroperitoneal fat through the defect [21]. Less commonly, kidney, colon, small bowel, liver, or spleen may also herniate through a Bochdalek hernia. On chest radiography, the differential diagnosis for a contour deformity in the posterior hemidiaphragm includes lipomas, lung or diaphragmatic masses, neurogenic tumors, pulmonary sequestrations, or intrathoracic kidneys.

9.17 Morgagni Hernia

In adults, less than 10% of congenital diaphragmatic hernias found are Morgagni hernias, found anteromedially, due to failure of fusion of the sternal and costal portions of the hemidiaphragm [20, 22]. Morgagni hernias are more common on the right, perhaps because of greater support provided by the pericardial attachments on the left. In adults, omentum is most commonly found, with bowel, stomach, or liver rarely passing through. On imaging, Morgagni hernias appear as low attenuation masses in the anterior cardiophrenic angle and can be difficult to differentiate from prominent epicardial fat pads or pericardial cysts on radiographs. Other differential diagnoses for masses in the anterior cardiophrenic region include lipoma, liposarcoma, thymoma, thymolipoma, or teratoma. Coronal plane reformatted CT or MR images can demonstrate displaced curvilinear omental vessels within the "mass" or coursing across the diaphragmatic defect, typical features of Morgagni hernia.

9.18 Diaphragmatic Eventration

Hemidiaphragmatic eventration occurs with congenital muscular aplasia or thinning of a portion of tendon, which bulges upward with abdominal contents, most commonly anteriorly, because of the pressure gradient between the peritoneum and the thorax [21]. Unlike true hernias, the chest and abdominal contents are still separated by a layer of pleura, diaphragmatic tendon or muscle, and peritoneum and are incidental findings [19]. Rare symptoms of eventration include dyspnea, tachypnea, recurrent pneumonia, and failure to thrive, and these cases can be treated with surgical plication (tucking or folding and suturing). Hemidiaphragm eventration is nearly always found on the right side anteromedially, and with increasing intra-abdominal pressure (such as from increased abdominal obesity), it can become more pronounced. On imaging in eventration, there is elevation of the anterior portion of the hemidiaphragm, with a normal posterior origin (takeoff point) and position. This differs from diaphragmatic paresis or paralysis, where the entire hemidiaphragm will be elevated, including the posterior portion and origin (takeoff point). Relative thickening of the muscle at the edge of the eventration may be seen or sometimes undercut edges with ballooning upward of the eventrated portion on CT [21].

9.19 Esophageal hiatus hernia

The esophageal hiatus lies at the level of the tenth thoracic vertebral body and conveys the esophagus, sympathetic nerve branches, and the vagus nerve [20]. This hiatus functions as an anatomic sphincter by constricting on inspiration and preventing gastroesophageal reflux. The esophageal hiatus can enlarge with increasing age, abdominal obesity, and with general weakening of the musculofascial structures, leading to hiatal hernia. Herniation of part of the stomach most commonly occurs, with occasionally other abdominal organs, bowel loops or fat, or, rarely, the entire stomach. Intrathoracic hiatal hernias are most commonly sliding (in 90% of cases), with displacement of the gastroesophageal junction and a portion of (or entire) stomach upward into the thoracic cavity and loss of the usual antireflux mechanism. Less commonly, intrathoracic hiatal hernias are the rolling (paraesophageal) type, with a portion of (or all) the stomach or other abdominal contents, such as spleen or intestines rolling up above the gastroesophageal junction to enter the thoracic cavity. A combination of the two types (sliding and rolling) can also occur. On chest radiography, herniation of stomach will be visible as opacification behind the heart on the lateral view and obliteration of the azygoesophageal line on a frontal view [23]. On CT imaging, one can evaluate the location of the stomach and intra-abdominal organs, bowel loops, and peritoneal fat.

9.20 Blunt Traumatic Diaphragmatic Rupture

In about 5% of patients with blunt trauma, diaphragmatic rupture occurs, with most associated with significant intra-abdominal injuries [24]. Injury mechanisms include frontal impact, causing increased intra-abdominal pressure and "blowing out" of the diaphragm, and lateral impact distorting the chest wall, causing shearing forces across the diaphragm. Diaphragmatic ruptures are thought to occur with equal frequency bilaterally, with ruptures on the right being clinically more occult due to protection from the liver. Consequently, left ruptures are reported in most (75–90%) cases, with most tears posterolaterally at the weakest portion, the musculotendinous junction. After blunt trauma, most diaphragmatic tears are longer than 2 cm and many left tears even more than 10 cm in length.

About half of diaphragmatic ruptures are complicated by visceral organ herniation with the stomach and colon most commonly herniating on the left, and occasionally small bowel, spleen and kidney. The liver most commonly herniates on the right and sometimes colon. Herniated organs can strangulate, leading to ischemia, infarction, or obstruction. Sometimes, herniation after diaphragmatic rupture is delayed, with the relatively increased intra-abdominal pressure gradually causing the defect to increase in size, increasing the likelihood of herniation of intra-abdominal contents into the thorax. The increase in size of the diaphragmatic defect may be slowed down or prevented if patients receive positive pressure ventilation after their injury as this eliminates or reverses the pressure gradient. The time delay between injury and herniation is known as the latent phase and last for months to years, but most cases of strangulation manifest clinically within 3 years of the trauma.

Secondary signs of herniation can be seen at radiography including apparent elevation of the hemidiaphragm; an altered, irregular, discontinuous, or obscured contour; mediastinal shift to the contralateral side; viscera containing air above the hemidiaphragm; and if present, the gastric tube tip may be elevated with a U-shaped configuration. Similar appearances can be seen with other entities, including atelectasis, lung contusion, posttraumatic lung cysts, pneumothorax, subpulmonic pleural effusion, hiatal hernia, and phrenic nerve paralysis. Diaphragmatic eventration can have similar appearances, and comparison with old studies may be helpful here.

Multiplanar CT is more sensitive and specific, with signs of diaphragmatic injury including focal hemidiaphragmatic discontinuity; difficulty seeing the hemidiaphragm; a large defect between the torn ends of the hemidiaphragm; thickening and curling at the torn ends (due to muscular contraction); herniation of intraperitoneal fat, omentum, bowel loops, or abdominal viscera; focal narrowing of an organ or loop of bowel at the muscular defect (the the dependent viscera sign sign and "the dependent viscera sign") (the unsupported herniated organs or bowel fall dependently, abutting the posterior ribs) (Fig. 9.3). Other accompanying signs include pneumothorax, hemothorax, pneumoperitoneum, and hemoperitoneum. Coronal T2-weighted MRI is an alternative modality that can be used to evaluate for diaphragmatic injuries in the non-acute setting.

Key Point

- Hemidiaphragmatic ruptures can go unnoticed initially, particularly in intensive care patients with positive end inspiratory pressure ventilation, due to equal intrathoracic and intra-abdominal pressures, but they usually progress later, due to the relatively increased intra-abdominal pressure, and therefore should be repaired.

9.21 Penetrating Diaphragmatic Injury

Penetrating injuries of the diaphragm are more common than blunt injuries. The site of injury depends on the location and trajectory of the penetrating object. Penetrating injuries tend to be smaller, related to the size of the penetrating object, with most less than 2 cm and many below 1 cm. Visceral herniation is uncommon with smaller penetrating injuries. Penetrating injuries are usually diagnosed clinically relying on the entry site and direction of the wound. Exploratory

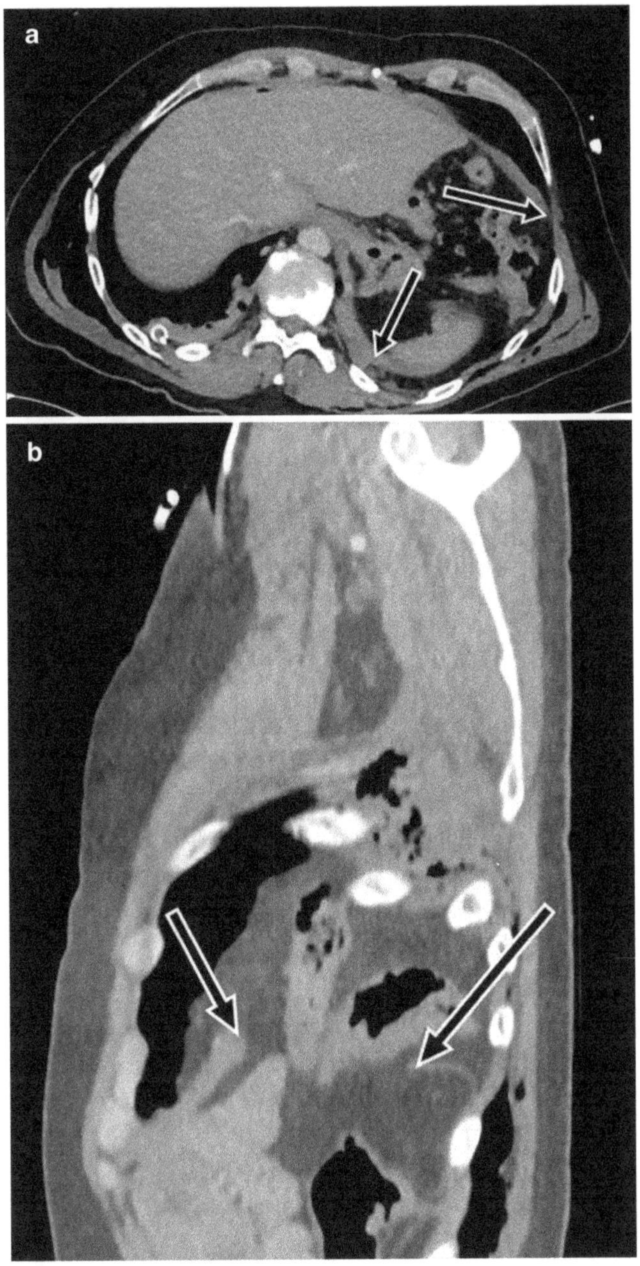

Fig. 9.3 (**a**, **b**): A 62-year-old woman who sustained blunt chest trauma in a road traffic accident. Axial contrast enhanced CT (**a**) shows diaphragmatic rupture, with thickened ends (black arrows) due to muscular contractions at the edge of the rupture. Note also the dependent location of the spleen (dependent viscera sign). There are also fractures of the right ribs and subcutaneous emphysema and a right basilar pleural drainage tube. Sagittal contrast-enhanced CT (**b**) demonstrates herniation of loops of colon through a large defect in the left hemidiaphragm, with thickening of the muscle at the margins (black arrows) of the defect, especially anteriorly

surgery is usually indicated in patients with penetrating injuries, at which time the diaphragmatic injury is diagnosed and repaired. CT imaging findings include pneumothorax, hemothorax, or radiopaque material associated with the projectile near the diaphragm or indicating the path through the diaphragm.

9.22 Diaphragmatic Paresis or Paralysis

Many processes result in diaphragmatic paresis or paralysis, including central nervous disease or local damage to the phrenic nerve from surgery or masses, but most cases are idiopathic, possibly caused by viral infection [25]. Thoracic imaging is usually unhelpful in determining etiologies for diaphragmatic paralysis, except in the case of direct invasion by intrathoracic tumors. Diaphragmatic paralysis is more commonly unilateral and often asymptomatic, being an incidental finding on imaging. Bilateral diaphragmatic paralysis is usually symptomatic, often presenting as respiratory compromise.

With bilateral diaphragmatic paralysis, frontal radiographs will demonstrate smooth elevation of the hemidiaphragms and decreased lung volumes and deep and narrow costophrenic and costovertebral recesses. The lateral view reveals a smooth contour and elevation of the entire diaphragm. Adjacent bibasilar linear atelectasis may be present. Apparent bilateral diaphragmatic elevation can also be seen with poor inspiratory effort, obesity, subpulmonic pleural effusions, subdiaphragmatic processes (like ascites, dilated bowel, and hepatomegaly), and pleural adhesions. With a unilateral elevated hemidiaphragm, the left may lie at a higher position compared to the right, or the right will lie more than one rib interspace higher than the left. A weak or paralyzed hemidiaphragm will show elevation in its entire course, including the posterior takeoff point, which helps differentiate it from hemidiaphragm eventration.

Fluoroscopic sniff testing can be helpful with unilateral diaphragmatic weakness or paralysis, by demonstrating slower downward (caudal) or paradoxical upward (with paralysis) movement during quiet inspiration, deep inspiration, and sniffing [25]. Sniff tests are not as useful for bilateral paralysis, may be falsely positive in normal individuals, and require user expertise. Ultrasonography can be used to diagnose paralysis, using the same principles as the fluoroscopic sniff test to assess diaphragmatic movement, but it requires operator experience. Chest and abdominal CT can be utilized to evaluate for processes that cause diaphragmatic elevation and simulate paralysis, including chronic obstructive airways disease, pleural effusions, subdiaphragmatic abscess, ascites, organomegaly, or ileus. Coronal (or sagittal) plane dynamic T2-weighted MRI imaging can be used to assess for paralysis (in centers with experience) with the diaphragm seen as a low T2 signal structure. Quantitative evaluation, including excursion, synchronicity, and velocity of diaphragmatic motion can also be performed with MRI.

9.23 Tumors of the Diaphragm

Primary tumors are rare, with more than half being benign, and the most common are lipomas [26]. Benign tumors are resected if there is diagnostic uncertainty or if they cause symptoms [26, 27]. Primary malignant lesions include rhabdomyosarcoma, followed by fibrosarcoma [2]. Secondary malignant lesions spread to the diaphragm by direct involvement from lung cancer, and other intrathoracic (mesothelioma, esophageal cancer) or intra-abdominal tumors (hepatic and adrenal cancer) more commonly occur. With malignant thymoma, drop metastases via the pleural space to the diaphragm can also occur as can intraperitoneal or serosal spread in ovarian cancer. Implants to the diaphragm can be found in benign processes such as endometriosis.

9.24 Conclusion

In evaluating the chest wall structures, the pleura, and the diaphragm, a combination of different imaging modalities can be employed, along with relevant clinical history (especially trauma and known primary malignancy). Previous imaging studies are particularly helpful in cases of suspected diaphragmatic trauma or paralysis. Comparing to the other (unaffected) side is helpful for chest wall pathology. Being familiar with image study techniques, coupled with knowledge of physics principles (air, water, blood, and soft tissue), can give valuable diagnostic clues.

Take-Home Messages

- Chest radiography has a major role in the evaluation of the chest wall, particularly for calcification and air but also to assess the skeletal structures.
- Certain fractures such as the sternum are extremely difficult to see on radiographs, and CT with contrast is indicated to evaluate for aortic and vascular injury, if sternal fracture is suspected.
- Remember the physical principles of fluid and air when assessing radiographs for pleural fluid or air. Pleural fluid will layer dependently in the supine position, posterior to the lungs. In the supine position, the pleural edge may not be seen with pneumothorax, and secondary signs, including the deep sulcus sign or a hemidiaphragm that is too clearly defined, should be looked for. Pleural implants are more commonly due to metastatic disease.
- Hemidiaphragmatic ruptures may not manifest initially, especially with positive end inspiratory pressure ventilation, which equalizes intrathoracic and intra-abdominal pressures, but defects will steadily progress after this, and therefore repair is indicated.

References

1. Hughes EK, James SL, Butt S, et al. Benign primary tumours of the ribs. Clin Radiol. 2006;61:314–22.
2. Tateishi U, Gladish GW, Kusumoto M, et al. Chest wall tumors: radiologic findings and pathologic correlation: part 2. Malignant tumors. Radiographics. 2003;23:1491–508.
3. Nam SJ, Kim S, Lim BJ, et al. Imaging of primary chest wall tumors with radiologic-pathologic correlation. Radiographics. 2011;31:749–70.
4. Carter BW, Benveniste MF, Betancourt SL, et al. Imaging evaluation of malignant chest wall neoplasms. Radiographics. 2016;36:1285–306.
5. Souza FF, de Angelo M, O'Regan K, et al. Malignant primary chest wall neoplasms: a pictorial review of imaging findings. Clin Imaging. 2013;37:8–17.
6. Bueno J, Lichtenberger JP 3rd, Rauch G, Carter BW. MR imaging of primary chest wall neoplasms. Top Magn Reson Imaging. 2018;27:83–93.
7. Schaub S, Sirkis HM, Kay J. Imaging for synovitis, acne, pustulosis, hyperostosis, and osteitis (SAPHO) syndrome. Rheum Dis Clin N Am. 2016;42:695–710.
8. Jeung MY, Gangi A, Gasser B, et al. Imaging of chest wall disorders. Radiographics. 1999;19:617–37.
9. Baez JC, Lee EY, Restrepo R, Eisenberg RL. Chest wall lesions in children. AJR Am J Roentgenol. 2013;200:W402–19.
10. Stewart VL, Herling P, Dalinka MK. Calcification in soft tissues. JAMA. 1983;250:78–81.
11. Donnelly LF. Use of three-dimensional reconstructed helical CT images in recognition and communication of chest wall anomalies in children. AJR Am J Roentgenol. 2001;177:441–5.
12. Miller LA. Chest wall, lung, and pleural space trauma. Radiol Clin North Am. 2006;44:213–24.
13. Orphanidou-Vlachou E, Tziakouri-Shiakalli C, Georgiades CS. Extramedullary hemopoiesis. Semin Ultrasound CT MR. 2014;35:255–62.
14. Woodring JH, Baker MD. Stark P (1996) Pneumothorax ex vacuo. Chest. 1996;110(4):1102–5.
15. Walker CM, Takasugi JE, Chung JH, et al. Tumor-like conditions of the pleura. Radiographics. 2012;32:971–85.
16. Rosado-de-Christenson ML, Abbott GF, McAdams HP, et al. From the archives of the AFIP: localized fibrous tumor of the pleura. Radiographics. 2003;23:759–83.
17. Wang ZJ, Reddy GP, Gotway MB, et al. Malignant pleural mesothelioma: evaluation with CT, MR imaging, and PET. Radiographics. 2004;24:105–19.
18. Truong MT, Viswanathan C, Godoy MB, et al. Malignant pleural mesothelioma: role of CT, MRI, and PET/CT in staging evaluation and treatment considerations. Semin Roentgenol. 2013;48:323–34.
19. Kharma N. Dysfunction of the diaphragm: imaging as a diagnostic tool. Curr Opin Pulm Med. 2013;19:394–8.
20. Nason LK, Walker CM, McNeeley MF, et al. Imaging of the diaphragm: anatomy and function. Radiographics. 2012;32:E51–70.
21. Sandstrom CK, Stern EJ. Diaphragmatic hernias: a spectrum of radiographic appearances. Curr Probl Diagn Radiol. 2011;40:95–115.
22. Taylor GA, Atalabi OM, Estroff JA. Imaging of congenital diaphragmatic hernias. Pediatr Radiol. 2009;39:1–16.
23. Anthes TB, Thoongsuwan N, Karmy-Jones R. Morgagni hernia: CT findings. Curr Probl Diagn Radiol. 2003;32:135–6.
24. Eren S, Ciriş F. Diaphragmatic hernia: diagnostic approaches with review of the literature. Eur J Radiol. 2005;54:448–59.

25. Eren S, Kantarci M, Okur A. Imaging of diaphragmatic rupture after trauma. Clin Radiol. 2006;61:467–77.
26. Kim MP, Hofstetter WL. Tumors of the diaphragm. Thorac Surg Clin. 2009;19:521–9.
27. Tateishi U, Gladish GW, Kusumoto M, et al. Chest wall tumors: radiologic findings and pathologic correlation: part 1. Benign tumors. Radiographics. 2003;23:1477–90.

10

Pediatric Chest Disorders: Practical Imaging Approach to Diagnosis

Alison Hart and Edward Y. Lee

> **Learning Objectives**
> - To apply an anatomical three-compartment model to some of the most commonly encountered pediatric chest pathologies including primary processes of the lung parenchyma, abnormalities of the large airway, and pathology originating in the mediastinum
> - To understand the advantages and disadvantages of current imaging modalities in imaging of the pediatric chest

10.1 Introduction

Symptomatology referable to the chest is one of the most common reasons for which pediatric patients present for clinical evaluation. While subsequent diagnosis widely varies depending upon the specific symptoms, clinical context, and age of the patient, imaging plays a critical role in elucidation of differential considerations. Furthermore, imaging provides valuable information in the evaluation of disease extent and associated abnormalities thereby directly impacting patient management decisions. Furthermore, diagnostic imaging provides a detailed assessment of treatment response.

Given the broad range of pathologies which affect the pediatric chest, anatomic localization is a useful classification approach and can be thought of in a three-compartment model, including primary processes of the lung parenchyma, abnormalities of the large airway, and pathology originating in the mediastinum. Here, we present this practical approach as it applies to some of the most commonly encountered pediatric chest pathologies. This chapter also reviews the advantages and disadvantages of current imaging modalities and characteristic imaging findings of pediatric thoracic disorders encountered in daily clinical practice.

A. Hart · E. Y. Lee (✉)
Department of Radiology, Boston Children's Hospital and Harvard Medical School, Boston, MA, USA
e-mail: Edward.Lee@childrens.harvard.edu

10.2 Advantages and Disadvantages of Imaging Modalities

Three most commonly used imaging modalities for evaluating pediatric thoracic disorders are chest radiography, computed tomography (CT), and magnetic resonance imaging (MRI). Their advantages and disadvantages are briefly summarized in the following section.

10.2.1 Chest Radiography

Chest radiography is the first-line and most commonly performed imaging examination in pediatric patients with potential thoracic disorders. Frequently, it is also the sole imaging study required for diagnosis. In thoracic pathologies unable to be fully characterized by chest radiography alone, such as those involving mediastinum or airway, it is often sufficient for appropriately tailoring subsequent imaging examinations. Given that ionizing radiation is required for the generation of chest radiography, its use must be weighed against the potential risk factor of radiation-induced malignancy. This is heightened in pediatric patients due to their increased susceptibility to the effects of ionizing radiation as well as their longer potential for repeated exposure as compared with adults. In the implementation of the ALARA principle, whereby radiation levels are maintained as low as reasonably achievable (ALARA), diagnostic chest radiography can be generated with very low radiation dose [1, 2]. This, thus, translates into a very low risk of the development of radiation-induced malignancy. Additionally, chest radiography offers the advantages of easy acquisition, low cost, and ready availability.

10.2.2 Computed Tomography

CT is the most common cross-sectional examination utilized in the evaluation of abnormalities of the lung parenchyma. This is due to its superior anatomic resolution and the high contrast between lung pathology and the adjacent air-filled lung parenchyma, a difference which can be further augmented with the use of intravenous contrast. Compared with chest radiography, CT provides superior characterization of abnormalities and aids in preprocedural evaluation by affording superior relational anatomy. Specialized CT techniques such as high-resolution acquisition, inspiratory and expiratory sequences, and volumetric 3D/4D image reconstruction can be used to answer specific clinical questions [3]. The rapid acquisition time afforded by the multidetector CT (MDCT) scanners currently in use is of further benefit, especially in the pediatric population, because it can diminish the need for sedation. While the benefits of CT are numerous, the most glaring disadvantage is the added ionizing radiation incurred over radiography, and, thus, the risk to benefit ratio must be weighed carefully. Tailored image acquisition parameters which account for patient body size as well as image optimization techniques such as iterative reconstruction in accordance with the principal of ALARA must be used for dose reduction [4].

10.2.3 Magnetic Resonance Imaging

MRI affords superior soft tissue contrast as compared to CT. Therefore, it is an ideal modality for characterization of extra-parenchymal soft tissue lesions such as those of the mediastinum or within the soft tissues of the chest wall. The lack of ionizing radiation, as compared with CT, is of added benefit especially in susceptible pediatric patients. Use of MRI in the evaluation of the lung parenchyma is hindered by the intrinsic paucity of photons within the air-filled alveoli which results in a small magnitude of MRI signal generation [5]. This generated signal is further degraded by increased susceptibility artifact which results from the many air-tissue interfaces within the lung. The decreased special resolution of MRI as compared with CT further limits its use in the evaluation of subtle pathologic changes of the lung parenchyma [6]. As such, MRI is of limited utility in the evaluation of lung parenchymal pathologies which result in an increase of air, the so-called negative pathologies, such as cystic lung disease or emphysema. However, recent development of improved MRI sequences has increased utilization of MRI for evaluation of the so-called plus pathologies which result in the deposition of material within the lung parenchyma [7, 8]. Because of this additive process, a larger number of photons are present within the lung parenchyma thereby increasing the magnitude of the MR signal generated. Disadvantages of MRI include availability and cost. In addition, because of long acquisition times, sedation is usually required as patient motion, in addition to the respiratory and cardiac motion intrinsic to imaging of the chest, can significantly degrade image quality and interfere with image interpretation.

10.3 Spectrum of Pediatric Thoracic Disorders

10.3.1 Pediatric Lung Disorders

10.3.1.1 Neonatal Lung Disorders

Surfactant Deficiency Syndrome due to Prematurity

Surfactant deficiency syndrome is the most common cause of death in premature infants, affecting 6.1/1000 live births [9], with incidence inversely related to gestational age. A lipoprotein produced by type II pneumocytes, surfactant production begins at 23 weeks gestation and maturation occurs at 35 weeks gestation [10]. Allowing for full opening of lung alveoli by reducing alveolar surface tension, surfactant increases lung compliance. In the absence of surfactant, lung compliance decreases leading to atelectasis and alveolar damage. Alveolar destruction results in the generation of cellular debris and fibrin which combine to form hyaline membranes which in turn impair oxygen exchange. Besides prematurity, other risk factors for developing surfactant deficiency syndrome include male gender, cesarean delivery, multiple gestations, and maternal diabetes due to decreased surfactant maturation at high serum insulin levels. Within minutes of birth, affected infants typically develop symptoms including grunting, nasal flaring, retractions, tachypnea, and cyanosis.

Chest radiography is the main imaging modality for evaluating surfactant deficiency syndrome [10] (Fig. 10.1). It classically demonstrates low lung volumes with diffuse fine granular/reticulogranular opacities or, in more severe cases, complete lung opacity. Air bronchograms may be variably present. In the absence of treatment, imaging findings progress reproducibly, being most severe at birth and normalizing over the course of days to weeks or progressing to chronic lung disease of prematurity (Fig. 10.2a). CT is infrequently utilized in surfactant deficiency syndrome but may help in the evaluation of long-term sequela (Fig. 10.2b).

Three currently available treatments include [1] delaying labor to allow for surfactant maturation to continue in utero, [2] administering antenatal maternal glucocorticoids which cross the placenta and stimulate surfactant production, and [3] providing surfactant replacement therapy at birth either in aerosolized or nebulized form. Although treatment advances have significantly decreased mortality from surfactant deficiency as a result of prematurity, the archetypal radiographic features have changed. Mechanical ventilator

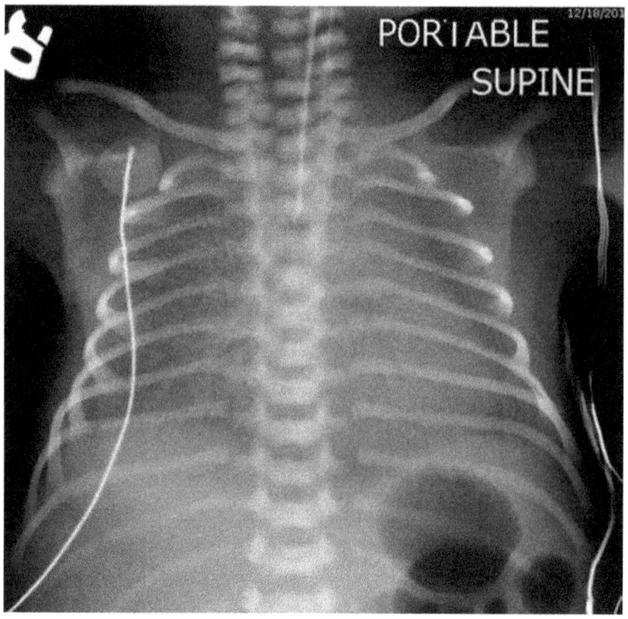

Fig. 10.1 A former 30-week gestation boy on the first day of life with surfactant deficiency of prematurity who presented with respiratory distress. Frontal chest radiograph shows diffuse symmetric hazy granular opacities in both lungs. Also noted is an endotracheal tube

support may artificially increase lung volumes or result in pneumothorax secondary to barotrauma. Inhomogeneous delivery of exogenous surfactant can result in variable aeration with areas of atelectasis distributed within persistent heterogeneous granular opacities which can mimic the appearance of meconium aspiration syndrome or neonatal pneumonia. Exogenous surfactant can also cause alveoli to hyper-expand creating bubbly lucencies that resemble the typical features of pulmonary interstitial emphysema. Additionally, antenatal maternal glucocorticoid administration can maintain patency of the ductus arteriosus resulting in pulmonary edema which manifests as diffuse pulmonary opacification with an enlarging heart radiographically.

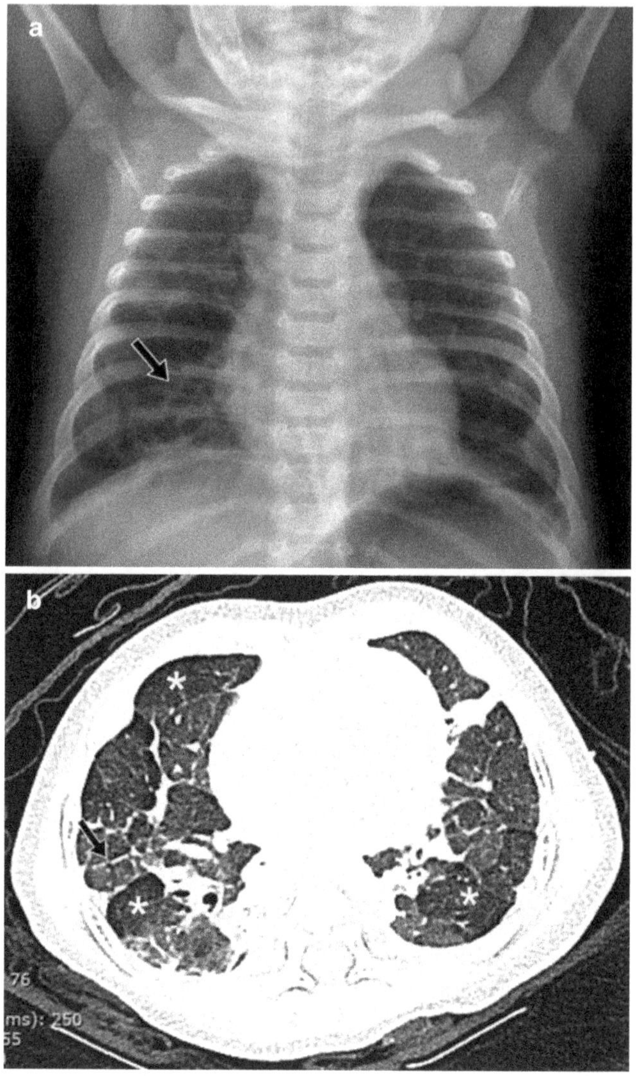

Fig. 10.2 A former 32-week gestation, now 71-day-old boy with chronic lung disease of prematurity. (**a**) Frontal chest radiograph shows bilateral hyperinflated lungs with coarse, reticular opacities (arrow) and architectural distortion. (**b**) Axial non-enhanced lung window setting CT image demonstrates coarse interstitial thickening (arrow), chronic appearing atelectasis, and areas of hyperinflation (asterisks)

Congenital Surfactant Deficiency

More rarely, surfactant deficiency can result from congenital genetic mutations in surfactant production and metabolism rather than solely on the basis of prematurity. Unlike surfactant disease of prematurity, congenital surfactant deficiency manifests most commonly in full-term infants who develop respiratory distress soon after birth without identifiable cause. Importantly, symptoms do not improve. Although a diverse variety of rare genetic mutations can result in surfactant deficiency, all ultimately lead to decreased oxygen exchange across the alveolar membrane.

Unlike the hyaline membranes generated in surfactant deficiency of prematurity, histologically, congenital surfactant deficiency results in diffuse alveolar hyperplasia and foamy macrophages. This histological appearance can sometimes mimic pulmonary alveolar proteinosis (PAP), although it is important to note that PAP is an acquired condition of children and adults rather than the result of inherent genetic mutation. Affected individuals may benefit from targeted genetic therapies for specific mutations but frequently require chronic ventilator dependence, infection prophylaxis, and long-term corticosteroids. Lung transplant may be necessary in severe cases.

Chest radiography typically demonstrates similar findings to surfactant deficiency syndrome due to prematurity including diffuse, hazy granular opacities with or without superimposed atelectasis (Fig. 10.3a). Unlike in surfactant deficiency syndrome due to prematurity, CT is more frequently utilized for initial evaluation and biopsy planning as pathological and

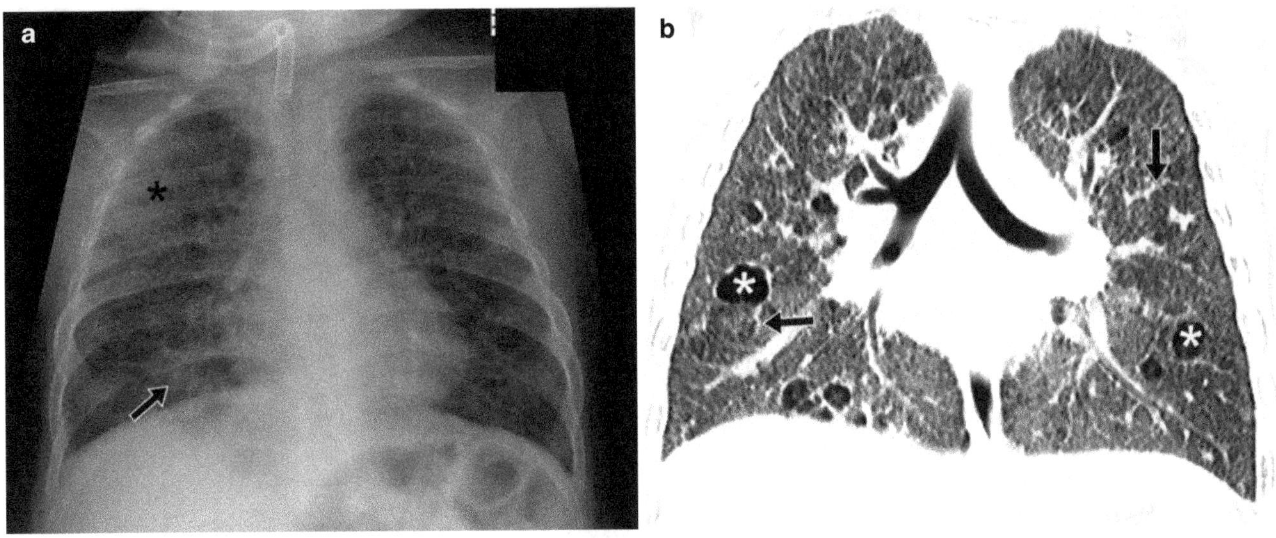

Fig. 10.3 A 13-month-old girl with congenital surfactant deficiency (ABCA3 mutation). The patient was born at term but with chronic respiratory failure since shortly after birth. Genetic testing and pathological analysis after lung biopsy confirmed the diagnosis of congenital surfactant deficiency (ABCA3 mutation). (**a**) Frontal chest radiograph shows diffuse interstitial thickening (arrow) and ground-glass opacity (asterisk). Also noted is a tracheostomy tube. (**b**) Coronal non-enhanced lung window CT image demonstrates multiple small bilateral lung cysts (asterisks) in addition to diffuse, bilateral ground-glass opacity and septal thickening (arrows)

genetic evaluation is required in pediatric patients with congenital surfactant deficiency. On CT, diffuse ground-glass opacities are observed which eventually coalesce into thin-walled cysts, the size and number of which increase over time. Intralobular septal thickening can also result, producing an imaging pattern similar to the crazing paving observed in PAP. Superimposed consolidative airspace disease may too be present (Fig. 10.3b).

Transient Tachypnea of Newborn

Transient tachypnea of newborn (TTN) is the most common cause of respiratory distress in full-term infants. Resulting from the delayed clearance of fetal lung fluid after birth, transient tachypnea of the newborn characteristically resolves within 48–72 h without long-term sequela [10]. Typically, affected infants are normal at birth and become increasingly tachypneic over the subsequent hours developing mild to moderate respiratory distress. Fluid within the fetal lungs is normally removed after birth via the tracheobronchial tree, interstitial lymphatics, and pulmonary capillaries aided by adrenergic sodium channel activation in labor and passage through the birth canal. Incidence of TTN, therefore, increases in cesarean delivery particularly those performed before the onset of labor. Other risk factors include fetal hypotonia, postnatal sedation, delivery prior to 38 weeks gestation, male gender, low birth weight, macrosomia, and maternal gestational diabetes or asthma [11]. Supportive treatment may be required in the initial hours to days of life with affected infants recovering fully.

Radiographic findings of TTN reflect increased fluid within the interstitium including perihilar prominence and

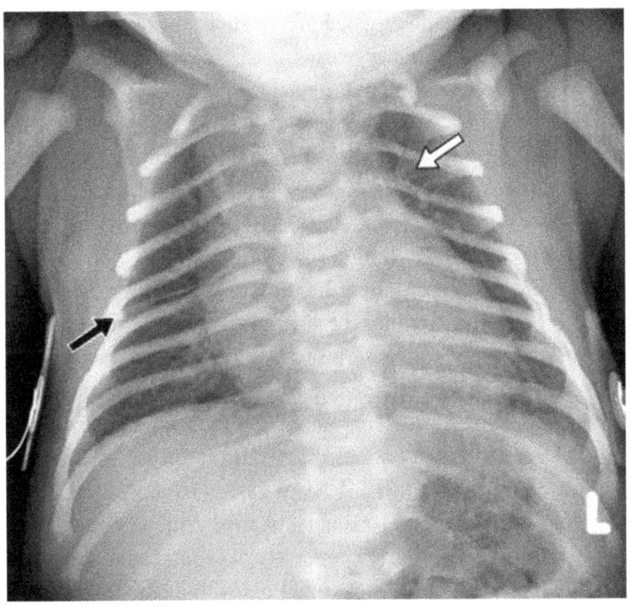

Fig. 10.4 An infant body on the first day of life born at term with transient tachypnea of newborn. The patient presented with respiratory distress. Frontal chest radiograph shows increased central interstitial markings (white arrow) and trace amount of fluid (black arrow) along the right minor fissure, suggestive of fetal lung fluid

trace fluid within the fissures [12] (Fig. 10.4). Lung volumes are typically normal to minimally increased and cardiac enlargement may be transiently present. The most specific imaging feature is improvement within 1–2 days. Infrequently, irregular bilateral opacities may be demonstrated mimicking meconium aspiration syndrome or neonatal pneumonia. Diffuse granular opacities may too be seen in a pattern similar to surfactant deficiency syndrome. In these cases, correlation with birth history and follow-up radiographs can aid in diagnosis.

Meconium Aspiration

Fetal inhalation of colonic material and subsequent aspiration is the most common cause of significant morbidity and mortality in full and postterm infants. Meconium is generally passed during the 24 h of antenatal life. Before 35 weeks gestation, however, approximately 10–15% of deliveries have meconium staining of amniotic fluid [10]. Aspiration, evidenced by the presence of meconium below the vocal cords, also increases with cesarean and postmaturity deliveries [13]. Additional risk factors include small for gestational age, intrauterine stress, and maternal factors such as hypertension, diabetes, or cardiovascular disease. The incidence of meconium aspiration has been improving in recent decades with closer fetal monitoring and improvement in obstetric practice of postterm mothers.

Aspiration of meconium produces both a mechanical obstruction secondary to plugging of small to medium airways and chemical pneumonitis which results in surfactant inactivation predisposing patients to superimposed infection. Additionally, pulmonary vasoconstriction in the setting of hypoxia may result in pulmonary hypertension. With supportive treatment, exogenous surfactant, deep suctioning, antibiotic prophylaxis, and mechanical ventilation, most patients recover within 2–3 days [10], although extracorporeal membrane oxygenation (ECMO) may be required in severe cases. Rarely, long-term complications such as pulmonary interstitial emphysema may result.

Radiographic findings of meconium aspiration vary on the severity of aspiration. Classically, lungs are hyperinflated with asymmetric, coarse, linear pulmonary opacities, frequently described as "ropelike," which radiate from the hilum. Pneumothorax should raise suspicion for meconium aspiration occurring in 10–40% of cases [10] (Fig. 10.5). Air trapping and segmental atelectasis are frequently seen concurrent findings. Although generally not required for diagnosis, CT may be helpful in atypical cases to evaluate for other etiologies of neonatal respiratory distress or to evaluate for sequela.

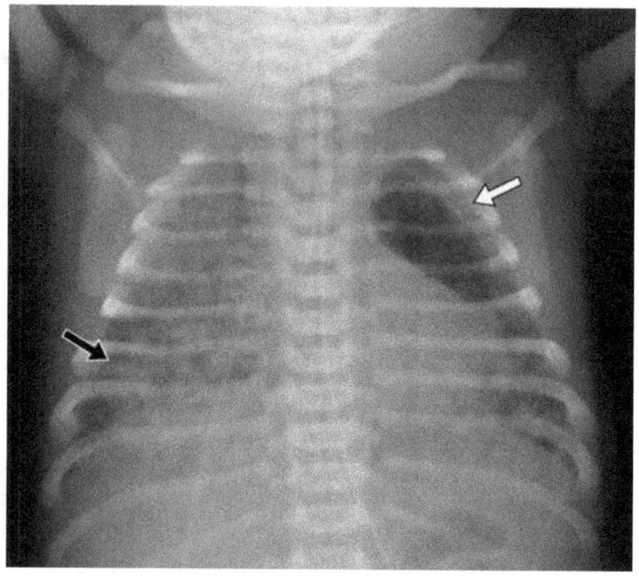

Fig. 10.5 An infant girl born at term on the first day of life who presented with respiratory distress due to meconium aspiration. She has history of meconium stained amniotic fluid at birth. Frontal chest radiograph shows hyperinflated lungs with asymmetric, coarse, linear, "rope-like" opacities (black arrow) which radiate from the hilum. An associated small left-sided pneumothorax (white arrow) is also noted

Neonatal Pneumonia

Neonatal pneumonia is defined as an infection of the lower respiratory tract occurring within the first 28 days of life [10] and is the most common cause of neonatal sepsis. One of the most frequently detected underlying infectious etiologies is *B. streptococcus*, the transmission of which occurs during passage through an affected birth canal. However, in utero or postnatal transmission can also occur. Risk factors of neonatal pneumonia include prolonged rupture of membranes, maternal infection, mechanical ventilation, prematurity, meconium aspiration syndrome, and therapeutic cooling. Although neonatal pneumonia is often associated with a significant morbidity and mortality, symptoms are frequently nonspecific including respiratory distress, labile temperature, and hypothermia. Screening mothers during the third trimester of pregnancy has decreased incidence. Empiric antibiotic therapy is the mainstay of treatment, in combination with supportive care, because blood and respiratory cultures are generally negative.

Radiographically, the imaging features of neonatal pneumonia are nonspecific, and thus a high clinical suspicion and corroborative history are required for accurate diagnosis. Diffuse and bilateral pulmonary opacities are the most frequent radiographic pattern, although focal airspace disease can also occur (Fig. 10.6). Neonatal pneumonia can also result in diffuse hazy opacities similar to surfactant deficiency syndrome or coarse irregular opacities similar to meconium aspiration syndrome. Pleural effusions are more frequently seen in neonatal pneumonia than in other causes of neonatal respiratory distress, a feature which can help differentiate these entities (Fig. 10.5a).

10.3.1.2 Pulmonary Infection in Children

Round Pneumonia

Pneumonia is the most common cause of illness in childhood and remains a significant cause of morbidity and mortality in both the developed and developing world [14]. While pediatric pneumonia can present as focal airspace opacity as is

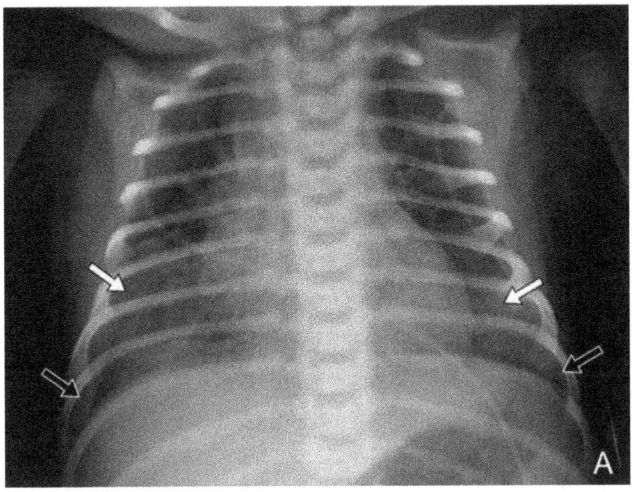

Fig. 10.6 An infant girl born at term on the third day of life with fever and respiratory distress due to neonatal pneumonia. Frontal chest radiograph shows bilateral diffuse and patchy opacities (white arrows) and trace of bilateral pleural effusions (black arrows)

classically observed in adults, round pneumonia is a distinct manifestation of lower respiratory tract infection in children less than 8 years of age [15]. Distinct differences in juvenile lung parenchyma including small alveoli, immature collateral pathways of air circulation via pores of Kohn and channels of Lambert, and closely opposed septa limit the spread of infection and round pneumonia results. Most commonly associated with *Streptococcus pneumoniae*, round pneumonia can also occur with *Klebsiella pneumoniae* and *Haemophilus influenzae*. Children with round pneumonia can present with more nonspecific clinical symptoms than demonstrated in adults including cough, rhinitis, vomiting, and high fever.

Radiographically, round pneumonia typically presents as a solitary, well-defined, round lesion measuring on average 3–4 cm usually located within the posterior lower lobes in contact with the adjacent pleura, hilum, or pulmonary fissure [15] (Fig. 10.7). Given the focality, size, and spherical appearance, round pneumonia may simulate a mass; although given appropriate clinical history, round pneumonia should be the primary differential consideration. Additionally, air bronchograms and satellite lesions may be present. While round pneumonia may evolve to demonstrate the more classic appearance of lobar pneumonia, with proper antibiotic treatment, 95% resolve without complications [16].

Cross-sectional imaging is unnecessary in classic cases of round pneumonia with appropriate clinical history. CT may be warranted if there is increased clinical risk for an underlying pulmonary mass, in the absence of appropriate clinical history, or in older children as larger alveoli and better developed collateral pathways prohibit the development of round pneumonia. A round airspace opacity in these populations should prompt alternative diagnostic considerations including atypical microorganism infection, immunodeficiency, and primary or secondary malignancy. Rarely, complications may result in round pneumonia necessitating cross-sectional imaging evaluation by CT including cavitation, calcification, or pleural effusion. Ultrasound can be a helpful imaging modality in the evaluation of pleural and parenchymal lung abnormalities in pediatric patients because it obviates the need for sedation and radiation. In addition, ultrasound may help to distinguish lung consolidation, as in the case with round pneumonia, from a solid pulmonary mass.

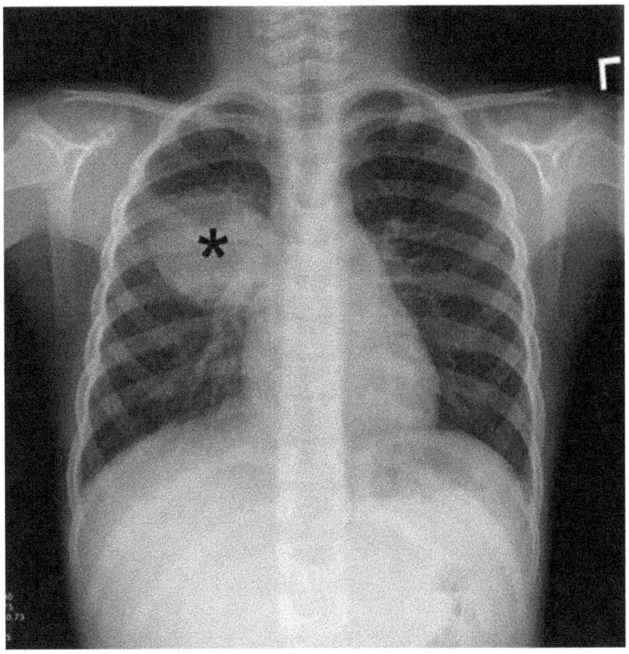

Fig. 10.7 A 5-year-old girl with cough and fever due to round pneumonia. Frontal chest radiograph shows a solitary, well-defined, and round opacity (asterisk) in the right upper to mid-lung zone adjacent to the minor fissure

10.3.2 Pediatric Large Airway Disorders

10.3.2.1 Large Airway Neoplasms

Subglottic Hemangioma

Subglottic hemangioma is a benign neoplasm of the subglottic airway and the most common obstructing subglottic soft tissue mass in the pediatric population. Characteristically arising along the posterior or lateral walls of the trachea, subglottic hemangioma accounts for 1.5% of congenital laryngeal malformations [17]. Although generally small, acute airway compromise can result with up to 50% mortality if untreated [17]. Symptoms typically develop at approximately 6–12 weeks of age due to postnatal lesional growth and include cough, inspiratory stridor, feeding difficulties, and hemoptysis [17]. Female, Caucasian infants are most commonly affected with up to 50% of patients also demonstrating cutaneous hemangiomas. Additional risk factors include low birth weight, prematurity, and multiple gestations [18].

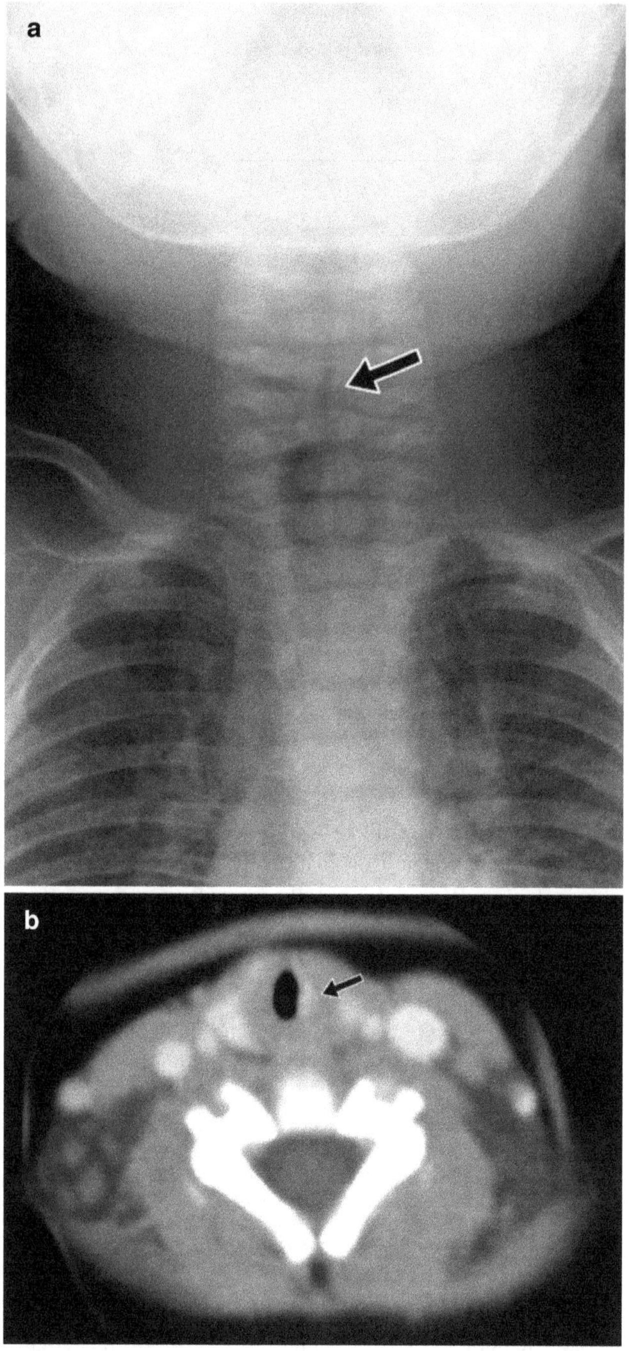

Fig. 10.8 A 3-month-old boy with subglottic hemangioma who presented with stridor. (**a**) Frontal soft tissue neck radiograph shows eccentric narrowing (arrow) of the left subglottic trachea. (**b**) Axial enhanced soft tissue window setting CT at the level of the subglottic trachea demonstrates a well-circumscribed, avidly enhancing soft tissue lesion (arrow) at the lateral aspect of the left subglottic trachea

The classic radiographic appearance of subglottic hemangioma is nonspecific, eccentric narrowing of the subglottic trachea on frontal views [19]. Such asymmetric appearance can help differentiate from other causes of subglottic tracheal narrowing such as croup (Fig. 10.8a). Following radiography, cross-sectional evaluation with CT or MRI is routinely performed for pretreatment planning with either modality typically demonstrates an avidly enhancing lesion at the posterolateral aspect of the subglottic trachea with soft tissue characteristics (Fig. 10.8b) [3, 20, 21].

Novel treatment techniques such as laser ablation, propranolol injection, or sclerotherapy have become the standard of care in the treatment of subglottic hemangioma, thereby reducing the morbidity associated with surgical excision.

Carcinoid Tumor

Carcinoid tumor is the primary neuroendocrine tumor of the lung. Although rare and less common than carcinoid tumor of the gastrointestinal tract, it is the most common primary lung tumor in the pediatric population with a mean age of presentation of 14 years [22]. A centrally located carcinoid tumor within a large airway is more likely to result in symptoms in comparison to a carcinoid tumor located more peripherally within the lung parenchyma. Affected children typically present with cough, shortness of breath, hemoptysis, or, most commonly, recurrent pneumonias. Histologically, carcinoid tumor can be classified as typical or atypical with typical lesions demonstrating fewer mitoses per high power field, lower likelihood of necrosis, and less malignant potential.

Radiographically, carcinoid tumor can present as a well-circumscribed, round, or ovoid lesion. However, if central in location, it may be obscured by hilar structures and only secondary signs observed such as atelectasis or pneumonia (Fig. 10.9a). The parallel sign has been described in the literature to describe the orientation of a non-spherical carcinoid tumor along axis of the nearest major bronchus or pulmonary artery. Cross-sectional imaging with CT or MRI is important for presurgical planning and typically demonstrates a well-defined or lobulated lesion with soft tissue attenuation characteristics and robust post-contrast enhancement (Fig. 10.9b) [23, 24]. Associated calcification may be demonstrated more commonly with central lesions versus those in the periphery. ^{111}In-labeled pentetreotide (Octreoscan) is suggested by the Pediatric Carcinoid Tumor Clinical Guidelines to assess for sites of metastatic disease.

Treatment is primarily surgical with low recurrence rates observed with segmentectomy or wedge resection. Chemotherapy or somatostatin-based therapies are reserved for unresectable cases.

10.3.2.2 Nonneoplastic Disorders of the Large Airway

Tracheomalacia

Tracheomalacia is defined as dynamic and disproportionate collapse of the tracheal lumen with expiration [25]. It results from weakening of the supporting cartilage, softening of the airway walls, or hypotonia of the supporting muscles [26]. Affecting both premature and term infants, tracheomalacia

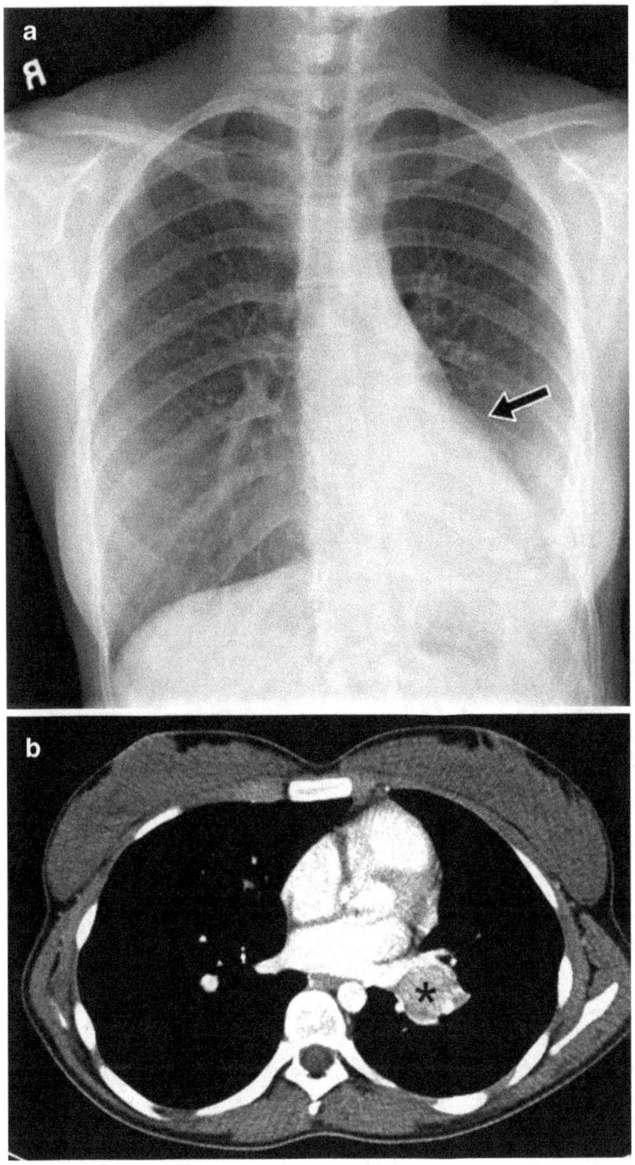

Fig. 10.9 A 16-year-old girl with endobronchial carcinoid who presented with cough and shortness of breath. The patient underwent surgical excision of the endobronchial mass in the left lower lobe bronchus and histological analysis confirmed the diagnosis of low-grade carcinoid tumor. (**a**) Frontal chest radiograph shows an opacity with volume loss in the left lower lobe (arrow) due to left lower lobe collapse. (**b**) Axial enhanced soft tissue window setting CT image, at the level of the left atrium, demonstrates a well-circumscribed, heterogeneously enhancing soft tissue mass (asterisk) near the left hilum

may be due to primary, congenital causes such as prematurity, tracheoesophageal fistula, or congenital cartilage disorder or may be acquired secondarily as a result of intubation, infection, surgery, extrinsic compression from vascular anomaly, cardiovascular defects, or neurologic causes. Typical symptoms include cough, recurrent lower airway infection due to decreased clearance, dyspnea, recurrent wheeze, or stridor with symptoms frequently worsening with activity or agitation.

Fluoroscopic measurement of the tracheal diameter has a limited role in the evaluation of tracheomalacia with a specificity of 96–100% but a sensitivity of only 23.8–62% because the trachea of a normal infant may collapse up to 50% with forceful crying [27]. A barium esophagram may help to evaluate causes of acquired tracheomalacia such as due to tracheoesophageal fistula or extrinsic compression due to vascular ring but with limited anatomic detail. In intubated infants using breath-hold technique as well as older children who can follow breathing instructions, CT with paired inspiratory and expiratory series can be used to evaluate precise localization, extent, and severity of tracheomalacia [28]. In recent years, with the availability of higher row multidetector CT (MDCT), real-time and dynamic 3D and 4D imaging of the large airway can be obtained even in infants and young children who cannot follow breathing instructions obviating the need for intubation (Fig. 10.10a–d). Additionally, CT allows for the identification of underlying causes as well as associated anomalies such as air trapping.

Cases of primary tracheomalacia due to prematurity and intrinsic weakness of the supporting cartilage may require only supportive care during the first 1–2 years of life after which normal stiffening of the cartilage occurs and the condition self-resolves [27]. In severe cases, aggressive treatment may be required including continuous positive airway pressure, tracheostomy, airway stenting, or surgical repair with pexy procedures. Recently, customized, bioresorbable 3D-printed splints have been used in cases of severe tracheomalacia with preliminary success in both pediatric and adult patients although larger and longer studies are necessary to evaluate long-term outcomes and complications [29].

Foreign Body Aspiration

Because infants and young children aged 6 months to 3 years lack molar teeth, have uncoordinated swallowing mechanisms, and, most importantly, engage with their surroundings by placing objects in their mouths, they are prone to foreign body aspiration [30]. Aspirate objects, most commonly peanuts, lodge with the highest frequency within the right main stem bronchus due to its larger size and more vertical alignment as compared with the left.

Chest radiography is the first-line imaging study in cases of suspected foreign body aspiration because it is readily available, low in cost, and associated with minimal radiation exposure [31]. As only 10% of aspirated foreign bodies are radiopaque [32], however, indirect signs of aspiration including air trapping, focal airspace disease, pleural effusion, mediastinal shift, pneumothorax, or subcutaneous emphysema are important imaging surrogates. Unilateral hyperinflation [33] is the most commonly identified indirect sign of aspiration [34] (Fig. 10.11a). This finding may be further evaluated with bilateral decubitus radiographs to assess for air trapping with the side of foreign body aspiration failing to deflate in the dependent position (Fig. 10.11b and c). Lateral

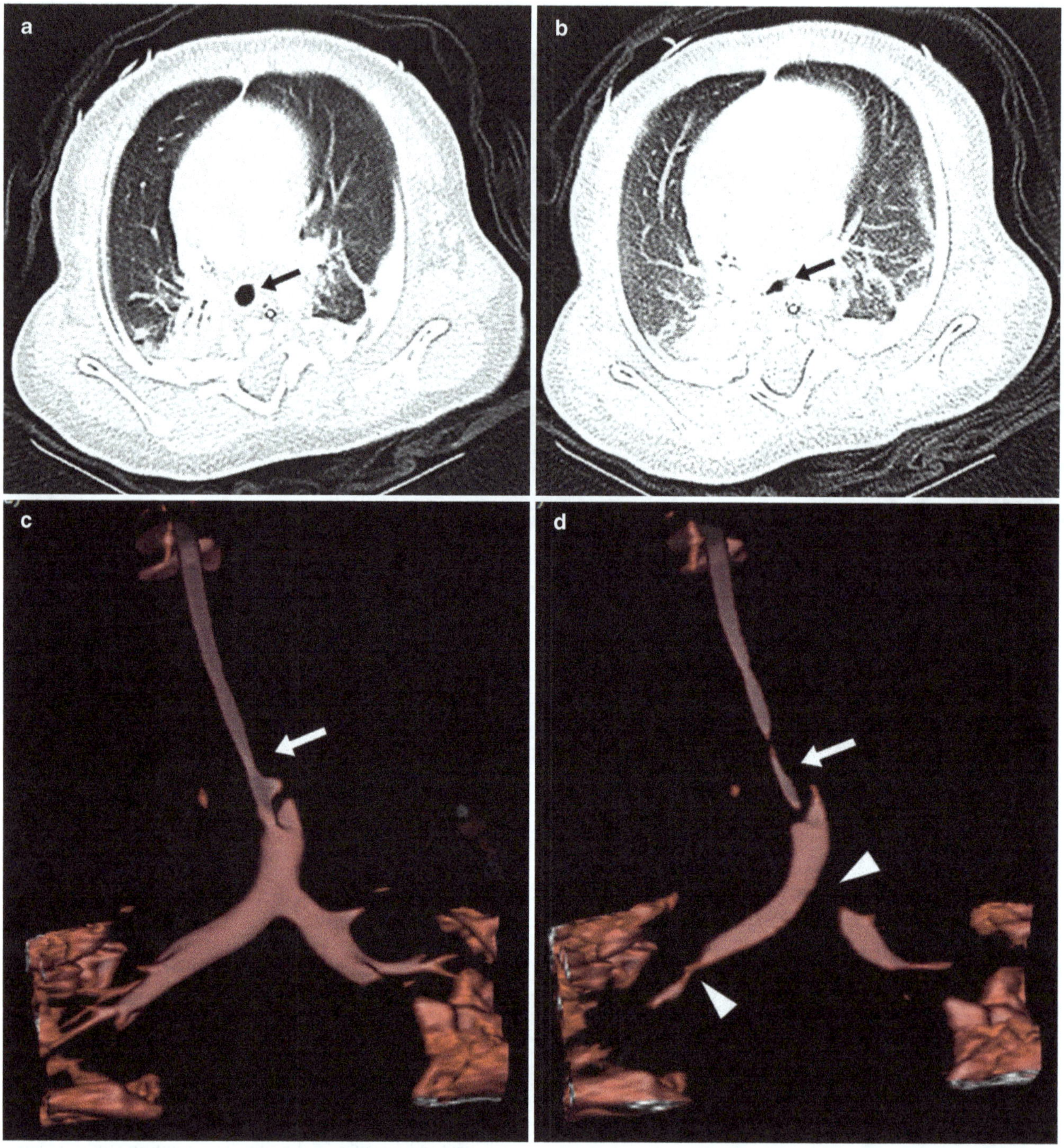

Fig. 10.10 A 3-month-old girl with tracheobronchomalacia who presented with recurrent wheezing and stridor. Subsequently obtained bronchoscopy confirmed the diagnosis of tracheobronchomalacia. (**a**) Axial non-enhanced lung window setting CT image, at the level of the mid-thoracic trachea, obtained at end-inspiration shows patent trachea (arrow). (**b**) Axial non-enhanced lung window setting CT image, at the level of the mid-thoracic trachea, obtained at end-expiration demonstrates focal collapse of the trachea (arrow) with greater than 50% decrease in cross-sectional area consistent with tracheomalacia. (**c**) 3D volume-rendered CT image of the large airways obtained at end-inspiration shows patent trachea (arrow). Patent bilateral main stem bronchi are also seen. (**d**) 3D volume-rendered CT image of the large airways obtained at end-expiration demonstrates focal marked collapse of the trachea (arrow) consistent with tracheomalacia. Also noted is similar focal marked collapse (arrowheads) of the distal right main stem bronchus and proximal left main stem bronchus, consistent with bilateral bronchomalacia

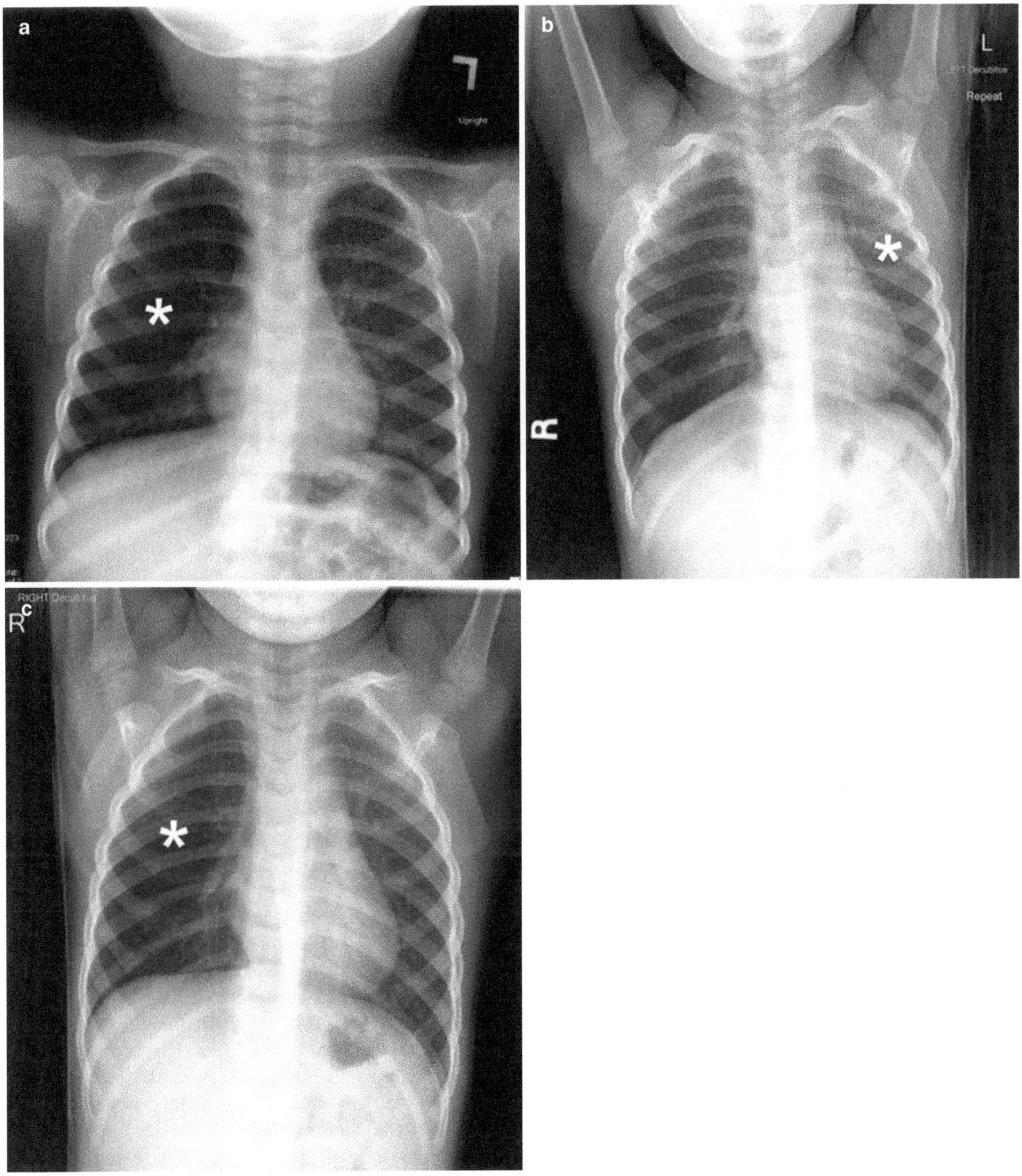

Fig. 10.11 A 30-month-old boy with an endobronchial non-radiopaque foreign body aspiration who presented with acute onset of wheezing and respiratory distress. (**a**) Frontal chest radiograph shows asymmetric hyperinflation of the right lung (asterisk) as compared with the normally aerated left lung. (**b**) Left lateral decubitus radiograph demonstrates expected deflation of the left lung (asterisk) in the dependent portion. (**c**) Right lateral decubitus radiograph shows persistent relative hyperinflation representing air trapping of the right lung (asterisk) despite dependent positioning. Radiographic findings suspicious for aspirated non-radiopaque foreign body in the right main stem bronchus. Subsequently obtained bronchoscopy demonstrated a nearly obstructive foreign body (likely almond) located within the right main stem bronchus

decubitus radiography, however, have only 68–74% sensitivity and 45–67% specificity [35]. Furthermore, it has been shown to increase false-positive rates without increasing the rate of true-positive identification. As such, a negative chest radiography in the setting of high clinical suspicion should prompt further evaluation with CT.

CT has an accuracy close to 100% for the detection of aspirated foreign body [35] able to identify both an endoluminal mass as well as secondary signs of aspiration. Because of the increased radiation exposure of CT as compared with radiography, study benefits must be weighed. 3D virtual bronchoscopy reconstructions can be utilized to assess foreign body aspiration and may be used for preprocedural planning. Additionally, following bronchoscopic removal, CT can be used to assess for residual aspirated foreign body [36].

10.3.3 Pediatric Mediastinal Disorders

10.3.3.1 Vascular Lesions

Vascular rings are congenital abnormalities of the aortic arch which result from abnormal development of the aortic arches formed during the fourth and fifth weeks of embryonic development. Depending upon the location of failed arch regression, various anomalous anatomic variants may result which encircle the trachea and esophagus to various degrees. While some remain asymptomatic and may be incidental findings later in life, others, namely, double aortic arch and right aortic arch with aberrant left subclavian artery, result in symptoms earlier in life and thus frequently present to clinical attention in early infancy. Abnormalities of aortic arch development may be associated with additional congenital cardiac anomalies, as is frequently the case with right aortic arch with mirror image branching, while others are isolated findings without additional congenital associations.

Double Aortic Arch

A double aortic arch is caused by persistence of the both the right and left embryonic arches which arise from the ascending aorta. Because a complete vascular ring encircling the trachea and esophagus is formed, affected pediatric patients generally develop symptoms early in life including wheezing, stridor, cyanosis, and dysphagia frequently exacerbated by activity or crying. In a double aortic arch, one arch is usually dominant with the descending aorta typically located on the side contralateral to the dominant arch, most commonly manifesting as a dominant right arch with left-sided descending aorta. A double aortic arch is rarely associated with additional congenital heart abnormalities.

Radiographically, a double aortic arch demonstrates bilateral aortic knobs on the frontal projection with displacement of the tracheal air column away from midline and indentation upon the right lateral tracheal border (Fig. 10.12a). On the lateral projection, the retrotracheal aorta may result in anterior displacement of the trachea. On barium esophagram, there may be bilateral indentations on the esophagus on frontal views and posterior indentation on the lateral view.

Whereas the presence of a double aortic arch may be inferred radiographically or fluoroscopically, cross-sectional imaging with CT or MRI has improved sensitivity and results in superior anatomic detail allowing for elucidation of relational anatomy to other mediastinal structures [37]. Characteristic of a double aortic arch is a symmetric vascular branching pattern demonstrated on single axial image at the level of the thoracic inlet consisting of the origins of the common carotid and subclavian arteries bilaterally, so-called the "four-vessel" sign (Fig. 10.12b). Cross-sectional imaging is also useful for planning of surgical approach with reformatted images offering important insight into arch size, position, and dominance (Fig. 10.12c).

The current management of double aortic arch involves surgical ligation of the nondominant arch usually via an ipsilateral thoracotomy.

Right Aortic Arch

In normal development, a left aortic arch forms from the involution of the right fourth arch and dorsal aorta. When there is involution of the left fourth arch and dorsal aorta, which occurs in 0.1% of the population [38], a right aortic arch results. Right aortic arch is the second most common aortic arch variant after double aortic arch. There are two main types of right aortic arch: right aortic arch with an aberrant subclavian artery and right aortic arch with mirror imaging branching. A right arch may be associated with an aberrant left subclavian artery arising from or independent to a Kommerell diverticulum occurring between the left common carotid and left subclavian arteries. A right aortic arch may also be associated with mirror imaging branching where the embryonic arch is interrupted just distal to the left ductus arteriosus. In addition, although the right aortic arch typically descends within the right aspect of the thoracic cavity, rarely the arch can cross to the midline posterior to the esophagus with the descending aorta located on the left as occurs in the case of right circumflex aorta. Such vascular anatomy creates a vascular ring which is completed by a left ductus or ligamentum arteriosum. Although a right aortic arch with an aberrant left subclavian artery is infrequently associated with additional congenital heart anomalies, a right arch with mirror image branching is highly associated with accompanying congenital heart anomalies (90–98%) most commonly Tetralogy of Fallot [39].

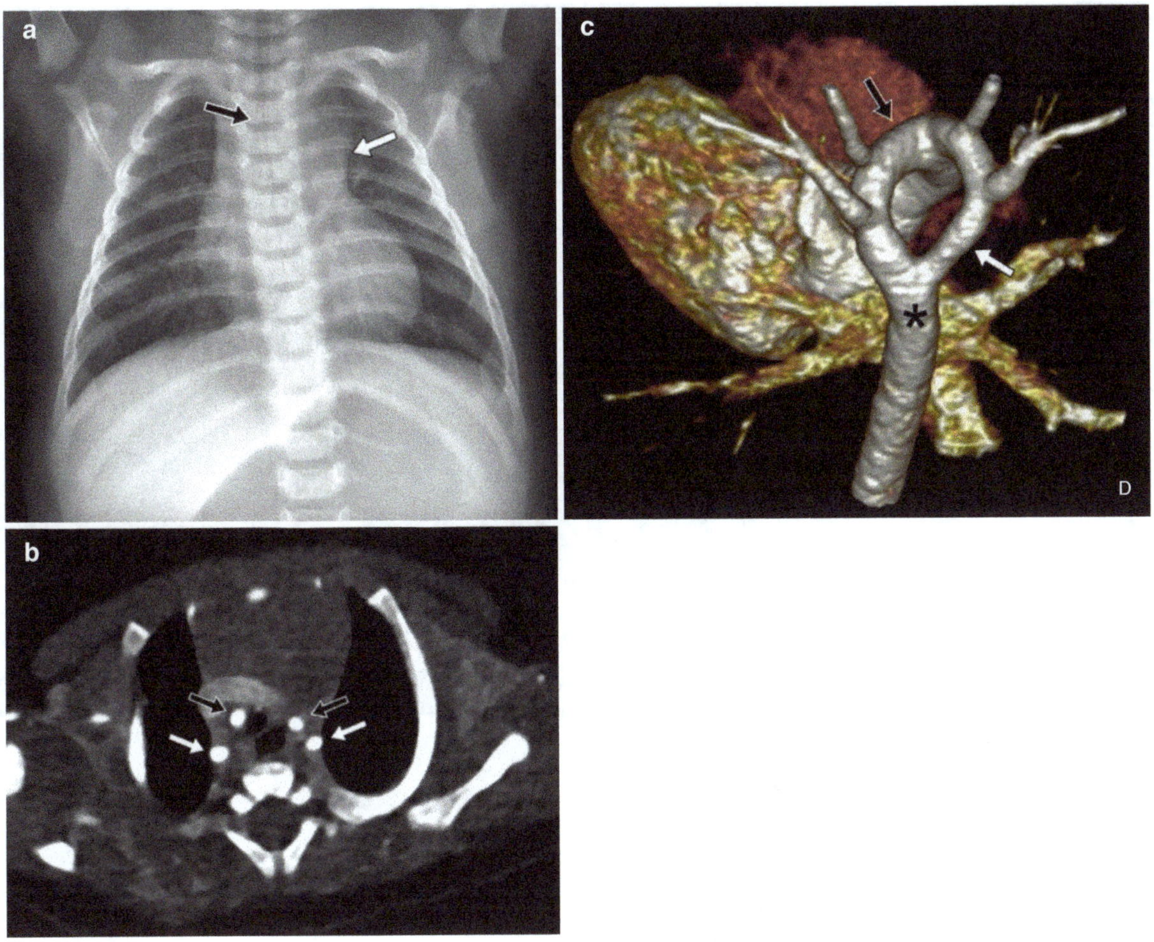

Fig. 10.12 A 74-day-old girl with double aortic arch who presented with wheezing and feeding difficulty. (**a**) Frontal chest radiograph shows minimal leftward deviation (black arrow) of thoracic trachea with indentation along the right lateral tracheal wall. There is also prominence (white arrow) of the superior mediastinum. (**b**) Axial enhanced soft tissue window setting CT image, at the level of thoracic inlet, demonstrates a symmetric vascular branching pattern comprised of the origins of the bilateral common carotid arteries (black arrows) and bilateral subclavian arteries (white arrows), the so-called the four-vessel sign. (**c**) Posterior view of 3D volume-rendered CT image shows double aortic arch anatomy including the left (black arrow) and right (white arrow) aortic arches which comprise a complete vascular ring. Right-sided descending aorta (asterisk) is also seen

Chest radiography characteristically demonstrates a right-sided aortic arch with variable positioning of the descending aorta (Fig. 10.13a). In cases of right aortic arch with mirror image branching, findings associated to the accompanying congenital heart disease may be present such as situs inversus or cardiac enlargement. As in cases of double aortic arch, cross-sectional evaluation with CT or MRI again provides superior anatomic resolution and allows for clarification of mediastinal relationships (Fig. 10.13b and c).

Management of right aortic arch depends on associated anomalies and symptomatology. An asymptomatic right arch with aberrant left subclavian artery requires no treatment. However, surgical ligation is required in symptomatic pediatric patients with right aortic arch constituting a vascular ring. Repair of underlying cardiac anomalies may be also needed in pediatric patients with right aortic arch with mirror imaging branching.

Pulmonary Artery Sling

A pulmonary artery sling results from failure of development of the left sixth aortic arch. As a result, there is anomalous origin of the left pulmonary artery from the right pulmonary artery with the left pulmonary artery then passing between the trachea and esophagus as it courses toward the left hilum. Consequently, compression of the trachea and right main stem bronchus may result with secondary development of tracheobronchomalacia or stenosis. A pulmonary artery sling is classified according to the associated airway abnormalities. Type I results in compression of the trachea and right main stem bronchus with normal airway branching. Type II often results in long segment tracheobronchial stenosis often with associated abnormal airway branching with development of a T-shaped carina.

Radiographically, a pulmonary sling may manifest as unilateral hyperinflation, low position of the left hilum, and anterior displacement of the trachea with posterior indenta-

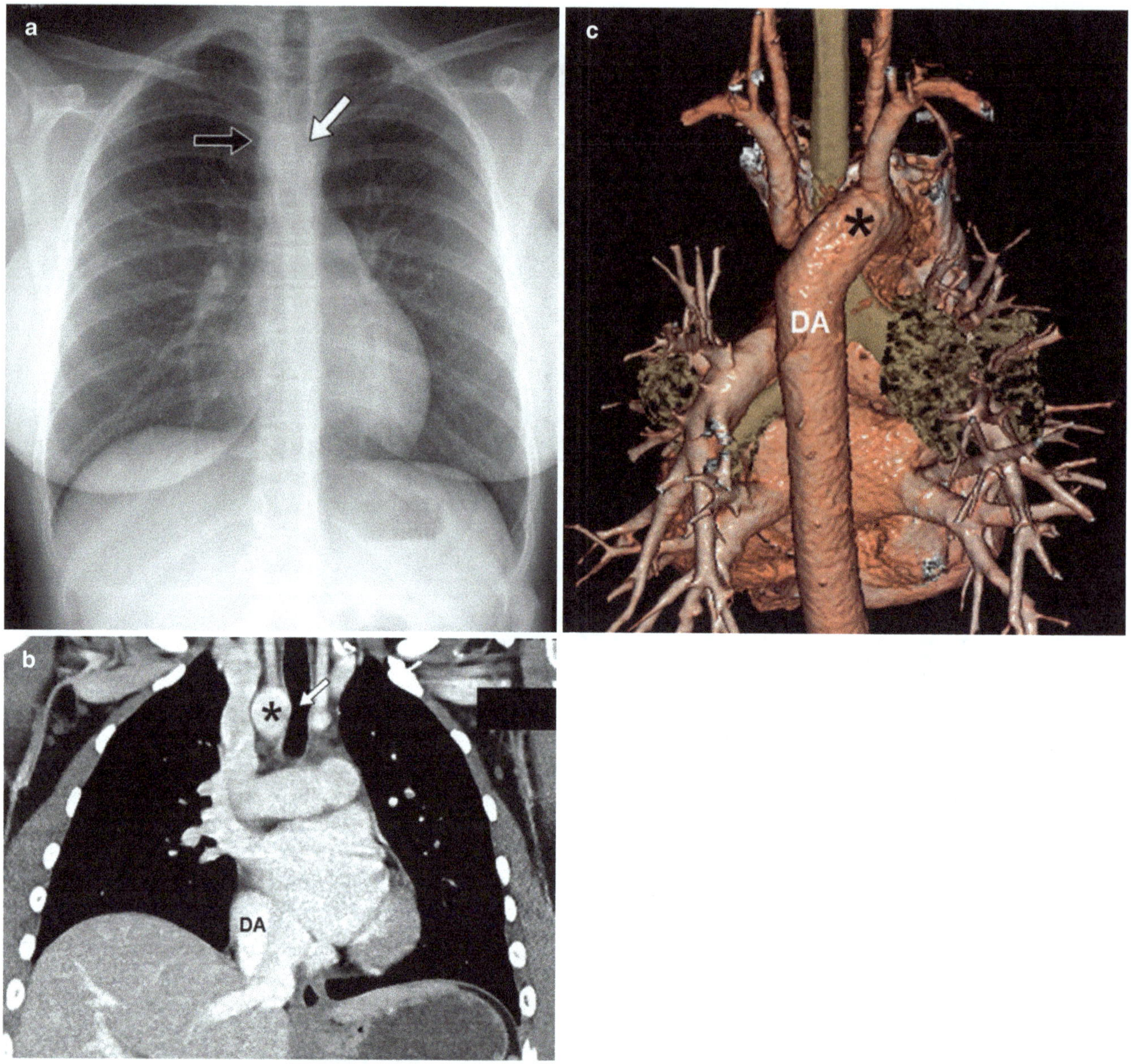

Fig. 10.13 A 15-year-old girl with a right aortic arch who presented with wheezing. (**a**) Frontal chest radiograph shows right-sided aortic knob (black arrow) which indents upon and leftward deviation (white arrow) of the thoracic trachea. (**b**) Coronal enhanced soft tissue window setting CT demonstrates a right-sided aortic arch (asterisk) and descending aorta (DA). Compression (arrow) of the trachea due to right aortic arch is also seen. (**c**) Posterior view of 3D volume-rendered CT image demonstrates right aortic arch anatomy with right-sided descending aortic arch (asterisk) and descending aorta (DA)

tion. Barium esophagram classically demonstrates anterior indentation on the esophagus. Cross-sectional imaging again better defines the vascular and airway anatomy while aiding in the exclusion of right pulmonary agenesis as a differential consideration. Additionally, CT can aid in the evaluation of secondary tracheobronchomalacia and stenosis. Cross-sectional imaging is also helpful for presurgical evaluation because treatment usually involves median sternotomy, cardiopulmonary bypass, reimplantation of the anomalous left pulmonary artery, and repair of large airway anomaly or abnormality if present (Fig. 10.14) [40].

10.3.3.2 Nonvascular Lesions

Foregut Duplication Cyst

Foregut duplication cyst is the most common primary mediastinal mass and comprises 11% of all mediastinal masses [41]. It is believed to arise from disturbances in embryologic differentiation of the primitive gut which typically develops into the pharynx, respiratory tract, esophagus, stomach, and the proximal duodenum [42]. In general, symptoms relate to the level of cyst, mass effect by the cyst on adjacent structures, and the specific cells involved in the cyst.

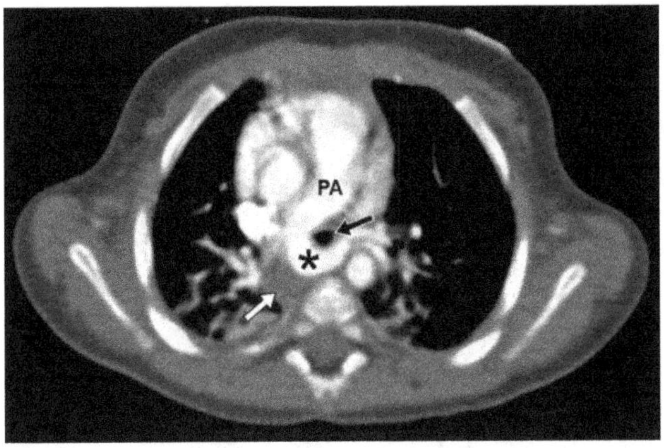

Fig. 10.14 A 2-month-old girl with pulmonary artery sling who presented with respiratory distress. Axial enhanced soft tissue window setting CT image demonstrates anomalous origin of the left pulmonary artery (asterisk) from the main pulmonary artery (PA). The left anomalous pulmonary artery (asterisk) passes between the trachea (black arrow) and esophagus (white arrow) as it courses toward the left hilum

Foregut duplication cyst can be broadly classified into three types which include bronchogenic cyst, esophageal duplication cyst, and neurenteric cyst. Bronchogenic cyst arises from abnormal lung budding during ventral foregut division and can occur anywhere along the tracheoesophageal tree, most commonly in the subcarinal or paratracheal regions. Although usually asymptomatic, if large, bronchogenic cyst can result in dyspnea from secondary compression of an adjacent airway. Esophageal duplication cyst is the result of abnormal division of the posterior embryonic foregut. It is most commonly associated with dysphagia as the duplication cyst may occur anywhere along the esophagus, though most arise in the upper one third. A failure of complete separation of the gastrointestinal tract from the primitive neural crest can result in a neurenteric cyst which is one variant of split notochord syndrome. Usually occurring in the posterior mediastinum, neurenteric cyst may communicate with the spinal cord resulting in pain as well as an associated cleft within the adjacent vertebral body.

Radiographically, foregut duplication cysts of all subtypes manifest as smooth, oval, or round middle or posterior mediastinal masses (Fig. 10.15a) requiring further cross-sectional imaging with CT or MRI evaluation prior to surgical removal [41, 43]. Although neurenteric cyst may have an associated vertebral body anomaly, other imaging features are less specific with a well-marginated cystic lesion most commonly identified. Uniform fluid attenuation or homogeneous T2 hyperintensity is demonstrated in up to one half of lesions (Fig. 10.15b). Heterogeneity, however, can result in the setting of prior hemorrhage, infection, or increased internal protein although most lesions still retain intrinsic T2 hyperintensity. After administration of contrast, irregular border and peripheral contrast enhancement may also be identified in the setting of prior or superimposed infection (Fig. 10.15c).

The current management of symptomatic pediatric patients with foregut duplication cysts is surgical resection.

Neuroblastoma

Thoracic neurogenic tumors may arise from any component of the nervous system within the chest. They are the most common posterior mediastinal masses in children, accounting for 90% of posterior mediastinal masses [41]. Mediastinal location of neuroblastoma is associated with more benign and mature subtype of neuroblastoma as compared with intra-abdominal location. Thoracic neurogenic tumors can be separated into two main categories based upon the origin of their precursor cell from either an autonomic nerve ganglia or the nerve sheath. Lesions of autonomic nerve ganglia origin are more commonly encountered in pediatric patients with differential consideration ranging from the benign ganglioneuroma to the malignant neuroblastoma with ganglioneuroblastoma having histological features of each and being of transitional malignant potential. Although imaging alone is not possible to differentiate these tumor types, imaging plays an important role in identifying and characterizing the mass and its extent.

Neuroblastoma is the most common posterior extracranial solid malignancy of childhood and most frequently occurs in patients less than 3 years of age. Depending on primary tumor location, presenting clinical symptoms may include Horner syndrome or heterochromia if the primary tumor is cervical or apical in location, paraplegia or loss of bladder/bowel function if there is spinal cord compression, or opsoclonus-myoclonus syndrome if circulating autoantibodies are present. In addition, associated nonspecific symptoms may be present including fever, irritability, weight loss, anemia, and pain. Levels of catecholamines or neurotransmitters, which are detected by blood or urine tests, are typically elevated in pediatric patients with neuroblastoma.

Classically included in the radiographic differential of a posterior mediastinal lesion, neuroblastomas frequently demonstrate associated calcification (50%) and may cause secondary osseous findings including rib erosion or enlargement of the neuroforamen [44] (Fig. 10.16a and b). Neuroblastoma usually lacks a well-defined capsule and may invade adjacent mediastinal structures or metastasize. Cross-sectional imaging with CT or MRI provides crucial staging information including location, lesion size, and the presence of metastatic disease (Fig. 10.16c). MRI is especially helpful in the classification of extradural disease due to the intrinsic high lipid and water content of these tumors which results in both T1 and T2 hyperintensity. MRI, in comparison to CT, can also better demonstrate the extension of thoracic neuroblastoma into the adjacent neural foramen.

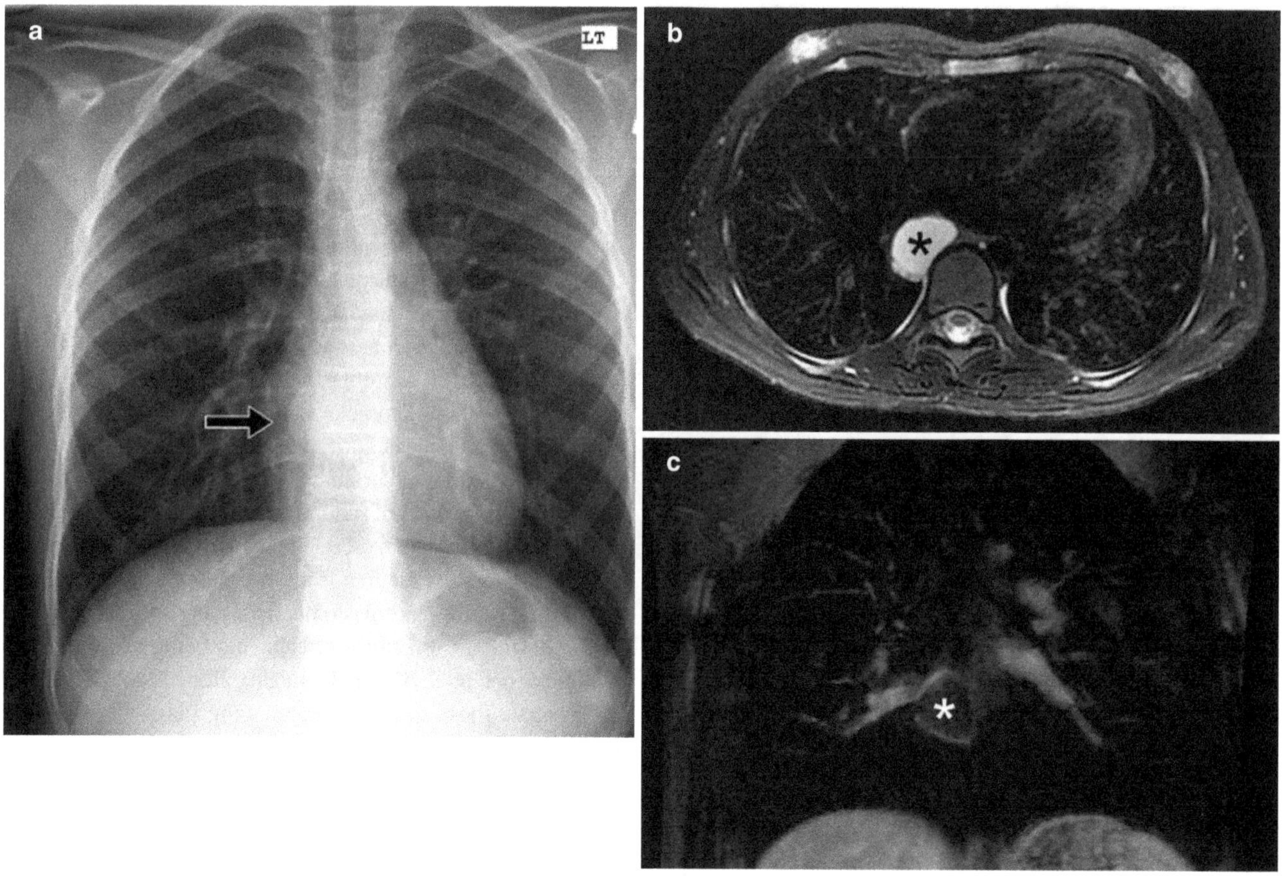

Fig. 10.15 A 14-year-old girl with esophageal duplication cyst who presented with dyspnea. The mediastinal mass was surgically excised and pathology was consistent with an esophageal duplication cyst. (**a**) Frontal chest radiograph demonstrates a well-circumscribed opacity (black arrow) overlying the right aspect of the heart. (**b**) Axial T2-weighted, fat-suppressed MR image shows a cystic lesion (asterisk) within the middle mediastinum. (**c**) Coronal enhanced T1-weighted, fat-suppressed MR image demonstrates a peripheral enhancement of the lesion (asterisk) within the right aspect of the middle mediastinum

Overall survival rate of thoracic neuroblastoma is superior to primary abdominal neuroblastoma with treatment usually involving a combination of surgical resection, chemotherapeutic agents, and radiation.

Lymphatic Malformation

Lymphatic malformation results from embryologic malformation of the lymphatic system. Such malformation results in lymph-containing smooth and skeletal muscle-lined channels with intervening fibro-connective tissue creating microcystic, macrocystic, or combined lesions of variable size. Intrathoracic lymphatic malformation in isolation is rare, accounting for less than 1% of all lymphatic malformations, and more generally results from extension of cervical, axillary, or mediastinal malformation. Typically present at birth, the majority of affected patients present to clinical attention before 2 years of age with an asymptomatic palpable mass although pain may occur with intralesional hemorrhage or infection. Large lesions, however, may produce symptoms such as dyspnea if there is secondary airway or vascular compression.

Intrathoracic lymphatic malformation, if small and asymptomatic, may be incidental findings on chest radiography performed for different indication. If located in the mediastinum, lymphatic malformation may present as a well-circumscribed mass or vague mediastinal fullness (Fig. 10.17a). If there is extension of the lymphatic malformation into the cervical region, deviation of the trachea may be identified on either the frontal or lateral radiography. MRI is currently considered the gold standard imaging modality in the evaluation of lymphatic malformations because it affords superior soft tissue contrast as compared with CT and enables evaluation of local extent and relationship to normal structures. As lymphatic malformations contain fluid, there is intrinsic T2 hyperintensity (Fig. 10.17b). Following contrast administration, there is variable enhancement of the

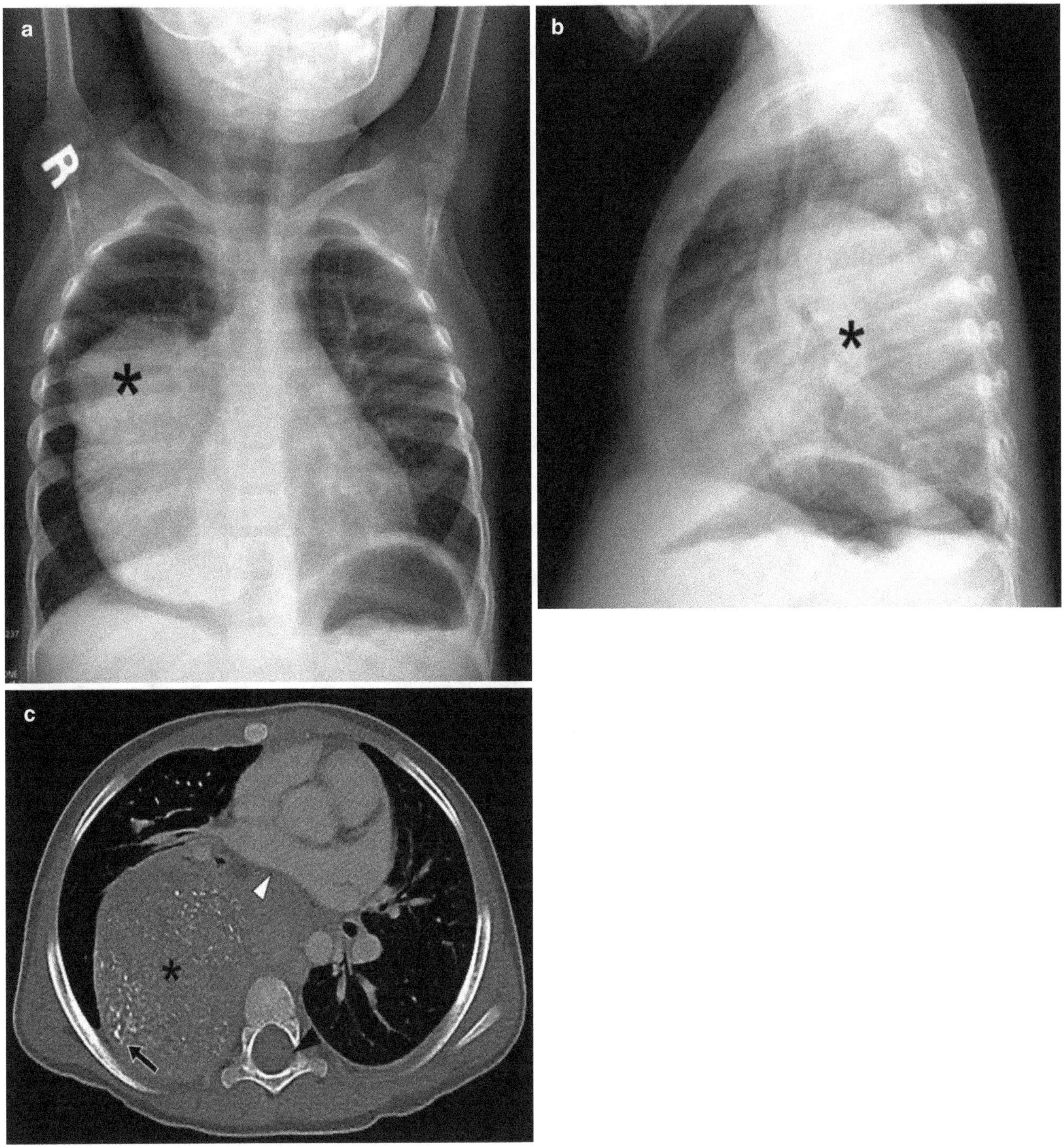

Fig. 10.16 A 2-year-old boy with thoracic neuroblastoma who presented with chest pain and paresthesia. (**a**) Frontal chest radiograph shows a well-circumscribed mass (asterisk) in the right hemithorax. Posterior mediastinal location of the mass is suspected by the presence of splaying of the right-sided posterior ribs. (**b**) Lateral chest radiograph confirms posterior mediastinal location of the mass (asterisk). (**c**) Axial enhanced bone window setting CT image demonstrates a large, well-circumscribed mass (asterisk) within the posterior mediastinum with associated punctate calcifications (arrow). The mass displaces the heart (white arrowhead) anteriorly. Lack of normal rim of cerebrospinal fluid surrounding the spinal cord (black arrowhead) and amorphous soft tissue attenuation within the spinal canal raise concern for intracanalicular invasion

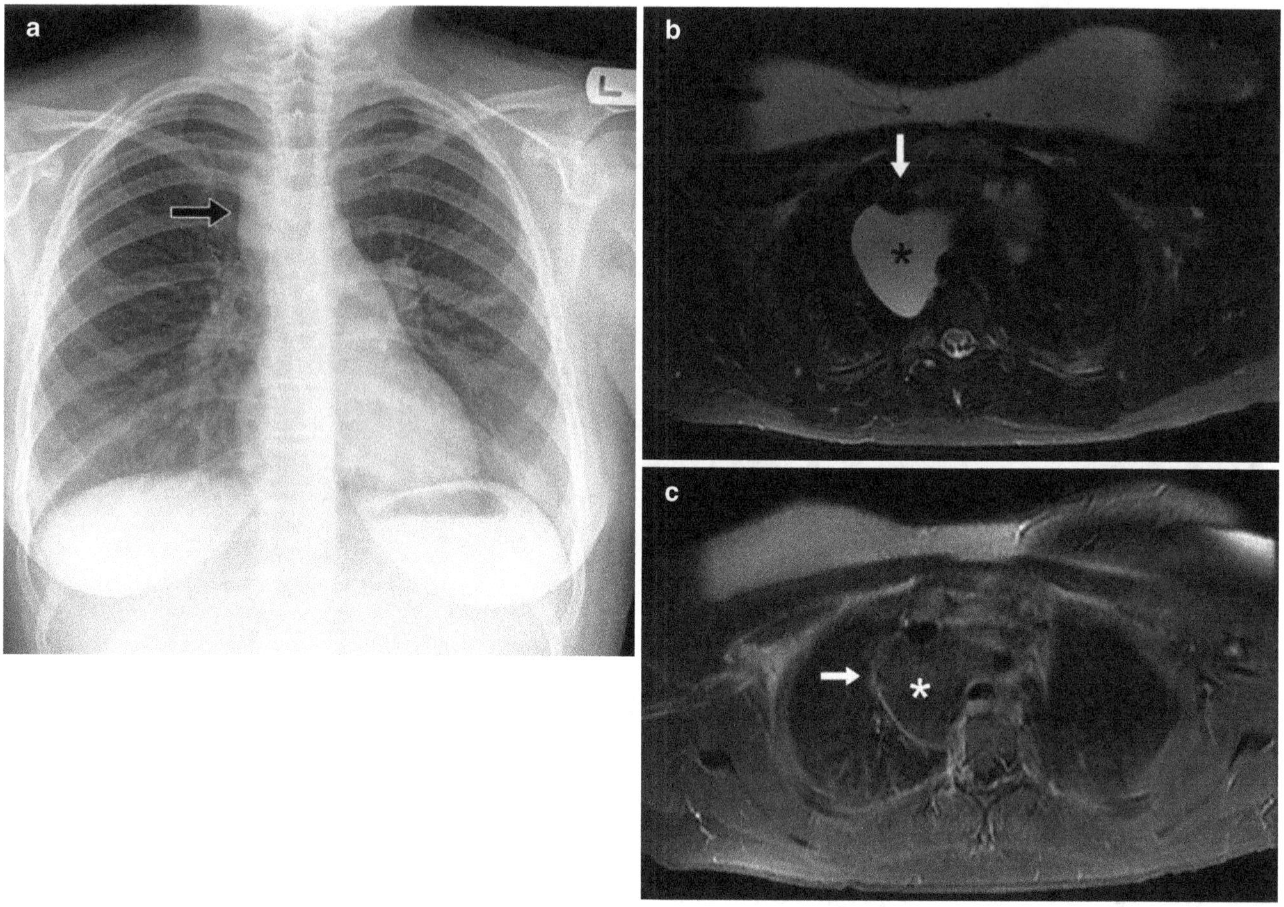

Fig. 10.17 A 14-year-old girl with thoracic lymphatic malformation who presented with cough. (**a**) Frontal chest radiograph shows prominence and undulating contour (arrow) of the right superior mediastinum. (**b**) Axial T2-weighted, fat-suppressed MR image demonstrates a cystic lesion (asterisk) located in the superior mediastinum posterior to the superior vena cava (arrow). (**c**) Axial enhanced T1-weighted, fat-suppressed MR image shows a peripheral enhancement (white arrow) of the lesion (asterisk) located within the superior mediastinum

intervening septa and surrounding walls, which may increase in the setting of prior hemorrhage or infection (Fig. 10.17c).

Surgical resection and localized sclerotherapy are the primary forms of treatment for thoracic lymphatic malformations although complete surgical resection may be limited in extensive, infiltrative lymphatic malformations. With either therapy, relapse is common. Recently, given the success of topical therapies in the treatment of facial angiofibromas and the capillary vascular malformations associated with Sturge-Weber syndrome, novel topical treatment modalities such as rapamycin have been described for lymphatic malformation with promising early results.

10.4 Conclusion

Thoracic disorders mainly arise from lung parenchyma, large airway, or the mediastinum in the pediatric population. Imaging assessment plays an important role for initial detection, preoperative assessment for surgical lesions, and follow-up evaluation. Clear understanding of advantages and disadvantages of currently available imaging modalities as well as characteristic imaging findings of thoracic disorders has a great potential for optimal care of the pediatric patient.

Key Points

- Chest radiography is the first-line and most commonly performed imaging examination in pediatric patients with potential thoracic disorders. CT provides superior characterization as compared with radiography though its use must be carefully weighed due to heighted susceptibility of pediatric patients to the harmful effects of ionizing radiation. Tailored acquisition parameters and image optimization techniques in accordance with the principal of ALARA must be used for dose reduction.
- Surfactant deficiency syndrome is the most common cause of death in premature infants, whereas transient tachypnea of the newborn is the most common cause of respiratory distress in full-term infants.
- Pneumonia is the most common cause of illness in childhood and is a significant cause of morbidity and mortality. Round pneumonia is a distinct manifestation of lower respiratory tract infection in children less than 8 years of age.
- Primary tracheomalacia secondary to prematurity and intrinsic weakness of the supporting cartilage is generally self-limiting and may require only supportive care in the first years of life.
- CT has an accuracy of close to 100% for the detection of aspirated foreign body and should be considered in the setting of high clinical suspicion with negative chest radiography.
- Neuroblastoma is the most common posterior mediastinal mass in pediatric patients and accounts for 90% of posterior mediastinal masses.

Take-Home Messages

- Differential considerations of commonly encountered pediatric chest radiology pathologies include both congenital conditions, such as surfactant deficiency syndrome due to prematurity and tracheomalacia, as well as acquired conditions, such as round pneumonia and neuroblastoma.
- Utilization of a three anatomic compartment model can help to narrow differential considerations in the imaging of pediatric chest pathologies.
- Chest radiography is the first-line and most commonly performed imaging examination in pediatric patients with potential thoracic disorders. The use of CT must be carefully weighed in pediatric chest radiology due to heighted susceptibility of pediatric patients to the harmful effects of ionizing radiation.

References

1. Sodhi KS, Lee EY. What all physicians should know about the potential radiation risk that computed tomography poses for paediatric patients. Acta Paediatr. 2014;103(8):807–11.
2. Sodhi KS, Krishna S, Saxena AK, Khandelwal N, Lee EY. Clinical application of "Justification" and "Optimization" principle of ALARA in pediatric CT imaging: "How many children can be protected from unnecessary radiation?". Eur J Radiol. 2015;84(9):1752–7.
3. Lee EY, Greenberg SB, Boiselle PM. Multidetector computed tomography of pediatric large airway diseases: state-of-the-art. Radiol Clin N Am. 2011;49(5):869–93.
4. Nogo AV, Winant AJ, Lee EY, Phillips GS. Strategies for reducing radiation dose in CT for pediatric patients: how we do it. Semin Roentgenol. 2018;53(2):124–31.
5. Ciet P, Tiddens HA, Wielopolski PA, Wild JM, Lee EY, Morana G, Lequin MH. Magnetic resonance imaging in children: common problems and possible solutions for lung and airways imaging. Pediatr Radiol. 2015;45(13):1901–15.
6. Baez JC, Ciet P, Mulkern R, Seethamraju RT, Lee EY. Pediatric chest MR imaging: lung and airways. Magn Reson Imaging Clin N Am. 2015;23(2):337–49.
7. Sodhi KS, Khandelwal N, Saxena AK, Singh M, Agarwal R, Bhatia A, Lee EY. Rapid lung MRI in children with pulmonary infections: time to change our diagnostic algorithms. J Magn Reson Imaging. 2016;43(5):1196–206.
8. Liszewski MC, Gorkem S, Sodhi KS, Lee EY. Lung magnetic resonance imaging for pneumonia in children. Pediatr Radiol. 2017a;47(11):1420–30.
9. Agrons GA, Courtney SE, Stocker JT, Markowitz RI. Lung disease in premature neonates: radiologic-pathologic correlation. Radiographics. 2005;25:1047–73.
10. Liszewski MC, Lee EY. Neonatal lung disorders: pattern recognition approach to diagnosis. AJR Am J Roentgenol. 2018;210(5):964–75.
11. Edwards MO, Kotecha SJ, Kotecha S. Respiratory distress of the term newborn infant. Paediatr Respir Rev. 2013;14(1):29–36.
12. Liszewski MC, Stanescu AL, Phillips GS, Lee EY. Respiratory distress in neonates: underlying causes and current imaging assessment. Radiol Clin N Am. 2017b;55(4):629–44.
13. Dargaville PA, Copnell B. The epidemiology of meconium aspiration syndrome: incidence, risk factors, therapies, and outcome. Pediatrics. 2006;117(5):1712–21.
14. Winant AJ, Schooler GR, Concepcion NDP, Lee EY. Current updates on pediatric pulmonary infections. Semin Roentgenol. 2017;52(1):35–42.
15. Restrepo R, Rajaneeshankar P, Matapathi UM, Wu Y. Imaging of round pneumonia and mimics in children. Pediatr Radiol. 2010;40:1931–40.
16. Kim YW, Donnelly LF. Round pneumonia: imaging findings in a large series of children. Pediatr Radiol. 2007;37(12):1235–40.. Epub 2007 Oct 19.
17. Raol N, Metry D, Edmonds J, et al. Propranolol for the treatment of subglottic hemangiomas. Int J Pediatr Otorhinolaryngol. 2011;75:1510–4.
18. Haggstrom AN, et al. Clinical spectrum and risk of PHACE syndrome in cutaneous and airway hemangiomas. Arch Otolaryngol Head Neck Surg. 2011;137(7):680–7.
19. Zapala MA, Ho-Fung VM, Lee EY. Thoracic neoplasms in children: contemporary prospectives and imaging assessment. Radiol Clin N Am. 2017;55(4):657–76.
20. Liszewski MC, Ciet P, Sodhi KS, Lee EY. Updates on MRI evaluation of pediatric large airways. AJR Am J Roentgenol. 2017c;208(5):971–81.
21. Amini B, Huang SY, Tsai J, Benveniste MF, Robledo HH, Lee EY. Primary lung and large airway neoplasm in children: current

imaging evaluation with multidetector computed tomography. Radiol Clin N Am. 2013;51(4):637–57.

22. Degnan AJ, Tocchio S, Kurtom W, Tadros SS. Pediatric neuroendocrine carcinoid tumors: management, pathology, and imaging findings in a pediatric referral center. Pediatr Blood Cancer. 2017;64(9).
23. Lee EY, Zucker EJ, Restrepo R, Daltro P, Boiselle PM. Advanced large airway CT imaging in children: evolution from axial to 4D assessment. Pediatr Radiol. 2013;43(3):285–97.
24. Tsai J, Lee EY, Restrepo R, Eisenberg RL. Focal large airway anomalies and abnormalities in pediatric patients. AJR Am J Roentgenol. 2013;201(2):W163–73.
25. Lee EY, Boiselle PM, Cleveland RH. Multidetector CT evaluation of congenital lung anomalies. Radiology. 2008a;247(3):632–48.
26. Lee EY, Litmanovich D, Boiselle PM. Multidetector CT evaluation of tracheobronchomalacia. Radiol Clin N Am. 2009;47(2):261–9.
27. Javia L, Harris MA, Fuller S. Rings, slings, and other tracheal disorders in the neonate. Semin Fetal Neonatal Med. 2016;21(4):277–84.
28. Lee EY, Mason KP, Zurakowski D, Waltz DA, Ralph A, Riaz F, Boiselle PM. MDCT assessment of tracheomalacia in symptomatic infants with mediastinal aortic vascular anomalies: preliminary technical experience. Pediatr Radiol. 2008b;38(1):82–8.
29. Shieh HF, Jennings RW. Three-dimensional printing of external airway splints for tracheomalacia. J Thorac Dis. 2017;9(3):414–6.
30. Green SS. Ingested and aspirated foreign bodies. Pediatr Rev. 2015;36(10):430–6.
31. Laya BF, Restrepo R, Lee EY. Practical imaging evaluation of foreign bodies in children: an update. Radiol Clin N Am. 2017;55(4):845–67.
32. Brian PS, Lim R, Avery LL. Review of ingested and aspirated foreign bodies in children and their clinical significance for radiologists. Radiographics. 2015;35(5):1528–38.
33. Wasilewska E, Lee EY, Esenberg RL. Unilateral hyperlucent lung in children. AJR Am J Roentgenol. 2012;198(5):W400–14.
34. Hegde SV, Hui PK, Lee EY. Tracheobronchial foreign bodies in children: imaging assessment. Semin Ultrasound CT MR. 2015;36(1):8–20.
35. Lee EY, Restrepo R, Dillman JR, Ridge CA, Boiselle PM. Imaging evaluation of pediatric trachea and bronchi: systematic review and updates. Semin Roentgenol. 2012;47(2):182–96.
36. Shin SM, Kim WS, Cheon JE, Jung AY, Youn BJ, Kim IO, Yeon KM. CT in children with suspected residual foreign body in airway after bronchoscopy. AJR Am J Roentgenol. 2009;192(6):1744–51.
37. Hellinger JC, Daubert M, Lee EY, Epleman M. Congenital thoracic vascular anomalies: evaluation with state-of-the-art MR imaging and MDCT. Radiol Clin N Am. 2011;49(5):969–96.
38. Etesami M, Ashwath R, Kanne J, Gilkeson RC, Rajiah P. Computed tomography in the evaluation of vascular rings and slings. Insights Imaging. 2014;5(4):507–21.
39. Hanneman K, Newman B, Chan F. Congenital variants and anomalies of the aortic arch. Radiographics. 2017;37(1):32–51.
40. Kondrachuk O, Yalynska T, Tammo R, Lee EY. Multidetector computed tomography evaluation of congenital mediastinal vascular anomalies in children. Semin Roentgenol. 2012;47(2):127–34.
41. Lee EY. Evaluation of non-vascular mediastinal masses in infants and children: an evidence-based practical approach. Pediatr Radiol. 2009;39(Suppl 2):S184–90.
42. Ranganath SH, Lee EY, Restrepo R, Eienberg RL. Mediastinal masses in children. AJR Am J Roentgenol. 2012;198(3):W197–216.
43. Hacker PG, Mahani MG, Heider A, Lee EY. Imaging evaluation of mediastinal masses in children and adults: practical diagnostic approach based on a new classification system. J Thorac Imaging. 2015;30(4):247–67.
44. Pavlus JD, Carter BW, Tolley MD, Keung ES, Khorashadi L, Lichtenberger JP. Imaging of thoracic neurogenic tumors. AJR Am J Roentgenol. 2016;207(3):552–61.

11

Pulmonary Manifestations of Systemic Diseases

Cornelia Schaefer-Prokop and Brett M. Elicker

Learning Objectives

- Discuss the typical lung manifestations of systemic diseases including sarcoidosis, connective tissue disease, and vasculitis.
- Understand the role of radiology, and in particular computed tomography, in the diagnosis and management of patients with systemic diseases.
- Identify typical CT findings and patterns of systemic diseases and their differential diagnoses.

11.1 Introduction

The diagnosis of systemic diseases involves an analysis of their characteristic clinical manifestations in different organ systems. Clinical features are often correlated with serologic abnormalities, radiologic findings, and, in some cases, histopathology. Systemic diseases may affect a variety of different compartments of the thorax including the lungs, pleura, pericardium, lymph nodes, vessels, and heart. This discussion will focus on their lung manifestations; however reference will also be made to their extrapulmonary manifestations, as these often provide important clues to diagnosis. The prevalence of lung involvement varies: while it is a predominant feature of certain systemic diseases, such as sarcoidosis or granulomatosis with polyangiitis (GPA, formerly Wegener's granulomatosis), it is only rarely present in others such as Henoch-Schönlein purpura.

The roles of imaging in systemic diseases vary somewhat depending upon the specific disorder. Radiology, and in particular computed tomography (CT), may be important in establishing a diagnosis. Sarcoidosis, as an example, is a disease for which typical CT findings are often critical in establishing an accurate diagnosis. Connective tissue disease, on the other hand, is often diagnosed primarily using clinical and serologic findings; thus imaging has a somewhat limited role in diagnosis. However, it is also seen in clinical practice that findings on CT such as signs of lung fibrosis (especially the NSIP pattern) represent the trigger for diagnostic workup for the presence of an underlying systemic disease. When imaging doesn't play a major role in diagnosis, it is still important in establishing the presence and pattern of lung disease as well as disease extent, all of which have an impact on treatment decisions. Imaging also has important roles in serial follow-up of lung abnormalities over time and evaluating patients with worsening or acute symptoms.

In the following we will focus on the more common systemic disorders that develop pulmonary abnormalities such as sarcoidosis, connective tissue diseases, and vasculitis. While a comprehensive review of the lung manifestations of all systemic diseases is not possible, a few selected rare disorders will also be discussed including inflammatory bowel disease, amyloidosis, Erdheim-Chester disease, and IgG4-related sclerosing disease.

11.2 Sarcoidosis

Sarcoidosis is a systemic disorder of unknown origin. A genetic predisposition to sarcoidosis is indicated by observations of familial clustering. Sarcoidosis is characterized by noncaseating epithelioid cell granulomas in multiple organs, but morbidity and mortality are closely related to pulmonary manifestations occurring in >90% of patients [1]. The CT appearance of pulmonary sarcoidosis varies greatly [2] and is known to masquerade many other diffuse infiltrative lung

C. Schaefer-Prokop (✉)
Department of Radiology, Meander Medical Centre, Amersfoort, Netherlands

Department of Radiology, Radboud University, Nijmegen, Netherlands

B. M. Elicker (✉)
Department of Radiology and Biomedical Imaging, University of California, San Francisco, CA, USA
e-mail: brett.elicker@ucsf.edu

diseases; conversely several diseases can resemble classical sarcoidosis.

The histology of pulmonary sarcoidosis consists of noncaseating granulomas with a rim of lymphocytes and fibroblasts in a perilymphatic distribution, which may resolve or cause fibrosis. The disease may occur at any age but mostly affects individuals between 20 and 40 years of age and only rarely occurs in over 65 years of age. The prognosis is mostly good with disease resolution often occurring in <2 years and mortality between 1% and 5%.

The three *criteria for diagnosis* are (1) typical clinical and radiological manifestations, (2) the presence of noncaseating granulomas, and (3) exclusion of alternative diseases. The respective weight of each criterion varies with individual presentation: while in some patients with suspected sarcoidosis typical findings on a chest radiograph can be sufficient in the correct context (i.e., uveitis, erythema nodosum), in other patients a classic nodular pattern on CT is necessary to establish diagnosis, and last there is a subgroup of patients in which controversial or nonspecific clinical and radiological findings make histological proof necessary (e.g., biopsy of skin lesions, endobronchial ultrasound-guided transbronchial needle aspiration for mediastinal or hilar lymphadenopathy).

Pulmonary findings on CT include small, well-defined *nodules in a characteristic perilymphatic distribution* in relation to the subpleural surface, adjacent to the major fissures, along thickened interlobular septa, and adjacent to vessels in the lobular core [3]. The nodules may be evenly distributed throughout both lungs with predominance of the upper and middle lung zones; however they may be also clustered in the perihilar and peribronchovascular regions with relative sparing of the lung periphery, or they may be grouped in small areas. Confluence of granulomas results in larger nodules (1–4 cm, nodular sarcoid, galaxy sign) or ill-defined opacities (ground glass or consolidations, up to 10 cm, alveolar sarcoidosis).

Lymphadenopathy is typically seen in a subcarinal, right paratracheal, aortopulmonary, and symmetric hilar distribution. In advanced stage CT calcifications are seen in lymph nodes with an eggshell or amorphous cloudlike ("icing sugar") pattern.

Up to 25% of patients develop irreversible pulmonary fibrosis with architectural distortion, displacement of the interlobular septa, traction bronchiectasis, honeycombing, and bullae (stage IV). Conglomerate masses, mostly in a perihilar location, represent areas of fibrosis with characteristic traction bronchiectasis. Volume loss of the upper lobes is associated with hilar retraction and septal displacement.

Airway abnormalities include airway compression caused by surrounding lymphadenopathy and traction bronchiectasis caused by surrounding fibrosis. Granulomas within the bronchial walls cause irregular bronchial wall thickening with narrowing of the large and small airways. Involvement of the small airways causes lobular air trapping more easily identifiable on expiratory CT scans.

Sarcoidosis may present with very characteristic HRCT features allowing for a secure diagnosis and obviating further invasive procedures. However, sarcoidosis is also known to present with less typical features (Table 11.1).

Especially in advanced disease with fibrosis, the differential diagnosis between sarcoidosis and other fibrosing diseases can be challenging. Table 11.2 summarizes imaging findings helpful for differentiating diseases.

Complications include the development of an aspergilloma and pulmonary hypertension.

Mycetomas are a typical complication of stage IV sarcoidosis: they present with a soft tissue mass located in a preexisting cavity in patients with fibrotic sarcoidosis. Life-threatening hemoptysis may require immediate interventional therapy (embolization of bronchial arteries).

Pulmonary hypertension occurs in patients with end-stage fibrosis but may be also caused by mediastinal fibrosis, extrinsic compression of the pulmonary arteries by lymphadenopathy, or intrinsic sarcoid vasculopathy including features of pulmonary veno-occlusive disease.

Staging based on chest radiography (Siltzbach classification, Table 11.3) was developed decades ago, before the broad use of CT; it is purely descriptive and does not indicate disease activity.

FDG-PET can be used to accurately assess inflammatory activity, for example, in patients with persistent disabling symptoms without serological inflammatory activity [4]. PET has also been described to be helpful to predict pulmonary deterioration at 1 year and to monitor therapy response.

Table 11.1 HRCT manifestations of Sarcoidosis

Typical features	
Lymphadenopathy:	hilar, mediastinal, bilateral symmetric, well defined
Nodules:	micronodules (2–4 mm), well-defined, larger coalescing nodules
Perilymphatic distribution:	subpleural, interlobular septa, peribronchovascular
Fibrosis:	reticular opacities, architectural distortion, bronchiectasis, volume loss
Distribution:	predominance of upper lobes and perihilar areas
Atypical features	
Lymphadenopathy:	unilateral, isolated, in atypical mediastinal locations
Airspace consolidations:	conglomerate masses, confluent alveolar opacities (alveolar sarcoidosis)
Linear opacities:	interlobular septal thickening
Fibrocystic changes:	cysts, bullae, honeycomb-like opacities, upper lobe predominance
Airway involvement:	atelectasis, mosaic pattern
Pleural disease:	effusion, pneumothorax, pleural plaques

Table 11.2 Diseases with imaging features that overlap with sarcoidosis

Differential diagnosis	Overlapping finding	Suggestive for sarcoidosis
Lymphangitic carcinomatosis	• Irregular "beaded" thickening of the interlobular septa	• Upper lobe predominance • Absence of pleural effusion • Less central bronchial cuffing
Silicosis/pneumoconiosis	• Pleural pseudoplaques • Egg shell calcifications of lymph nodes • Perihilar fibrotic masses	• No calcifications in pseudoplaques, • Pseudoplaques consist of confluent nodules • The perihilar fibrotic masses extend directly from the hilar structures and move posteriorly (volume loss upper lobe)
Chronic EAA/chronic HP and UIP/IPF	• Honeycombing • Traction bronchiectasis • Architectural distortion • Lobular distribution of areas with air trapping (in the presence of obliterative bronchiolitis) and fibrosis	• UIP pattern predominantly in upper lobes or perihilar region • Thickened interlobular septa • Lymph node calcifications • Fibrosis and traction bronchiectasis tend to run from the hilar structures dorsolaterally
Lymphoproliferative disorders	• Lymphadenopathy	• Usually but not always symmetric • Presence of typical parenchymal findings (caveat: biopsy may be necessary)
Chronic beryllium disease	• Nodular pattern	• Large hilar lymphadenopathy • No exposure to beryllium • Other organ involvement
Tuberculosis	• Nodular pattern (normally random versus perilymphatic nodules; however, sarcoidosis may occasionally show a random pattern)	• Egg shell or disperse calcifications as opposed to rough TB calcifications • Symmetric calcifications (in Tb frequently asymmetric) • Clinical symptoms of acute infection in patients with military TB
Common variable immune deficiency (CVID)	• Nodules in perilymphatic distribution • Ill-defined nodules in mid-lower predominance	• Different clinical histories (in CVID recurrent bacterial infection) • Different histological features

EAA, exogenic allergic alveolitis; HP, hypersensitivity pneumonitis
see also *Spagnolo P, Sverzellati N, Wells AU, and Hansell D. Eur Radiol 2014;24: 807*

Table 11.3 Siltzbach classification of sarcoidosis

	CXR findings	Stage at diagnosis	Spontaneous remission in
Stage 0	Normal chest radiograph	5–10%	
Stage 1	Bilateral hilar and paratracheal lymphadenopathy	50%	60–90%
Stage 2	Lymphadenopathy and nodular opacities	25–30%	40–70%
Stage 3	Nodular opacities without lymphadenopathy or signs of fibrosis	10–12%	10–20%
Stage 4	Fibrosis	5%, in up to 25% progression to stage 4 during course of disease	0%

Inhibition of the physiological myocardial FDG uptake, e.g., by appropriate diets, enables the detection of cardiac sarcoidosis active lesions.

Recently an integrated clinicoradiological staging system [5] has been proposed to identify patients with poor prognosis and at risk for mortality (50% in 5.5 years): while initial separation between the two prognostic groups was done by applying a weighted combination of lung function parameters, further separation was yielded if extent of fibrosis on CT exceeded 20% and/or a pathological diameter ratio of the main pulmonary and ascending aorta (>1) was seen.

> **Key Point**
> - The typical CT findings of sarcoidosis include (1) perilymphatic nodules located predominantly in the peribronchovascular and subpleural interstitium, (2) symmetric bilateral hilar and mediastinal lymphadenopathy, and (3) upper lobe and peribronchovascular fibrosis.

11.3 Connective Tissue Disease

Connective tissue diseases (CTDs) are characterized primary upon clinical grounds, namely, typical clinical complaints and physical examination findings. The presence of specific autoantibodies also assists in making a specific diagnosis. While imaging has an important role in determining the presence and pattern of lung disease present, its role in diagnosis is limited. It is important to note, however, that lung abnormalities may precede the other clinical manifestations, sometimes by more than 5 years. In these cases, imaging may suggest the possibility of CTD, even when a patient doesn't meet the criteria for a specific one (see interstitial pneumonia with autoimmune features below).

CTD can affect different compartments of the thorax including the lung, pleura, pericardium, lymphatics, vasculature, and heart. Commonly, more than one compartment is involved. Involvement of the respiratory system is common in CTDs and results in significant morbidity and mortality. Many of the lung manifestations of CTD [6] are similar to the idiopathic interstitial pneumonias and can be classified using the same system [7].

Lung biopsy is rarely obtained in patients with a defined CTD. For this reason, high-resolution CT often determines the predominant pattern of injury present. This pattern is important in determining treatment and prognosis. While many possible patterns of injury are associated with each specific CTD [8], certain patterns are more common than others (Table 11.4). For instance, organizing pneumonia is most commonly seen in association with polymyositis or dermatomyositis. It is also important to note that more than one pattern of injury may be present in the same patient.

Table 11.4 Different connective tissue diseases and their primary pulmonary manifestations

Connective tissue disease	Most common pattern(s)	Less common pattern(s)
Rheumatoid arthritis	• Usual interstitial pneumonia • Nonspecific interstitial pneumonia	• Airways disease
Scleroderma	• Nonspecific interstitial pneumonia • Pulmonary hypertension	• Usual interstitial pneumonia
Systemic lupus erythematosus	• Pulmonary hemorrhage • Diffuse alveolar damage	• Pulmonary hypertension • Pulmonary thromboembolism
Myositis	• Nonspecific interstitial pneumonia • Organizing pneumonia	• Diffuse alveolar damage
Sjögren syndrome	• Nonspecific interstitial pneumonia • Lymphoid interstitial pneumonia • Airways disease	
Mixed connective tissue disease	• Nonspecific interstitial pneumonia • Usual interstitial pneumonia	

> **Key Point**
> - The diagnosis of CTD is made predominantly using clinical and serologic findings. Imaging is important in the detection and characterization of lung disease, particularly given that pathology is not usually obtained.

11.3.1 Rheumatoid Arthritis

Most patients with rheumatoid arthritis (RA) have abnormalities on high-resolution chest CT; however they are commonly asymptomatic. The most common CT findings in the lungs include bronchial wall thickening (12–92%), bronchial dilation (30–40%), reticulation (10–20%), ground-glass opacity (15–25%), honeycombing (10%), and consolidation (5%) [9].

Airways disease appears to be the earliest manifestation of RA in the lung [10]. Bronchiectasis and air trapping are common findings [11]. There is a recognized association between RA and obliterative bronchiolitis (constrictive bronchiolitis) in which bronchioles are destroyed and replaced by scar tissue. The characteristic CT finding is mosaic perfusion with expiratory air trapping often associated with bronchial dilation. Follicular bronchiolitis is a second type of small airway disorder recognized in rheumatoid lung disease. The major CT finding is centrilobular nodules and areas of ground-glass opacity.

RA lung fibrosis is substantially more common in men than in women. The two most common patterns of lung fibrosis are UIP and NSIP [12]. Of all CTDs, RA is the most common to present with a UIP pattern. CT findings in interstitial pneumonia associated with RA are often indistinguishable from the idiopathic varieties; however other findings such as nodules, pulmonary arterial enlargement, or pleural abnormality may provide a clue to the underlying diagnosis. UIP and NSIP both typically demonstrate a subpleural and basilar distribution of findings. A confident diagnosis of UIP may be made when honeycombing and reticulation is present in this distribution. A confident diagnosis of NSIP may be made when there is an absence of honeycombing and subpleural sparing is present.

The new generation of biologic agents used to treat RA has resulted in a new array of potential pulmonary side effects. The most important of these is impaired immunity related to use of anti-TNFα antibodies (etanercept, infliximab, and adalimumab), which results in a substantially increased incidence of tuberculosis (sometimes disseminated or extra-articular) and nontuberculous mycobacterial infection.

Low-dose methotrexate [13] may be associated with subacute hypersensitivity pneumonitis in 2–5% of cases. Preexisting radiographic evidence of interstitial lung disease probably predisposes to the development of methotrexate pneumonitis in patients with RA. Infections, such as pneumocystis pneumonia, are also a potential complication of therapy.

11.3.2 Scleroderma (Progressive Systemic Sclerosis)

Parenchymal lung involvement is very common in patients with scleroderma. Scleroderma is, in fact, the only CTD in which lung disease is a component of the defining criteria. At autopsy, the lungs are abnormal in at least 80% of cases. Lung fibrosis is the most common pattern of abnormality, with NSIP being much more common (>90%) than UIP [14]. Pulmonary hypertension is also common, either as an isolated finding or in association with lung fibrosis. Pulmonary hypertension is particularly common in patients with limited scleroderma (CREST syndrome) [15]. Esophageal dilation is found in up to 80% of cases on CT.

CT findings in scleroderma reflect the dominant NSIP histology. Cellular NSIP presents with ground-glass opacity, often in a posterior and subpleural distribution. Fibrotic NSIP shows irregular reticulation and traction bronchiectasis as the predominant findings. Honeycombing is often absent, but when present, it is limited in extent [16]. Cellular and fibrotic NSIP often coexist, so findings may overlap. Subpleural sparing is particularly suggestive of a NSIP pattern.

The lung fibrosis associated with scleroderma is associated with a much better prognosis than that found in idiopathic lung fibrosis [17], most likely due in part to the predominant NSIP histology [18]. Fibrotic changes may stay stable for many years.

Pulmonary arterial hypertension usually causes enlargement of the main and proximal pulmonary arteries on chest radiograph or CT; however normal-sized pulmonary arteries do not exclude the diagnosis, and the presence of pericardial thickening or fluid in patients with scleroderma is also a strong predictor of echocardiographic pulmonary hypertension.

There is an increased prevalence of lung cancer in scleroderma, with relative risk of malignancy ranging from 1.8 to 6.5. Lung cancer in this condition often occurs in individuals with lung fibrosis.

11.3.3 Systemic Lupus Erythematosus (SLE)

Pleuritis is the most common pleuropulmonary manifestation of SLE, found in 40–60% of patients, and may or may not be associated with pleural effusion.

Fibrotic interstitial lung disease [19] is less common in SLE than in the other CTDs. While pulmonary infection is said to be the most common pulmonary complication of SLE, acute pulmonary hemorrhage is also an important pulmonary complication of this condition, characterized radiologically by diffuse or patchy consolidation and ground-glass opacity [20].

Acute lupus pneumonitis is a poorly defined entity, characterized by a variable degree of respiratory impairment accompanied by focal or diffuse pulmonary consolidation, occurring in patients with lupus. It is now believed that most cases previously identified as lupus pneumonitis probably represented diffuse alveolar damage with or without pulmonary hemorrhage.

Other complications of lupus may include diaphragmatic dysfunction, pulmonary hypertension, and pulmonary thromboembolism [21], which may be related to antiphospholipid antibodies. Diaphragmatic dysfunction, thought to be due to a diaphragmatic myopathy, is manifested by reduced lung volumes ("shrinking lungs" with platelike atelectasis).

Key Point

- Fibrotic lung disease is much less common with SLE compared to other CTDs. Hemorrhage, diffuse alveolar damage, and pulmonary hypertension are more common findings.

11.3.4 Polymyositis/Dermatomyositis (PM/DM)

The presence of interstitial lung disease (ILD) in PM/DM correlates strongly with the presence of anti-Jo-1. About 50–70% of patients who are anti-Jo-1 positive have ILD, whereas the frequency of ILD falls to about 10% if antibodies are absent. ILD may antedate myositis in patients with anti-Jo-1 antibodies.

The most common pathologic findings are NSIP [22] and OP, often occurring in combination. As with other CTDs, the occurrence of interstitial pneumonia may precede the development of clinical myositis.

Lung disease associated with PM/DM or with the antisynthetase syndrome, a closely related entity, is often associated with a characteristic CT appearance [23]. Confluent ground-glass opacity and consolidation in the lower lobes is superimposed on a background of traction bronchiectasis. This pattern reflects the characteristic histologic combination of organizing pneumonia and NSIP. On serial evaluation after treatment, consolidation often shows significant improvement or resolution; however fibrosis, manifested by reticulation and traction bronchiectasis, usually persists.

Diffuse alveolar damage is another pattern that may be seen in patients with PM/DM. Patients present with acute symptoms, as opposed to the subacute or chronic symptoms of NSIP and/or organizing pneumonia. Typical CT features of diffuse alveolar damage include symmetric bilateral ground-glass opacity and/or consolidation.

There is an increased risk for malignancy (especially for breast, lung, ovary, and stomach malignancies) that is concurrently diagnosed within 1 year follow-up in up to 20% of patients.

11.3.5 Sjögren Syndrome

CT provides substantial information regarding the pattern of pulmonary involvement in Sjögren syndrome. The patterns may be divided into airway abnormalities, interstitial fibrosis, pulmonary hypertension, and lymphoid interstitial pneumonia [24].

Airway-related abnormalities are common and consist of bronchial wall thickening, bronchiectasis, bronchiolectasis, and tree-in-bud opacities. Small airway disease may manifest by mosaic attenuation on inspiratory CT and air trapping on expiratory air trapping [25].

Nonspecific (NSIP) and lymphoid (LIP) interstitial pneumonia are the most common patterns of parenchymal lung disease. NSIP resembles that seen in scleroderma as above. LIP is characterized by ground-glass opacity due to the homogenous lymphocytic infiltration. Perilymphatic or centrilobular nodules may also be seen. Cysts measuring 5–30 mm may be seen in isolation or associated with other findings. These changes are ascribed to bronchiolar obstruction on the basis of lymphocytic wall infiltration. Cysts are helpful in distinguishing LIP from lymphoma.

Lymphoma should be suspected if consolidation, large nodules (>1 cm), mediastinal lymphadenopathy, or effusions are present. However, similar large "pseudo-alveolar" nodules can be found in combined amyloidosis and LIP. In contrast to other cystic lung diseases such as lymphangioleiomyomatosis, the cysts of LIP are fewer in number and show a peribronchovascular and lower lung predominance.

11.3.6 Mixed Connective Tissue Disease

Mixed connective tissue disease (MCTD) is an overlap syndrome that is a distinct clinicopathological entity. The principal characteristics are the presence of (1) features of SLE, scleroderma, and PM/DM, occurring together or evolving sequentially during observation and (2) antibodies to an extractable nuclear antigen (RNP).

Pulmonary involvement is common in MCTD with infiltrative lung disease present in as many as two thirds of patients. Many affected patients are asymptomatic. The pulmonary abnormalities resemble those seen in SLE, SS, and PM/DM. Thus, pleural thickening and pleural and pericardial effusions are common. Ground-glass attenuation is the commonest parenchymal abnormality [26]. The CT pattern corresponds most closely to NSIP. Less common findings include honeycombing, consolidation, and poorly defined centrilobular nodules.

Other important complications of MCTD include pulmonary arterial hypertension and esophageal dysmotility with sequelae of recurrent aspiration in the lungs.

11.3.7 Interstitial Pneumonia with Autoimmune Features

There is growing attention in the literature toward patients with interstitial lung disease that have some, but not all, features of a CTD. Multiple studies retrospectively identified subgroups of patients with one or multiple serological features of an autoimmune process in patients with histologically proven UIP or NSIP that were originally diagnosed as idiopathic because they did not fulfill the criteria of one of the stablished CTDs. Several terms have been suggested as a description for these subgroups including interstitial pneumonia with autoimmune features, undifferentiated CTD (UCTD), or lung-dominant CTD.

The term *interstitial pneumonia with autoimmune features* (IPAF) has been proposed for a subgroup of patients with findings suggestive but not diagnostic of a CTD [27]. To meet criteria for IPAF, patients must demonstrate specific features in two of the three following domains: (1) clinical, (2) serologic, and (3) anatomic. The anatomic domain may be satisfied by either typical patterns on CT or pathology. The CT patterns that are suggestive of CTD include nonspecific interstitial pneumonia (NSIP), organizing pneumonia (OP), an overlap of NSIP and OP, or lymphoid interstitial pneumonia. The presence of multi-compartmental findings is also suggestive including the combination of an interstitial pneumonia with any of the following: unexplained pleural effusion or thickening, pericardial effusion or thickening, airways disease, or pulmonary vasculopathy.

Key Point

- IPAF is a term used to describe patients who have some, but not all features, of a specific CTD. CT patterns that are suggestive of this diagnosis include NSIP, OP, an overlap of NSIP and OP, LIP, and multi-compartmental disease (e.g., interstitial pneumonia with pleural thickening).

11.3.8 Pulmonary Vasculitis/Diffuse Alveolar Hemorrhage

The term "vasculitis" refers to disorders characterized by inflammation of blood vessel walls. Pathology includes the presence of leucocytes and fibrinoid necrosis in the vessel wall with consequent compromise of vessel integrity and hemorrhage, narrowing of vessel lumen with consequent downstream ischemia, and necrosis.

Classification of systemic vasculitis (Table 11.5) remains controversial. The current classification dated from the Chapel Hill Consensus Conference (CHCC) in 2012 continued to consider the predominant vascular size involved and distinguishes large-, medium-, or small-vessel vasculitis (LVV, MVV, or SVV, respectively). For the first time, ANCA (antineutrophil cytoplasmic antibody) was included in the classification.

Pulmonary involvement is typically seen with small-vessel vasculitis (SVV). SVV affects arterioles, venules, and capillaries. It is divided into antineutrophil cytoplasmic antibody (ANCA)-associated vasculitis (AAV) that includes microscopic polyangiitis, granulomatosis with polyangiitis (formerly Wegener), and eosinophilic granulomatosis with polyangiitis (formerly Churg-Strauss) [28]. The second group refers to immune complex SVV comprising among others antiglomerular basement membrane disease (Goodpasture) as the only one with regularly seen lung involvement. Behcet disease also belongs to immune complex-mediated vasculitis but involves variable vessel sizes (variable vessel vasculitis).

Clinical symptoms and radiologic signs [29] suggestive of pulmonary vasculitis include diffuse alveolar hemorrhage (DAH), acute glomerulonephritis, upper airway disease, lung nodules or cavitary nodules, mononeuritis multiplex, and palpable purpura [30]. Combined involvement of the lungs and kidneys by some of these diseases is also described as pulmonary-renal syndrome.

In addition to the abovementioned "primary pulmonary vasculitis," there is pulmonary vasculitis associated with connective tissue disorders such as rheumatoid arthritis, SLE, and systemic sclerosis as well as sarcoidosis and relapsing polychondritis. This type of vasculitis is considered "secondary vasculitis," though the differentiation between primary and secondary becomes increasing "blurry" as more and more etiologies for secondary vasculitis are discovered (e.g., drug-associated immune complex vasculitis). Nevertheless they all have in common the involvement of the small vessels (>100 μm and <1 mm).

Diffuse alveolar hemorrhage (DAH) consisting of hemoptysis, diffuse alveolar infiltrates, and drop in hematocrit is a clinical syndrome and not a disease in itself. It occurs in all primary and secondary small-vessel vasculitides with capillaritis (GPA, EGPA, MPA, Henoch-Schonlein purpura, Behcet, SLE, and Goodpasture). It has to be differentiated from other conditions such as bland pulmonary hemorrhage (e.g., coagulation disorders, mitral stenosis, drug-induced, etc.) and hemorrhage associated with diffuse alveolar damage (drug-induced, ARDS, bone marrow transplantation, or cocaine inhalation).

Key Point

- Small-vessel vasculitis is the most common to affect the lungs and primarily includes three diseases: microscopic polyangiitis, granulomatosis with polyangiitis (formerly Wegener), and eosinophilic granulomatosis with polyangiitis (formerly Churg-Strauss) [28]. Typical CT findings include multiple cavitating nodules and diffuse alveolar hemorrhage characterized by bilateral groundglass and consolidations.

11.3.9 ANCA-Associated Granulomatous Vasculitis with Polyangiitis (GPA, Former Wegener's Disease)

GPA is the most common of the AAV. It affects the sinuses, kidneys, and lungs resulting in the classic triad of symptoms comprising upper airway diseases (sinusitis, otitis, ulcerations, subglottis, and bronchial stenosis), lower respiratory tract involvement (clinically presenting as hemoptysis, chest pain, dyspnea, and cough), and glomerulonephritis (presenting as hematuria and azotemia). However, at initial presentation patients may not have the full spectrum (limited expressions of GPA); on the other hand, any part of the body may be affected in the course of disease. Females and males are affected equally and at any age (mostly age 40–55). Airway involvement is more frequent in men. The most common cause of death is renal failure. With treatment, the 24 months survival is 80%. The factors initiating disease are unknown; current data support the involvement of (recurrent) infection for GPA. Up to 80% of patients are (in the course of disease) ANCA positive (mostly PR3-ANCA). Histologic findings include necrotizing granulomatous vasculitis of small to medium vessels without associated infection.

Though a number of attempts have been made to define diagnostic criteria (e.g., ACR criteria, CCHC nomenclature), it can be difficult to reliably distinguish GPA from MPA. Patients are usually included in the GPA category, if they are ANCA positive and if they have respiratory tract involvement supporting GPA, even though there is lack of identifiable evidence of systemic vasculitis (no renal involvement).

The most frequently seen pulmonary abnormalities are multiple nodules or masses of varying size with or without a CT halo sign (perinodular hemorrhage). They tend to involve

Table 11.5 Classification of vasculitis according to the 2012 Chapel Hill Consensus conference (CHCC)

	Vasculitis	Pulmonary-renal syndrome	Pulmonary hemorrhage	Pulmonary hypertension
Small-vessel vasculitisANCA-associated	Granulomatous vasculitis with polyangiitis(GPA)(former Wegener's)	Pulmonary involvement 90% Renal involvement 80%	In about 10%	–
	Eosinophilic granulomatous vasculitis with polyangiitisGPA(Church Strauss)	Up to 25%	Rare	–
	Microscopic polyangiitis	Frequently associated with necrotizing glomerulonephritis	Frequent	
Small-vessel vasculitisImmune complex type	Cryoglobulinemic IgA(Henoch-Schonlein)			
	HUV(hypocomplementemic urticarial vasculitis)			
	Anti-GBM)		40–60%	
Medium-vessel vasculitis (MVV)	Polyarteritis nodosa(PAN)	–	Very rarely idiopathic, associated with hepatitis Bpart of RA, SLE	–
Large-vessel vasculitis (LVV)	Kawasaki syndrome			
	Giant cell arteritis (GCA)	–	Rare, focal	Rare
	Takayasu	–	Rare, focal	Rare
Connective tissue disorders	RA	–	Very rare, diffuse	Up to 60%
	SSc	–	Rare, diffusewith necr. vasculitis	10–60%
	MCTD	–	Rare, diffuse	Up to 45%
	SLE	Up to 60%, late	In 4%, diffuse(potentially more frequent)	5–45%

the subpleural regions; there is no predilection for upper or lower lung zones. Lesions can be as large as 10 cm; however most are smaller. Lesions are often cavitary and have thick walls. Peripheral wedge-shaped areas of consolidation resemble infarcts and may also cavitate. Diffuse consolidation or ground-glass opacity is present in patients with pulmonary hemorrhage. Focal fibrotic changes reflect prior episodes of active disease, although diffuse lung fibrosis may occasionally be seen (mostly UIP pattern). Superinfection of cavitating nodules is not uncommon. A reverse halo sign may also be seen, reflecting organizing pneumonia. A key feature of GPA is the rapid temporal evolution of the nodules and airspace opacities.

In addition there may be a concentric thickening of tracheal or bronchial walls (in about 70%) with a reduction in the luminal diameter and associated with atelectasis (seen in about 15%). Bronchial abnormalities mainly involve the segmental and subsegmental bronchi. Involvement of the subglottic trachea is most typical.

The differential diagnosis depends upon the predominant manifestation. When nodules are the predominant feature, the differential diagnosis includes neoplasms (adenocarcinoma, metastases, and lymphoma) and certain infections (fungal and mycobacterial infections). In the setting of airspace consolidation, infection is also considered. When airway thickening is present, other considerations include amyloidosis, granulomatous disease, and relapsing polychondritis for airway disease.

11.3.9.1 Eosinophilic Granulomatosis with Polyangiitis (EGPA, Former Churg-Strauss)

Eosinophilic granulomatous disease with polyangiitis (formerly called Churg-Strauss syndrome) is caused by a SVV that almost exclusively occurs in patients with asthma and is characterized by a marked serum eosinophilia. Clinically, radiologically, and pathologically, it combines features of GPA and eosinophilic pneumonia (allergic granulomatosis and angiitis) [31]. Many other organs may be involved including the heart (up to 47%), the skin (up to 40%), and the musculoskeletal system (up to 50%). Involvement of the peripheral nerves (in up to 75%) is more frequent, while renal involvement and pulmonary hemorrhage are less common than in GPA.

Up to 30% are ANCA positive mostly MPO-ANCA; ANCA positivity is higher in active disease. Biopsy confirmation is recommended in case of ANCA negativity (in up to 40%) and the presence of easily accessible lesions (e.g., skin). Histology demonstrates small-vessel (arteries and veins) vasculitis with eosinophilic infiltrates and vascular and extravascular granulomas. The 5-year survival is reported in up to 80% of patients; 50% of deaths are related to cardiac involvement. Clinically EGPA presents in three distinct phases (asthmatic, eosinophilic, and vasculitis phase), although these are not necessarily seen in that order. The asthmatic phase precedes the vasculitic phase by 8–10 years.

Upper airway disease and pulmonary abnormalities are seen in up to 70% of patients with EGPA. The most common pulmonary findings include transient, multifocal, and non-segmental consolidations or ground-glass opacifications without zonal predilection [32]. The presence of (non-cavitating) small nodules or diffuse reticular opacities has also been reported. If located subpleurally, the consolidations mimic eosinophilic pneumonia. Pleural effusions are seen in about one third of patients due to cardiomyopathy or eosinophilic pleuritis. Interlobular thickening is seen in about 50% and is secondary to cardiogenic pulmonary edema, eosinophilic septal infiltration, or mild fibrosis.

Airway abnormalities are also an important thoracic manifestation and include wall thickening, dilatation, small centrilobular nodules, and mosaic perfusion. Bronchial wall thickening refers to eosinophilic and lymphocytic infiltration of the airway wall (the clinical symptom of asthma some time during disease course is obligatory for the diagnosis). Increased interlobular septa may reflect edema caused by cardiac and/or renal involvement or eosinophilic infiltration of the septa. Eosinophilic pleural effusion is seen in up to 50% of patients.

Airway changes consisting tree-in-bud, bronchial wall thickening and bronchial dilatation are likely to be related to asthma and are seen in almost patients; the wall thickening can also be caused by eosinophilic involvement.

The differential diagnosis includes chronic eosinophilic pneumonia, organizing pneumonia, and simple eosinophilic pneumonia (Löffler syndrome) in airspace disease. In airway-dominant disease, the list is longer and includes EAA, MPA, SLE, infectious bronchiolitis, and asthma.

11.3.9.2 Microscopic Polyangiitis (MPA)

Microscopic polyangiitis (MPA) is a systemic necrotizing small-vessel vasculitis without granulomatous inflammation. Clinically it is characterized by a long prodromal phase with weight loss and fever followed by a rapidly progressive glomerulonephritis. Microscopic polyangiitis is the most common cause of pulmonary-renal syndrome: rapidly progressive glomerulonephritis is seen in up to 90% and pulmonary involvement in up to 30–50%. More than 75% of patients are ANCA positive in the course of disease, mostly MPO ANCA (in 35–65%).

Microscopic polyangiitis is characterized by the combination of glomerulonephritis and diffuse alveolar hemorrhage (DAH). Imaging findings include patchy, bilateral, or diffuse airspace opacities. The opacity can show both features of consolidations and ground glass dependent on the amount of alveolar filling by blood. Typically DAH is more extensive in the perihilar areas, sparing lung apices, and the costophrenic angles. A halo surrounding a consolidation or nodule underlines the character of hemorrhage. During the phase of resorption, interlobular lines (crazy paving) may become more apparent.

Repeated hemorrhage leads to fibrosis with honeycombing, reticulation, and traction bronchiectasis. Interstitial lung disease may be seen in some patients, more frequently in MPA than in GPA.

11.3.10 Antiglomerular Basement Membrane Disease (Anti-GBM Disease)

Anti-GBM disease belongs to the group of immune complex SVV and is characterized by circulating antibodies against an antigen intrinsic to the glomerular basement membrane. It results in necrotizing glomerulonephritis with acute renal failure. The diagnosis is usually made via renal biopsy. Diffuse alveolar hemorrhage (DAH) occurs in about 40–60%; isolated pulmonary involvement is extremely rare. The term Goodpasture syndrome is used for patients with glomerulonephritis and pulmonary hemorrhage irrespective of underlying cause, while the term Goodpasture disease is restricted to the combination of DAG, glomerulonephritis, and anti-GBM antibodies.

The serology comprises c-ANCA or p-ANCA positivity in 30% and anti-basement membrane antibodies in >90%. Young men are more often affected than women (M:F = 9:1), though it may also be seen in elderly women. With treatment the prognosis is good. Underlying pulmonary injury, e.g., by smoking or cocaine inhalation, is thought to predispose to pulmonary involvement. Recurrent episodes cause pulmonary fibrosis.

Imaging features consist of diffuse or patchy ground glass or consolidation, due to the alveolar hemorrhage, that typically resolve within days. Typically there is sparing of the subpleural space with predominance of the perihilar areas in the mid- and lower lung zones. Pleural effusion is uncommon. After recurrent episodes traction bronchiectasis, reticular opacities and honeycombing may evolve.

11.4 Miscellaneous Systemic Disorders

11.4.1 Inflammatory Bowel Disease

Ulcerative colitis and Crohn's disease are associated with a wide variety of pulmonary complications [33]. Pulmonary complications may precede the diagnosis of inflammatory bowel disease or may occur years after the initial diagnosis and even after complete colectomy for ulcerative colitis. Indeed there is some suggestion that pulmonary complications may be more common after surgical treatment, perhaps because anti-inflammatory treatment is withdrawn. Both Crohn's disease and ulcerative colitis can be associated with tracheobronchitis and airway stenosis [34]. Bronchiectasis and bronchial wall thickening are also common. Parenchymal abnormalities associated with inflammatory bowel disease include organizing pneumonia, pulmonary hemorrhage, and granulomatous infiltration in Crohn's disease.

11.4.2 Amyloidosis and Light Chain Deposition Disease

Amyloidosis and light chain deposition disease are rare disorders characterized by the extracellular deposition of proteins in one or more organs. They both share clinical, radiographic, and pathologic features. The main difference between these two entities is the Congo red staining and fibrillar structure on electron microscopy of amyloidosis. Both entities may be associated with a plasma cell dyscrasia.

Three radiographic manifestations of amyloidosis are described: nodular parenchymal, diffuse alveolar septal, and tracheobronchial [35]. The nodular parenchymal form presents radiographically as one or more solid lung nodules, often found incidentally. These may be confused with malignancy, particularly when spiculated borders are present. A slow growth rate is typical, and calcification may be present. The diffuse alveolar septal form is characterized by the presence of widespread deposits throughout the lungs. The most common findings are small nodules (typically in a perilymphatic distribution), consolidation, ground-glass opacity, and reticulation. The presence of calcification associated with these abnormalities may be particularly suggestive. The tracheobronchial form shows extensive thickening of the trachea and/or bronchi with or without calcification.

The imaging findings of light chain deposition disease are less well described. There are two types: nodular and diffuse [36]. The nodular type presents with scattered solid nodules, often associated with cysts. The nodules are typically located within or adjacent to the wall of the cysts. The diffuse type may show diffuse small nodules, resembling the diffuse alveolar septal type of amyloidosis.

11.4.3 Erdheim-Chester Disease

Erdheim-Chester disease is an infiltrative disorder in which non-Langerhans' cell histiocytes are found in one or more organ systems. The primary organs affected include bones, brain, kidneys, and the cardiovascular system. Middle-aged males are most commonly affected. While pathology is helpful in excluding lymphoproliferative malignancies, the pathologic findings may be nonspecific; thus typical radiographic features are a key to appropriate diagnosis. Characteristic imaging findings [37] in the chest include periadventitial aortic soft tissue thickening. This thickening may involve the aorta and its main branches diffusely, giving rise to the term "coating" of the aorta. The most common lung finding seen is smooth interlobular septal thickening, resembling pulmonary edema. The most characteristic finding outside of the chest is circumferential perinephric soft tissue, resembling lymphoma.

11.4.4 IgG4-Related Sclerosing Disease

IgG4-related sclerosing disease is a disorder originally thought to be isolated to the pancreas and previously called lymphoplasmacytic sclerosing pancreatitis. It is now recognized as a systemic order associated with IgG4 plasma cells and fibrosclerosis in multiple organ systems. The primary organs involved include the pancreas, hepatobiliary system, salivary glands, and lymph nodes. The findings in the chest are variable and may include nodules, lymphadenopathy, airway thickening, and pleural abnormalities [38]. Also, it is possible that IgG4-related sclerosing disease may account for a proportion of cases of idiopathic interstitial pneumonias.

11.5 Conclusions

Systemic disorders demonstrate a wide variety of manifestations in the chest. Imaging, and in particular computed tomography, plays a critical role in the diagnosis of these disorders, however the imaging findings must be correlated with the typical clinical manifestations affecting multiple organ systems. An in-depth knowledge of both typical and atypical imaging features is critical in the multidisciplinary diagnosis and follow-up of patients with these diseases.

Take-Home Messages

- The classic imaging features of sarcoidosis include (1) clustered nodules in the peribronchovascular and subpleural interstitium (a perilymphatic distribution), (2) symmetric bilateral hilar and mediastinal lymphadenopathy, and/or (3) peribronchovascular and upper lung fibrosis.
- Diagnosis in CTDs is made predominantly using clinical and serologic criteria; however imaging is critical in determining the predominant pattern of imaging present.
- The most typical patterns of lung disease seen with CTD include nonspecific interstitial pneumonia, organizing pneumonia, and lymphoid interstitial pneumonia. These patterns not infrequently overlap.
- Vasculitis is classified by the size of vessels involved, and lung disease is most commonly seen with small-vessel vasculitis including granulomatosis with polyangiitis, microscopic polyangiitis, and eosinophilic granulomatosis with polyangiitis.
- The most typical CT appearances of vasculitis include multiple cavitary nodules of varying sizes and alveolar hemorrhage characterized by bilateral ground-glass opacity and consolidation.

References

1. Valeyre D, Prasse A, Nunes H, Uzunhan Y, Brillet P-Y, Müller-Quernheim J. Sarcoidosis. Lancet. 2014;383:1155–67.
2. Spagnolo P, Sverzellati N, Wells AU, Hansell DM. Imaging aspects of the diagnosis of sarcoidosis. Eur Radiol. 2014;24:807–16. Springer Berlin Heidelberg.
3. Criado E, Sánchez M, Ramírez J, et al. Pulmonary sarcoidosis: typical and atypical manifestations at high-resolution CT with pathologic correlation. Radiographics. 2010;30:1567–86.
4. Treglia G, Annunziata S, Sobic-Saranovic D, Bertagna F, Caldarella C, Giovanella L. The role of 18F-FDG-PET and PET/CT in patients with sarcoidosis: an updated evidence-based review. Acad Radiol. 2014;21:675–84.
5. Walsh SL, Wells AU, Sverzellati N, et al. An integrated clinicoradiological staging system for pulmonary sarcoidosis: a case-cohort study. Lancet Respir Med. 2014;2:123–30.
6. Fischer A, Bois du R. Interstitial lung disease in connective tissue disorders. Lancet. 2012;380:689–98.
7. Travis WD, Costabel U, Hansell DM, et al. An official American Thoracic Society/European Respiratory Society statement: update of the international multidisciplinary classification of the idiopathic interstitial pneumonias. Am J Respir Crit Care Med. 2013;188:733–48. American Thoracic Society.
8. Kim EA, Lee KS, Johkoh T, et al. Interstitial lung diseases associated with collagen vascular diseases: radiologic and histopathologic findings. Radiographics. 2002;22:S151–65.
9. Mori S, Cho I, Koga Y, Sugimoto M. Comparison of pulmonary abnormalities on high-resolution computed tomography in patients with early versus longstanding rheumatoid arthritis. J Rheumatol. 2008;35:1513–21.
10. Remy-Jardin M, Remy J, Cortet B, Mauri F, Delcambre B. Lung changes in rheumatoid arthritis: CT findings. Radiology. 1994;193:375–82.
11. Perez T, Remy-Jardin M, Cortet B. Airways involvement in rheumatoid arthritis: clinical, functional, and HRCT findings. Am J Respir Crit Care Med. 1998;157:1658–65. American Thoracic Society, New York, NY.
12. Tanaka N, Kim JS, Newell JD, et al. Rheumatoid arthritis-related lung diseases: CT findings. Radiology. 2004;232:81–91.
13. Hilliquin P, Renoux M, Perrot S, Puéchal X, Menkès CJ. Occurrence of pulmonary complications during methotrexate therapy in rheumatoid arthritis. Br J Rheumatol. 1996;35:441–5.
14. Kim DS, Yoo B, Lee JS, et al. The major histopathologic pattern of pulmonary fibrosis in scleroderma is nonspecific interstitial pneumonia. Sarcoidosis Vasc Diffuse Lung Dis. 2002;19:121–7.
15. Fagan KA, Badesch DB. Pulmonary hypertension associated with connective tissue disease. Prog Cardiovasc Dis. 2002;45:225–34.
16. Remy-Jardin M, Remy J, Wallaert B, Bataille D, Hatron PY. Pulmonary involvement in progressive systemic sclerosis: sequential evaluation with CT, pulmonary function tests, and bronchoalveolar lavage. Radiology. 1993;188:499–506.
17. Wells AU, Cullinan P, Hansell DM, et al. Fibrosing alveolitis associated with systemic sclerosis has a better prognosis than lone cryptogenic fibrosing alveolitis. Am J Respir Crit Care Med. 1994;149:1583–90. American Public Health Association.
18. Bouros D, Wells AU, Nicholson AG, et al. Histopathologic subsets of fibrosing alveolitis in patients with systemic sclerosis and their relationship to outcome. Am J Respir Crit Care Med. 2002;165:1581–6. American Thoracic Society.
19. Fenlon HM, Doran M, Sant SM, Breatnach E. High-resolution chest CT in systemic lupus erythematosus. AJR Am J Roentgenol. 1996;166:301–7. American Public Health Association.
20. Wiedemann HP, Matthay RA. Pulmonary manifestations of systemic lupus erythematosus. J Thorac Imaging. 1992;7:1–18.
21. Swigris JJ, Fischer A, Gillis J, Gilles J, Meehan RT, Brown KK. Pulmonary and thrombotic manifestations of systemic lupus erythematosus. Chest. 2008;133:271–80.
22. Arakawa H, Yamada H, Kurihara Y, et al. Nonspecific interstitial pneumonia associated with polymyositis and dermatomyositis: serial high-resolution CT findings and functional correlation. Chest. 2003;123:1096–103.
23. Fischer A, Swigris JJ, Bois du RM, et al. Anti-synthetase syndrome in ANA and anti-Jo-1 negative patients presenting with idiopathic interstitial pneumonia. Respir Med. 2009;103:1719–24.
24. Taouli B, Brauner MW, Mourey I, Lemouchi D, Grenier PA. Thin-section chest CT findings of primary Sjögren's syndrome: correlation with pulmonary function. Eur Radiol. 2002;12:1504–11. Springer-Verlag.
25. Franquet T, Giménez A, Monill JM, Díaz C, Geli C. Primary Sjögren's syndrome and associated lung disease: CT findings in 50 patients. AJR Am J Roentgenol. 1997;169:655–8. American Public Health Association.
26. Saito Y, Terada M, Takada T, et al. Pulmonary involvement in mixed connective tissue disease: comparison with other collagen vascular diseases using high resolution CT. J Comput Assist Tomogr. 2002;26:349–57.
27. Fischer A, Antoniou KM, Brown KK, et al. An official European Respiratory Society/American Thoracic Society research state-

ment: interstitial pneumonia with autoimmune features. Eur Respir J. 2015;46:976–87.
28. Khan I, Watts RA. Classification of ANCA-associated vasculitis. Curr Rheumatol Rep. 2013;15:383. Springer US.
29. Chung MP, Yi CA, Lee HY, Han J, Lee KS. Imaging of pulmonary vasculitis. Radiology. 2010;255:322–41. Radiological Society of North America, Inc.
30. Marten K, Schnyder P, Schirg E, Prokop M, Rummeny EJ, Engelke C. Pattern-based differential diagnosis in pulmonary vasculitis using volumetric CT. AJR Am J Roentgenol. 2005;184:720–33.
31. Specks U, DeRemee RA. Granulomatous vasculitis. Wegener's granulomatosis and Churg-Strauss syndrome. Rheum Dis Clin N Am. 1990;16:377–97.
32. Worthy SA, Müller NL, Hansell DM, Flower CD. Churg-Strauss syndrome: the spectrum of pulmonary CT findings in 17 patients. AJR Am J Roentgenol. 1998;170:297–300. American Public Health Association.
33. Camus P, Piard F, Ashcroft T, Gal AA, Colby TV. The lung in inflammatory bowel disease. Medicine (Baltimore). 1993;72:151–83.
34. Garg K, Lynch DA, Newell JD. Inflammatory airways disease in ulcerative colitis: CT and high-resolution CT features. J Thorac Imaging. 1993;8:159–63.
35. Urban BA, Fishman EK, Goldman SM, et al. CT evaluation of amyloidosis: spectrum of disease. Radiographics. 1993;13:1295–308.
36. Bhargava P, Rushin JM, Rusnock EJ, et al. Pulmonary light chain deposition disease: report of five cases and review of the literature. Am J Surg Pathol. 2007;31:267–76.
37. Brun A-L, Touitou-Gottenberg D, Haroche J, et al. Erdheim-Chester disease: CT findings of thoracic involvement. Eur Radiol. 2010;20:2579–87.
38. Ryu JH, Sekiguchi H, Yi ES. Pulmonary manifestations of immunoglobulin G4-related sclerosing disease. Eur Respir J. 2012;39:180–6. European Respiratory Society.

12

Thoracic Trauma

Loren Ketai and Steven L. Primack

Learning Objectives

- Understand how the CT spectrum of ATAI influences treatment decisions.
- Know the imaging appearance of the most common survivable cardiac injuries.
- Describe the differences in imaging findings between blunt and penetrating diaphragm injuries.
- Know the coexisting injury patterns associated with fractures and dislocations involving the sternum and shoulder girdle.

Both blunt and penetrating traumas commonly affect the thorax, blunt trauma occurring predominantly as the result of motor vehicle collisions. The thorax is the fourth most injured area in unrestrained motor vehicle passengers but is the most commonly injured area in individuals who are restrained by a seat belt [1]. Other common causes of blunt thoracic trauma include falls from heights of greater than 10 feet and motor vehicle collisions involving pedestrians/bicyclists.

While not as common as blunt thoracic injury, penetrating thoracic trauma is not rare. Records from the Centers for Disease control (CDC) show that in 2016, the deaths from gunshot wounds in the United States were comparable to the number of deaths from motor vehicle accidents (MVAs). Tissue damage from these injuries may be complex and is dependent not only on the trajectory of the projectile but upon the pressure gradient that radiates laterally from the tract causing temporary cavitation within adjacent tissue [2]. In both blunt and penetrating trauma, radiologists' familiarity with typical injury patterns assists with rapid diagnosis and treatment.

While the initial screening test in thoracic trauma is the frontal chest radiograph obtained in the trauma bay, in many emergency rooms, this is accompanied by E-FAST (extended focused assessment with sonography in trauma) performed by non-radiologists. In addition to detecting intraabdominal trauma, this study can detect important thoracic injuries, specifically pneumothoraces, hemothoraces, and hemopericardium. Patients with large hemothoraces or hemopericardium can be directed to emergent surgery, while the remaining patients with significant trauma mechanism should usually be further evaluated by CT [3]. Among patients with penetrating trauma, CT with multiplanar reconstructions is particularly useful to determine the trajectory of a bullet through the chest and identify injured organs. Used in hemodynamically stable patients, CT can accurately identify those patients that can be managed nonoperatively, reported negative predictive values as high as 99% [4].

12.1 Acute Traumatic Aortic Injury

Acute traumatic aortic injury (ATAI) is a common cause of prehospital mortality in MVAs, accounting for approximately 15–20% of deaths in high-speed collisions. Of individuals with ATAI, 70–90% die at the trauma scene [5]. Most of the surviving 10–20% individuals with ATAI from blunt trauma undergo CT imaging. Patients with penetrating aortic trauma who reach the hospital usually proceed to surgery without intervening imaging.

Decision rules using clinical parameters for predicting ATAI have had very limited success. An initial case control study restricted true positive cases to those confirmed by surgery or conventional angiography. In that population, the

L. Ketai
Department of Radiology, University of New Mexico HSC, Albuquerque, NM, USA
e-mail: lketai@unm.edu

S. L. Primack (✉)
Department of Diagnostic Radiology, Oregon Health and Science University, Portland, OR, USA
e-mail: primacks@ohsu.edu

likelihood of ATAI was approximately 5% if three clinical predictors were present and 30% if four or more predictors were present. A more recent case control validation study performed by the same group in the era of CT angiography identified only four composite clinical criteria that were predictive of ATAI (abdominopelvic injury, thoracic injury, hypotension, and history of MVA while unrestrained). The likelihood of ATAI in patients with three or four of these criteria was only 2%, much lower than the derivation study, and is probably more relevant to current clinical practice [6].

Among patients surviving to reach the hospital, 90% of blunt aortic injuries are seen at the level of the aortic isthmus, which extends from the origin of the subclavian artery approximately 2 cm to the insertion of the ligamentum arteriosum. The propensity for injury to occur at this location is incompletely understood, and multiple mechanisms have been proposed. The ascending aorta is injured in less than 5% of blunt ATAI victims who survive transport, but injuries at that site are more common at autopsy series [5]. Ascending aorta injuries are frequently (80%) associated with significant cardiac damage, including damage to the aortic valve or pericardial tamponade. Traumatic aortic injuries located at the diaphragmatic hiatus account for less than 2% of cases.

The continuous motion of the heart during cross-sectional scanning leads to motion artifacts of the ascending aorta that can have the appearance of aortic dissection or pseudoaneurysm in non-cardiac-gated acquisitions, even with current rapid acquisition multidetector CT scanners. These artifacts can often be differentiated from intimal flaps, appearing less distinct and sometimes extending outside the vessel wall.

Because less than 5% of surviving patients will have an ascending aortic injury, the benefit of gated cardiac CT at initial presentation is limited. Most patients with ATAI are too unstable to undergo prolonged imaging, and thus evaluation of the aorta with standard, nongated contrast-enhanced CT is generally preferred. In patients whose initial CT contains artifacts closely mimicking aortic root injury, cardiac-gated CT can be performed.

Transesophageal echocardiography is a potential alternative to CTA for exclusion of ATAI if there are no contraindications, such as vertebral body fracture or severe maxillofacial injury. The disadvantages of transesophageal echocardiography include the logistical time required to perform the study and its user dependence as well as inability to evaluate the remainder of the thorax.

ATAI ranges from intimal hemorrhage to complete transection. The adventitia may be injured in up to 40% of cases and is almost universally fatal because of rapid exsanguination, although in rare cases, temporary tamponade may be achieved by surrounding mediastinal soft tissues. Historically, of those patients who survive to the hospital after aortic rupture, 22% die during initial resuscitation, 28% die during or shortly after surgical repair, and 14% develop subsequent paraplegia [7]. Shift of current practice to endovascular stenting has been associated with post-procedure mortality rates <10% and a decrease in the incidence of paraplegia to <2% [8].

12.1.1 Radiography

Although the principal purpose of the trauma bay chest radiograph is the rapid detection of pneumothorax and hemothorax, it can also be assessed for evidence of a mediastinal bleeding. This bleeding can be seen secondary to ATAI, sternal/thoracic spine fracture, or small artery or vein damage within the mediastinum. The resulting mediastinal blood can be free or partially free flowing (associated with small mediastinal vessel rupture) or form a contained hematoma which is more concerning for an ATAI.

The negative predictive value of a properly obtained chest radiograph may be as high as 93–98%, but consideration of mechanism severity is important before ATAI can be excluded. The positive predictive value of an abnormal radiograph remains low, only 15%. Specificity of mediastinal widening is degraded by mediastinal fat, vascular congestion, anomalous vessels, and rotation. When the right paratracheal region is equal to or more opaque than the aortic arch or a left apical cap is present, mediastinal widening is more likely to represent a free-flowing mediastinal blood [9].

Radiographic findings more suggestive of a contained aortic rupture include rightward deviation of an enteric tube, rightward deviation of the trachea, downward displacement of the left main bronchus, loss of aortic arch definition, increased aortic arch opacity, and increased width and opacity of the descending aorta [9].

12.1.2 Computed Tomography

Multidetector helical CT is a very sensitive diagnostic tool for exclusion of ATAI, often quoted as the gold standard for ATAI detection [10]. A morphologically normal aorta with no mediastinal hematoma has a 100% negative predictive value for exclusion of ATAI. The positive predictive value of an equivocal study (i.e., para-aortic hematoma only) is uncertain; these studies require additional imaging or clinical follow-up. Mediastinal hematomas not in contact with the aorta, but located in the anterior or posterior mediastinum, are more likely to be related to chest wall or spinal fractures [11]. If the patient is a victim of penetrating trauma with a wound trajectory passing near the aorta, a repeat CTA should be obtained in 24–48 h.

The direct signs of ATAI on CT include aortic wall or contour abnormality (pseudoaneurysm) contrast extravasation (Fig. 12.1), polypoid intraluminal clot or low-density filling

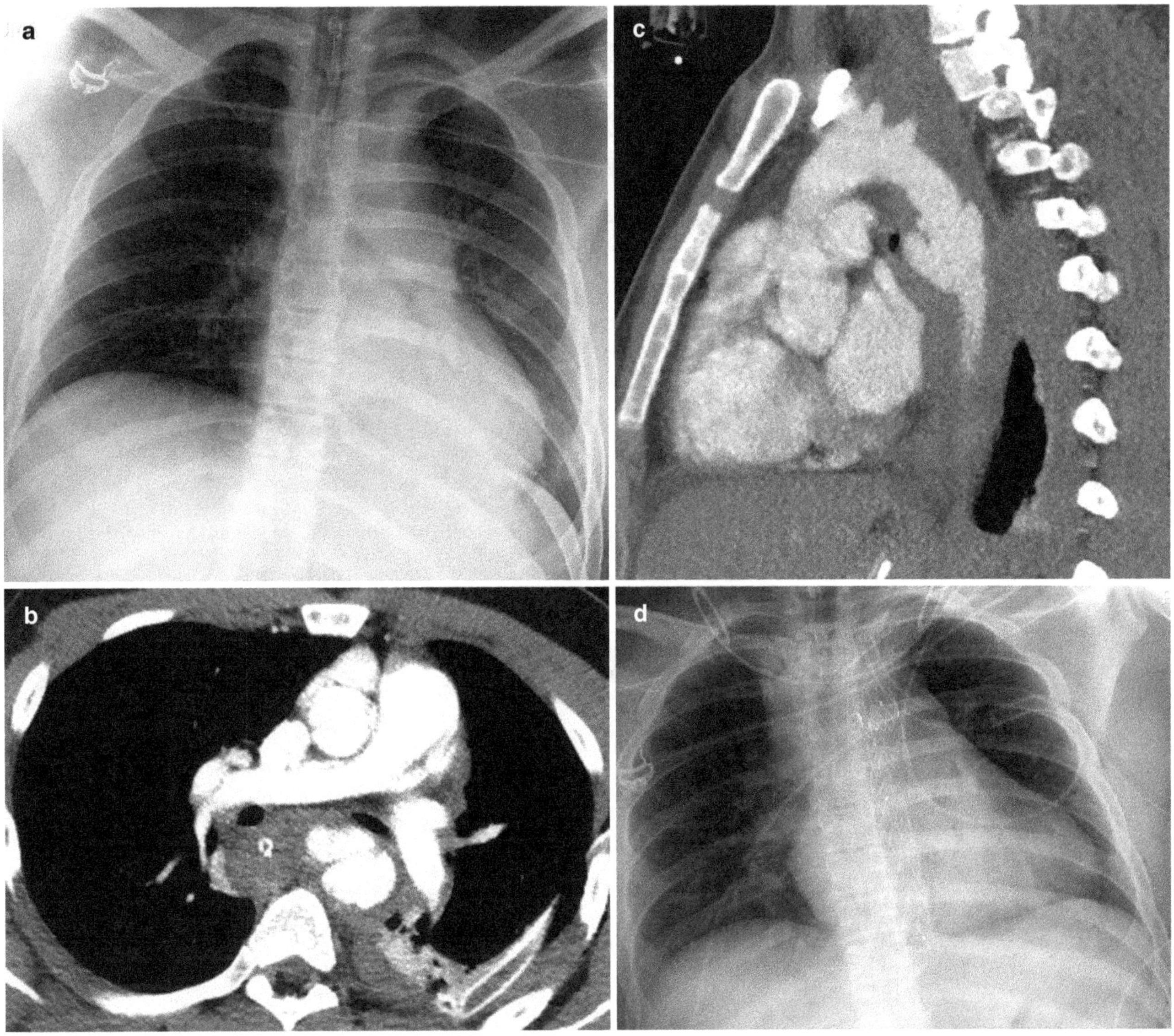

Fig. 12.1 Traumatic aortic injury. (**a**) AP chest radiograph shows widened mediastinum and indistinctness of aortic arch contour. (**b, c**) Axial (**b**) and sagittal (**c**) contrast-enhanced CT demonstrates disruption of the proximal descending thoracic aortic wall contour with contrast extravasation indicating aortic rupture. (**d**) AP chest radiograph following intervention with aortic stent

defect, change in caliber of the aorta (i.e., pseudocoarctation), and dissection [10]. The least severe injury, intimal tear, appears on contrast-enhanced CT as either a rounded or triangular intraluminal filling defect attached to the wall of the aorta.

Recently the surgical treatment of ATAI has become more nuanced, and reporting of ATAI should include details useful for surgical decision-making. Initially nonoperative therapy was focused on "minimal" aortic injuries that were sometimes described as small (<1 cm) intimal flaps (Fig. 12.2). More recently initial nonoperative therapy has been extended to intimal injuries extending over more than 1 cm and to intramural hematomas [12]. These intramural hematomas may involve the entire circumference of the aortic wall or occur within a portion of the aortic wall, such that the high-attenuation thrombus appears crescentic in shape. Neither intimal injuries nor intramural hematomas, classified as grade I and II in the surgical literature, are accompanied by an abnormal outer contour of the aorta. If initial management is nonoperative, follow-up CT imaging is necessary. Exact timing of follow-up is not well established, but a reasonable approach would be a repeat CT in 36–72 h and then again in several weeks if stable [13]. A minority of these injuries demonstrate progression on follow-up CT imaging, at which time endovascular stenting can be performed if necessary.

Unlike lower-grade injuries described above, pseudoaneurysm do cause an abnormal outer contour abnormality. Small pseudoaneurysms (less than 1 cm in length and less than 50% of the aortic diameter) may also be initially treated nonoperatively in hemodynamically stable patients

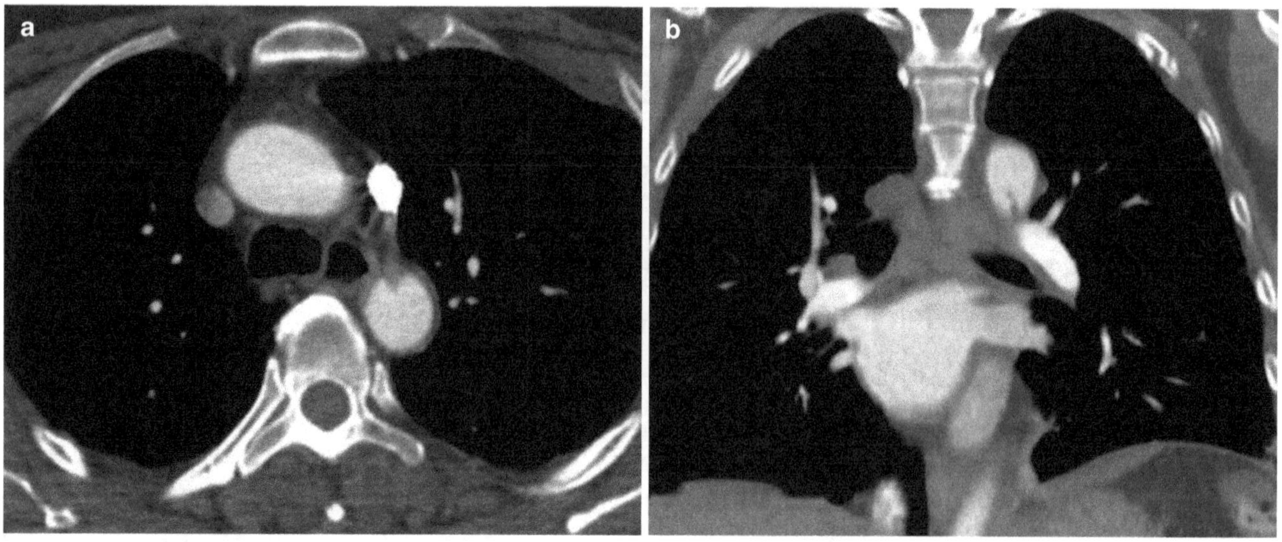

Fig. 12.2 Minimal traumatic aortic injury. (**a**, **b**) Axial (**a**) and coronal (**b**) contrast-enhanced CT demonstrates an intimal flap involving the proximal descending thoracic aorta

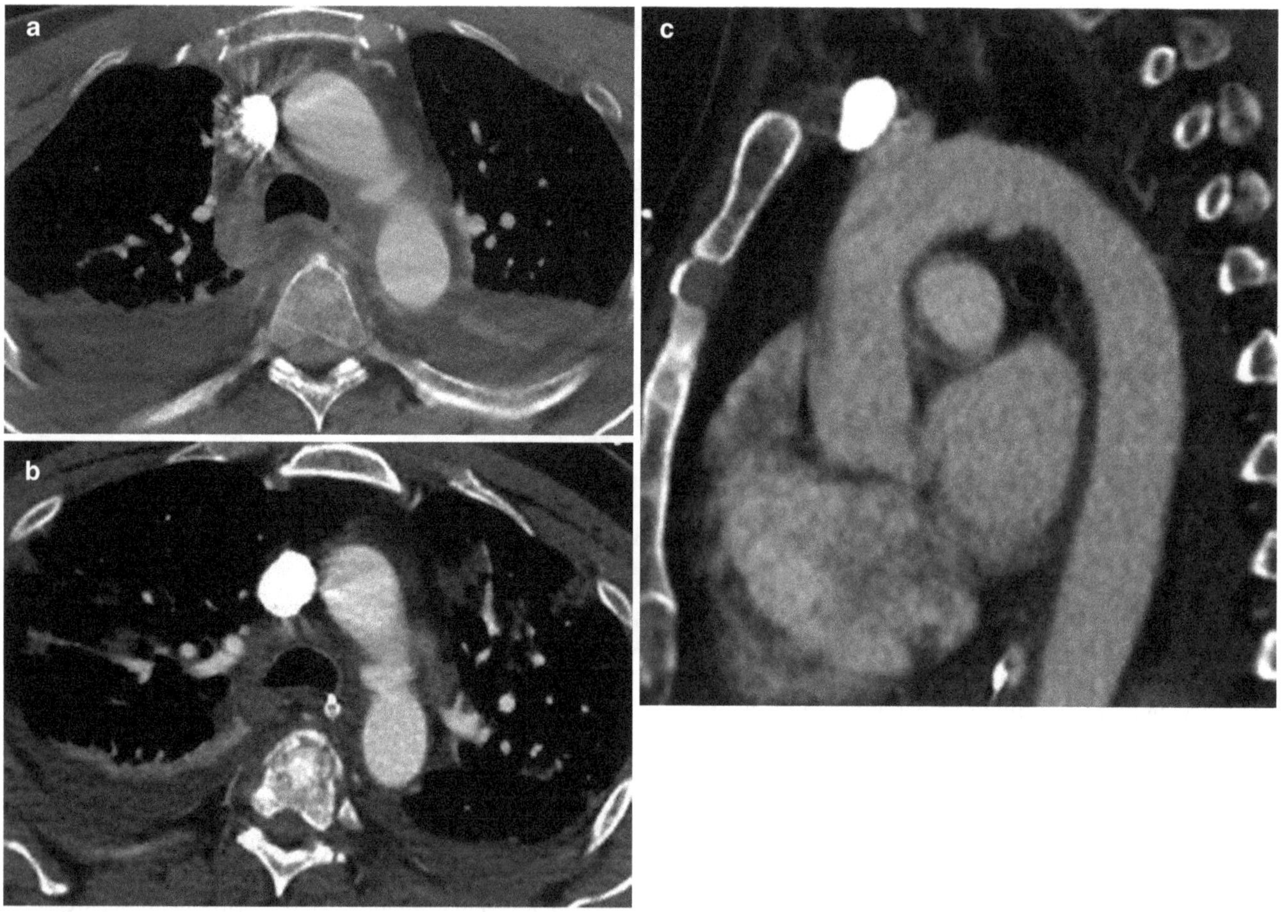

Fig. 12.3 Minimal traumatic aortic injury. (**a**) Axial contrast-enhanced CT demonstrates a small pseudoaneurysm arising from the undersurface of the aortic arch. (**b**, **c**) 2 weeks following presentation, axial (**b**) and sagittal (**c**) contrast-enhanced CT show no change in small pseudoaneurysm

(Fig. 12.3). Those pseudoaneurysms that involve greater than 50% of the aortic circumference or are accompanied by an adjacent mediastinal hematoma >15 mm thick are at higher risk for progression and may be difficult to differentiate from aortic ruptures. These injuries warrant more urgent intervention. True thoracic aortic rupture/transection remains a surgical emergency.

Key Points

Report Elements to Include on CTAs Positive for TAI

- Presence of intimal flap and its length
- Presence of endoluminal thrombus
- Presence of outer contour abnormality
  - Extent of involvement of the aortic circumference (e.g., <50%)
  - Length of abnormality along the axis of the aorta (e.g., <1 cm)
- Distance of proximal extent of injury from the subclavian artery (relevant for TEVAR)

12.2 Great Vessel and Supra-aortic Branch Vessel Injury

Injuries to the superior and inferior vena cava, the pulmonary artery, and the pulmonary veins are commonly associated with other severe, non-survivable injuries and therefore are rarely imaged. When encountered, SVC ruptures are associated with right atrial rupture and azygous vein ruptures and are accompanied by mediastinal hematoma [14]. Blunt trauma injuries to the supra-aortic branch vessels, the brachiocephalic artery (right subclavian/right common carotid), left common carotid artery, and the left subclavian artery are also uncommon. In one retrospective series of blunt trauma, ATAI made up 84% of the vascular injuries, isolated branch vessel injury 14%, and combined injuries only 4% [15].

Penetrating trauma with potential injury to the great vessels and supra-aortic vessels often involves a transmediastinal trajectory of the projectile. These are frequently severe injuries, and hemodynamically unstable patients usually proceed to surgery with minimal imaging. Patients who are hemodynamically stable may undergo echocardiography or E-Fast exam followed by CTA. Since transmediastinal penetrating trauma can involve the esophagus and tracheobronchial tree, exams optimally include upper alimentary tract contrast (see below).

12.2.1 Radiography

The screening trauma radiograph is unlikely to aid in the diagnosis of great vessel and supra-aortic branch vessel injury, other than to identify ballistic trajectory in the setting of penetrating trauma. As in ATAI, a mediastinal hematoma is usually present.

12.2.2 Computed Tomography

Similar to the setting of ATAI, CT may demonstrate intimal flaps and pseudoaneurysms. Alternatively, subtle findings, such as asymmetric vascular caliber or decreased contrast enhancement, may provide evidence of vascular injury. Although multidetector CT scans are likely to detect a traumatic injury to the supra-aortic branch vessel, catheter angiography maintains a role in confirming injury [15].

CT findings caused by penetrating vascular trauma include those signs of injury described above, as well formation of arteriovenous fistula. Additional indirect findings include proximity to ballistic fragments and end organ infarcts due to peripheral embolization of intraluminal thrombus. As for blunt injuries, many vessel abnormalities seen on CTA warrant catheter-directed angiography for confirmation and possible treatment.

12.3 Cardiac Injury

Significant cardiac injuries are uncommon in blunt trauma victims surviving to reach the emergency department. Autopsy data indicate that numerous prehospital deaths result from traumatic cardiac or valvular rupture. Penetrating injury to the heart is traditionally suspected when wounds penetrate the "cardiac box," an area on the anterior thorax bounded by the clavicles, the midclavicular lines, and the costal margin where intersected by the midclavicular lines. Recent literature has defined the cardiac box in three dimensions, extending anterior-posterior, particularly in the left hemithorax.

Blunt cardiac injury can cause cardiac contusion and more critical injuries specifically pericardial, myocardial, or valvular rupture. Myocardial injuries most commonly involve the right ventricular free wall, while valvular injuries more commonly occur in the left-sided chambers, likely related to higher transvalvular pressures. The most innocuous and most common of these injuries, cardiac contusion, is usually diagnosed based on troponin levels and ECG findings. Although CT can reveal multiple ancillary signs of cardiac contusion, myocardial enhancement is an insensitive indicator and should not be used to rule out cardiac injury [16]. Echocardiogram and occasionally MRI may aid diagnosis of cardiac contusion by evaluating for wall motion abnormalities.

Hemopericardium may be the result of cardiac chamber rupture (usually fatal prior to arrival in the hospital), myocardial contusion, aortic root injury, coronary lacerations, or damage to the small surrounding pericardial vessels such as those damaged from displaced rib fractures. Pericardial rupture is a rare injury. It commonly occurs on the left side, often along the course of the phrenic nerve, and can be accompanied by tears of the adjacent pleura or diaphragm. Such injuries become hemodynamically significant when the heart herniates through the tear, impeding cardiac filling and potentially causing coronary vessel occlusion. The proposed mechanism of injury for pericardial rupture likens the injury to a pendulum since the inferior portion of the heart is free floating without significant attachments. In the setting of a lateral deceleration injury, the heart presumably collides with the adjacent pericardium, creating the rupture [17]. Cardiac herniation through a pericardial defect may not be present initially and may occur after the administration or discontinuation of positive-pressure ventilation.

The most commonly ruptured cardiac chamber in the autopsy of blunt trauma victims is the right ventricle, while the atria are the most commonly ruptured chambers in individuals who survive to hospitalization. Penetrating trauma most commonly affects the right ventricle, followed in frequency by the left ventricle. Right ventricle and right atrial wounds are more likely to be survivable than left-sided chambers. Unfortunately, the increased relative incidence of gunshot wounds compared to stabbing injuries over the last two decades has been associated with multichamber cardiac injuries, which have a much lower survival rate.

12.3.1 Radiography

Hemopericardium may or may not be evident on chest radiograph at presentation. Chest radiography may show an unusual position or configuration of the heart if cardiac herniation is present. As noted above, in the setting of penetrating trauma, chest radiographs can yield important clues to the projectile's trajectory.

12.3.2 Computed Tomography

Most patients who have a mechanism of injury sufficient to produce hemopericardium are imaged with CT if stable. Simple fluid should demonstrate attenuation values of 0–10 HU, whereas hemopericardium will have attenuation values in the 35 HU range. The rapid accumulation of hemopericardium may result in cardiac tamponade, the diagnosis suggested when CT demonstrates a triad of high-attenuation pericardial effusion, distention of the inferior vena cava and renal veins, and periportal low-attenuation fluid. Hemopericardium is visible on nearly all CT scans in cases of pericardial rupture. Not all pericardial tears are associated with cardiac herniation; the chest radiograph and CT scan may be unrevealing. Pericardial rupture is diagnosed on CT by the presence of a focal pericardial defect with a collar sign of herniated cardiac tissue. The presence of adjacent pneumothorax, pneumomediastinum, or both may complicate the diagnosis if the pericardium is mistaken for the pleura.

CT does not play a diagnostic role in patients with penetrating injury that are either hemodynamically unstable or demonstrate hemopericardium on ultrasound. As with transmediastinal penetrating injuries, CT may be useful in establishing bullet trajectory in hemodynamically stable patients and suggest occult cardiac injury based on the projectile track or the presence of ballistic fragments. CT may demonstrate occult cardiac trauma in 3–4% of hemodynamically stable patients with penetrating thoracic trauma, usually by demonstrating hemopericardium or pneumopericardium [18].

12.4 Pneumomediastinum

Pneumomediastinum is present in 10% of patients with blunt thoracic injury and is most commonly secondary to the Macklin effect [19]. This is the process by which air dissects along bronchovascular bundles after alveolar rupture and spreads to the mediastinum. Mediastinal air may also occur from the extension of subcutaneous or deep cervical emphysema. Direct extension of retroperitoneal air to the mediastinum occurs via periesophageal and periaortic fascial planes and at the level of the sternocostal attachment of the diaphragm [9].

12.4.1 Radiography

Pneumomediastinum can be identified on the chest radiograph by visualization of lucency along the pericardium and lateral mediastinum outlined laterally by the pleura [9]. Pneumomediastinum may be difficult to differentiate from medial pneumothorax; this can best be done by searching for other manifestations of the two entities. Air within the mediastinum characteristically outlines other structures so that they are more conspicuous than usual. These include the "ring around the artery sign" (air surrounds right pulmonary artery), "tubular artery sign" (air outlines supra-aortic vessels), and "double bronchial wall sign" (air outlines the outer contour of a major bronchus) [20]. Air posterior to the pericardium yields the continuous diaphragm.

Differentiation of pneumomediastinum from pneumopericardium on radiography relies on recognition that air is not confined to the limits of the pericardium, an assessment most

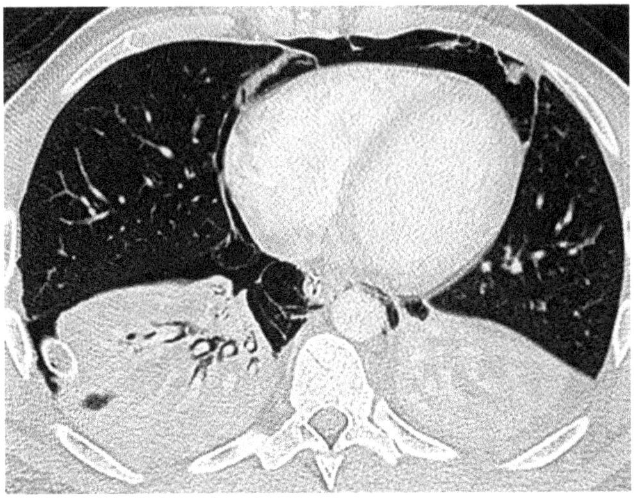

Fig. 12.4 Pneumomediastinum due to Macklin effect following gunshot wound to the right lung. Axial CT demonstrates extensive pneumomediastinum secondary to alveolar rupture. Note peribronchovascular interstitial air in the right lower lobe. Macklin effect is most commonly related to blunt trauma or barotrauma

commonly confirmed by identifying subcutaneous emphysema in the neck. An additional pitfall is the error in perception caused by Mach effect, which causes an apparent lucency surrounding the convexity of the heart border that mimics pneumomediastinum. The absence of an adjacent opaque pleural line usually differentiates this from true pneumomediastinum.

Pneumomediastinum typically resolves with time. Serious complications, such as tension pneumomediastinum, are rare. Failure of resolution or lack of improvement with time raises the suspicion of tracheobronchial or penetrating esophageal injury. Esophageal rupture from blunt trauma is rare.

12.4.2 Computed Tomography

CT can prove the presence of Macklin effect by demonstrating the triad of a bronchus, a pulmonary vessel, and an additional adjacent air collection (Fig. 12.4). The presence of Macklin effect does not exclude the possibility of a tracheobronchial or esophageal injury, though both are unlikely if the resulting pneumomediastinum is confined to the anterior compartment. The absence of the Macklin effect calls for increased scrutiny of the CT images to identify signs of esophageal or airway injury (see below).

12.5 Esophageal Injury

Esophageal injuries caused by non-iatrogenic trauma are rare but potentially catastrophic. Mortality for undiagnosed rupture after 24 h is 10–40%. Chest radiograph findings include pneumomediastinum and pleura effusions, left sided if the lower third of the esophagus is injured, right side if upper two thirds is injured. Fluoroscopic esophagography is moderately sensitive, e.g., 75%, and very specific but can be technically difficult to perform in critically ill patients. CT esophagography (CTE) performed after ingestion or instillation of contrast and effervescent granules was shown to be 100% sensitive in detecting injury in a small group of patients. A more recent study following a similar protocol with the exception of effervescent granules has reported a sensitivity near 80%. In the setting of penetrating trauma, concomitant performance of CTA and CTE may diminish specificity [21].

12.6 Airway Injury

Tracheobronchial injuries include mucosal tears and complete transection of the airway. These are uncommon injuries, occurring in 1–3% of patients with blunt thoracic trauma.

12.6.1 Radiography

The radiographic manifestations of tracheobronchial injury are usually nonspecific and include pneumomediastinum, pneumothorax, deep cervical emphysema, and subcutaneous emphysema. Injuries to the trachea or proximal left main bronchus typically result in pneumomediastinum but not pneumothorax. The fallen lung sign is specific to bronchial fracture. This sign describes the lung "falling" dependently, rather than collapsing centrally toward the hilum in the presence of a pneumothorax.

Tracheal or bronchial tear should be suspected with persistent or increasing soft tissue emphysema, or if pneumothorax persists despite continuous chest tube drainage. Extraluminal position of the endotracheal tube and cuff overinflation also indicate tracheal injury [22].

12.6.2 Computed Tomography

Approximately 75% of tracheobronchial injuries occur within 2 cm of the carina. Right main bronchus injuries generally occur closer to the carina (usually within 2.5 cm) than injuries to the left main bronchus, and the right main bronchus is injured more frequently than either the trachea or the left main bronchus. While CT can readily demonstrate secondary signs of trachea bronchial injury (pneumomediastinum and pneumothorax), older literature demonstrated relatively low sensitivity in detection of direct evidence of

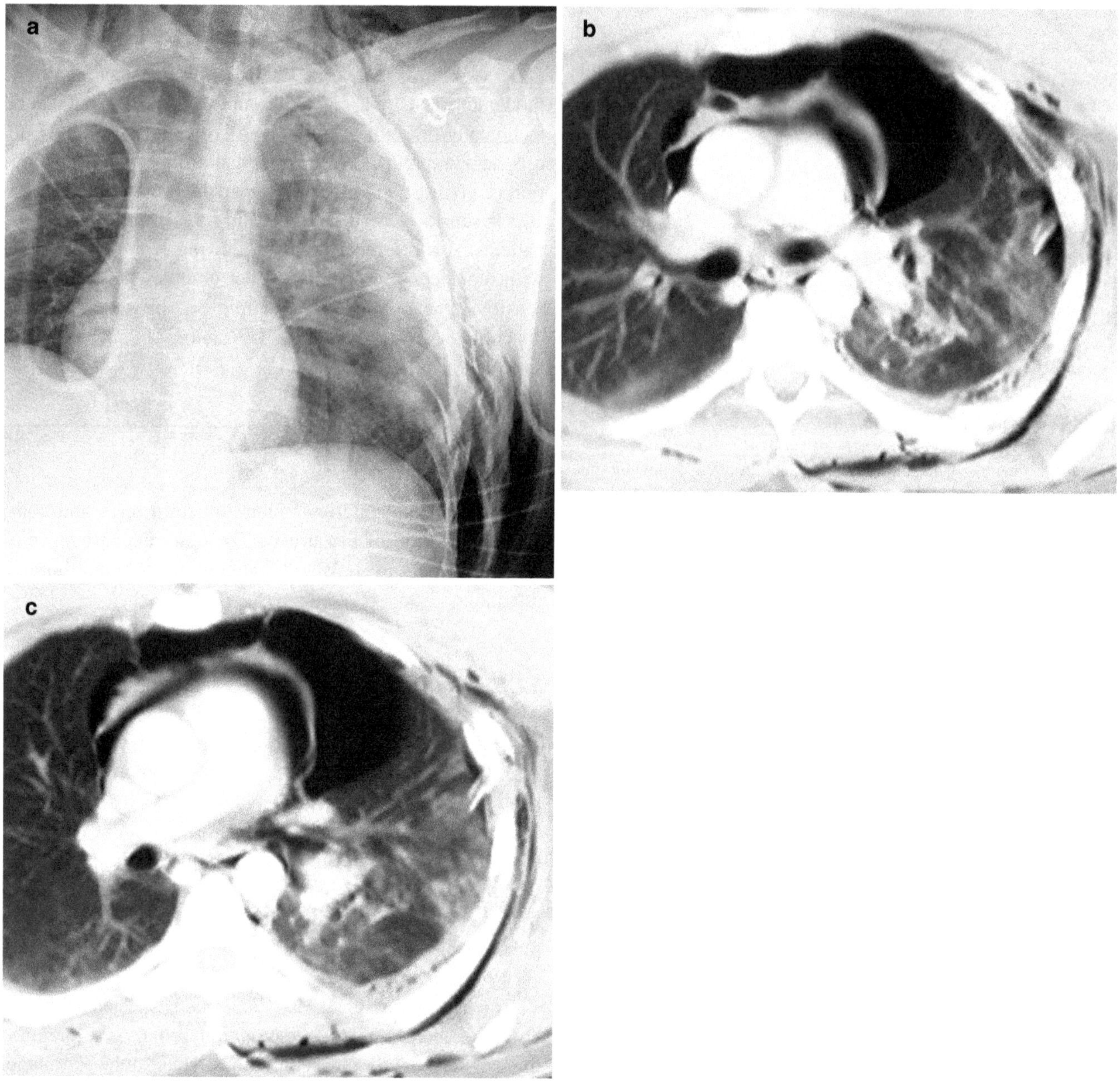

Fig. 12.5 Left bronchial tear. (**a**) AP chest radiograph shows extensive predominantly left-sided subcutaneous air, pneumomediastinum and left rib fractures. (**b**) CT at the level of the main bronchi shows extensive pneumomediastinum, left pneumothorax and subcutaneous air. (**c**) CT inferior to the level of (**b**) demonstrates complete disruption of left-sided airways. At surgery, there was near complete disruption of the distal left main bronchus with tear extending into the left upper and lobe bronchi

tracheobronchial injuries [23]. Direct visualization of a tear on CT can be difficult and best accomplished using thin (<3-mm) collimation (Fig. 12.5). More recent small series using thinner collimation have reported sensitivities >90% [24]. Nevertheless complications of tracheobronchial injury can be severe, including bronchopleural and tracheoesophageal fistulas, and chronic tracheal or bronchial stenosis leading to postobstructive pneumonia and bronchiectasis. Accordingly, a high index of suspicion and liberal use of bronchoscopy are important for the prompt diagnosis of tracheobronchial injury.

12.7 Pulmonary Contusion

Pulmonary contusion is seen in 30–70% of patients with blunt thoracic injury [1, 25]. It is the most common cause of pulmonary parenchymal opacification on chest radiography in blunt thoracic trauma. Short-term morbidity is substantial, and clinical signs and symptoms include hypoxia, mild fever, hemoptysis, and dyspnea. Acute respiratory failure may develop, requiring intubation and mechanical ventilation. Contusion may also be associated with long-term respiratory dysfunction.

Pulmonary contusion represents pulmonary hemorrhage and edema from disruption of the alveolar capillary membrane [9]. It is often caused by a direct blow to the chest wall with injury of the adjacent lung and may be accompanied by contrecoup injuries. Contusion is frequently seen where the lungs have been compressed against the denser heart, liver, chest wall, and spine. In deceleration injuries, such as motor vehicle accidents, the alveolar capillary membrane is disrupted as the lower-density alveoli shear from the higher-density bronchovascular bundles [9, 26].

12.7.1 Radiography

Pulmonary contusions can manifest as focal, patchy, or diffuse ground-glass opacities or parenchymal consolidation. These opacities cross fissural boundaries and are often present at the site of impaction and adjacent to rib fractures. The lung bases are most frequently affected secondary to increased basilar mobility [9]. Air bronchograms are usually absent owing to blood filling the airways.

Pulmonary parenchymal contusion follows a predictable temporal pattern on imaging. Contused lung may not be apparent on initial chest radiography but is usually present within 6 h after the inciting injury. Conspicuity of pulmonary opacities peaks at 24–72 h and gradually diminishes over 1 week although severe contusions may be radiographically evident for 2 weeks. Persistence beyond this duration should prompt consideration of other pulmonary diseases, such as pneumonia, atelectasis, aspiration pneumonitis, and hydrostatic or noncardiogenic pulmonary edema.

12.7.2 Computed Tomography

CT is superior to chest radiography in the detection of pulmonary contusion, but the clinical utility of this higher sensitivity is likely low. Contusions visible on CT but not on chest radiograph are associated with low mortality and low likelihood of requiring mechanical ventilation, both <5%. CT-based quantification of more extensive contusions may be helpful in predicting respiratory complications [27]. For example, the likelihood of development of ARDS is much higher in those patients with contusion involving >20% of the lung. CT may also be helpful in distinguishing acute aspiration from contusion, tree in bud opacities being present in the former and absent in pulmonary contusions. CT demonstration of subpleural sparing by parenchymal opacities (Fig. 12.6) has been shown to accurately differentiate pulmonary contusions from pneumonia and atelectasis in children.

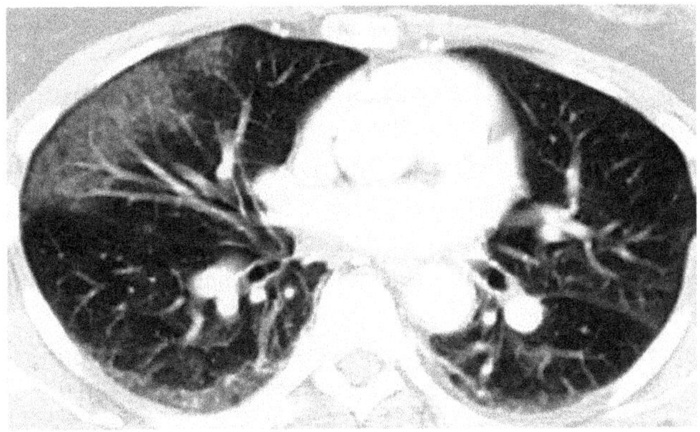

Fig. 12.6 Pulmonary contusion. Axial CT demonstrates peripheral homogeneous ground-glass opacity anteriorly in the right middle lobe. Note the thin region of subpleural sparing

12.8 Pulmonary Laceration and Traumatic Lung Cyst

Lacerations of the lung parenchyma cause traumatic lung cysts that may be filled with air (pneumatocele), blood (hematoma), or both. Several mechanisms of injury in blunt trauma have been proposed based on CT and surgical findings. Type 1, the most common type, occurs when a sudden compressive force causes alveolar rupture. Type 2 results from shear injury of the lower lung near the spine as a compressive force causes the lung to shift across the vertebral column. Type 3 manifests as lung cysts near the chest wall adjacent to a rib fracture fragment that has directly punctured the pulmonary parenchyma. Type 4 occurs when previously formed pleuropulmonary adhesions tear the lung after sudden movement or fracture of the attached chest wall.

12.8.1 Radiography

In approximately half of the cases, pulmonary lacerations are obscured by the consolidation related to pulmonary contusion on the initial chest radiograph. As the lung contusion resolves, pulmonary lacerations become visible as thin-walled cystic spaces or as soft tissue nodules (pulmonary hematomas). Radiographic resolution of traumatic lung cysts occurs over weeks to months. Uncommonly, the cysts persist for years. If clot remains in the cavity, these cysts can be mistaken for pulmonary nodules, and air-filled cavities may mimic other forms of cystic lung disease. Knowledge of previous trauma is important in correctly differentiating between these entities.

12.8.2 Computed Tomography

On CT imaging, traumatic lung cysts manifest as ovoid structures secondary to the elastic recoil of the lung [9]. Blood may completely fill the cavity causing an ovoid pulmonary hematoma or can partially fill the cavity, causing an air-fluid level is present. Large cystic spaces may be present, or blunt trauma can create multiple, small, air-filled lung cysts sometimes referred as "pulverized" or "Swiss cheese" appearance of the lungs [26]. The most common complication associated with a pulmonary laceration from blunt is a pneumothorax, and, while rare, other complications of traumatic lung cysts include infection with formation of a pulmonary abscess and the development of a bronchopleural fistula.

Lung lacerations commonly occur secondary to penetrating trauma and can manifest as linear lung defects along the projectile track or as round or oval air cysts. Like blunt trauma, penetrating trauma to the lungs usually can be managed with chest tube placement. Occasionally treatment of bronchopleural fistula or hemorrhage requires surgery, most commonly pneumonorraphy, tractotomy, or wedge resection, rarely lobectomy or pneumonectomy [28].

Key Points
Acute Lung Parenchymal Trauma

- Pulmonary contusion
  - Peak extent in 24–72 h
  - Peripheral, nonanatomic opacities, sometimes with immediate subpleural sparing
- Lung lacerations
  - Pneumatoceles appear as thin-walled cystic spaces.
    Unilocular or multilocular
    With or without air-fluid levels
  - Hematomas manifest as soft tissue masses that may persist for months.
- Acute aspiration
  - Tree in bud opacities, dependent lung or diffuse
  - May progress to ARDS

12.9 Hemothorax

Hemothorax occurs in approximately 50% of blunt thoracic trauma. Intrathoracic blood may arise from any surrounding structures, including the lung, mediastinum, thoracic wall, and diaphragm [26]. Hemothoraces may be large and increase rapidly if the bleeding source is arterial. Delayed hemothorax occurs rarely but is more common in patients with multiple rib fractures and/or flail chest. It presents as new onset sharp pleuritic chest pain and dyspnea. Occasionally, intraperitoneal blood migrates to the pleural space via diaphragmatic defects or rupture of the diaphragm.

12.9.1 Radiography

Small hemothoraces may be missed easily on chest radiography. On the supine radiograph, the apex is the most dependent portion of the pleural space, and fluid should be suspected if an apical cap is seen. Larger amounts of fluid will extend inferiorly along the lateral chest wall. On supine radiographs fluid also may manifest as a hazy opacity of the lower or entire hemithorax.

12.9.2 Computed Tomography

Hemorrhage within the pleural space typically can be differentiated from simple fluid or chyle by its relatively high, and often heterogeneous, attenuation, usually 35–70 HU. On contrast-enhanced CT, fluid with attenuation within 10–15 HU of vascular structures suggests active extravasation. Occasional findings include fluid-hematocrit levels and coalescence of blood clots that may mimic pleural-based tumors. CT can also be useful in quantifying retained hemothoraces, which are associated with high rates of pneumonia and empyema. Volume of residual hemothorax can be estimated by the following formula: volume = maximal length × (maximal distance from lung to pleural surface) [2]. Residual hemothorax >300 cc usually requires video-assisted thoracoscopy (VATS) or thoracotomy [29].

12.10 Pneumothorax

Pneumothorax is a common sequela of blunt chest trauma. Mechanisms include rupture of the alveoli and dissection through the interstitium to the pleural space, lung puncture from rib fracture fragments, tracheobronchial injury, and extension of pneumomediastinum through a tear in the parietal pleura [9, 25]. Small pneumothoraces can expand rapidly in patients receiving positive-pressure ventilation.

12.10.1 Radiography

The definitive radiographic finding of pneumothorax, a thin pleural line seen when air is present on either side of the visceral pleura, is often absent on supine radiographs. On supine radiographs air often accumulates in the anteromedial recess, the least dependent aspect of the pleural space and in the subpulmonic recess. Signs of anteromedial pneumothorax include sharp delineation of the mediastinal structures, outlining of the medial diaphragm beneath the heart, and a deep anterior cardiophrenic sulcus. A subpulmonic pneumothorax manifests as a hyperlucent upper abdominal quadrant, deep lateral costophrenic sulcus, and visualization of the anterior costophrenic sulcus and inferior surface of the lung. Subcutaneous air coupled with rib fractures indicates the presence of pneumothorax even if pleural air is radiographically occult.

Tension pneumothorax is a life-threatening condition that occurs when intrathoracic pressure exceeds atmospheric pressure, causing hemodynamic compromise. Mild mediastinal shift is commonly present in the absence of tension, since the negative pleural pressure in the unaffected hemithorax will always be lower than in the pleural space affected by the pneumothorax. The most specific radiographic finding of tension pneumothorax is depression or inversion of the diaphragm, which indicates that pleural pressure has exceeded subdiaphragmatic pressure [9].

12.10.2 Computed Tomography

CT is much more sensitive than radiography in the detection of pneumothoraces, 30% of which are missed on supine and semirecumbent chest radiographs [9]. Prospective study has suggested that many pneumothoraces seen on CT only may be managed without tube thoracostomy, even if on positive pressure ventilation [30]. Risk of tension pneumothorax has diminished with the current use of lower tidal volumes for mechanical ventilation, but this complication can still occur.

12.11 Traumatic Diaphragmatic Injury

Traumatic diaphragmatic tears can result from penetrating or blunt injury. Penetrating diaphragmatic injury is twice as common as blunt injury. Diaphragmatic rupture occurs in 0.8–8% of all patients with major blunt trauma [9]. Detection of diaphragmatic injury requires a high index of suspicion since masking of the injury by pleural fluid or pulmonary contusion may delay diagnosis. In addition, diaphragmatic injury is associated with other major traumatic injuries, including pneumothorax, hepatic and splenic lacerations, and pelvic fractures, which may distract from identification of diaphragmatic injury [31].

12.12 Mechanism of Injury

Blunt frontal impact can cause sufficient increase in intraabdominal pressure to rupture the diaphragm. Shearing injury may occur when a lateral blow distorts the chest wall [31]. Diaphragmatic tears associated with blunt trauma are usually 10 cm or greater. Injury is most frequently left-sided (75%) owing to the protective cushioning effect of the liver. Relative difficulty in detection of right-sided injury may contribute to its underdiagnosis and underrepresentation in the literature.

Penetrating injury results from shootings, stabbings, and, less commonly, iatrogenic causes such as a malpositioned chest tube. Stabbings and shootings usually result in left-sided diaphragmatic damage, presumably because most assailants are right-handed and facing their victims. Entrance wound occurring anywhere between the level of the nipples and inferior costal margin have the potential to cross the diaphragm. The resulting focal diaphragmatic injury often produces a small tear in the diaphragm (usually <1 cm in length). CT detection of penetrating diaphragm injury has increased in importance as more patients with penetrating trauma (most commonly stabbing victims) undergo nonoperative management, such that laparotomy cannot be relied upon to discover small diaphragm defects. Occult diaphragm injury has been found in up to 20% of patients with penetrating trauma who would otherwise be managed nonoperatively [32].

12.12.1 Radiography

The chest radiograph, although a useful screening tool, is relatively insensitive in the detection of diaphragmatic rupture. Overall sensitivity ranges from 17% to 64%, although serial radiographs can increase sensitivity by 12% [10]. Radiographic signs of diaphragmatic injury include obscuration of the hemidiaphragm, elevation of the hemidiaphragm, and contralateral shift of the mediastinum [31]. The most specific radiographic finding of diaphragmatic injury is the presence of gas-containing stomach or bowel within the thorax. Termination of a nasogastric tube within the left hemithorax is another specific finding.

12.12.2 Computed Tomography

CT using thin collimation and thin reconstruction images (1- to 2-mm-thick slices) is the imaging modality of choice in the evaluation of suspected diaphragmatic injury in patients with blunt or penetrating trauma. Sagittal and coronal reformations have been shown to increase sensitivity and confidence of interpretation. Sensitivities of 70–90% are reported.

A constellation of CT findings has been evaluated for the detection of diaphragmatic rupture. The most frequently cited are direct discontinuity or focal defect of the diaphragm, intrathoracic herniation of abdominal viscera, the collar sign, and the dependent viscera sign (Fig. 12.7). Visualization of a focal discontinuity of the diaphragm is 73–82% sensitive and 90% specific for diaphragmatic injury. Bochdalek hernias, focal defects in the posterolateral dia-

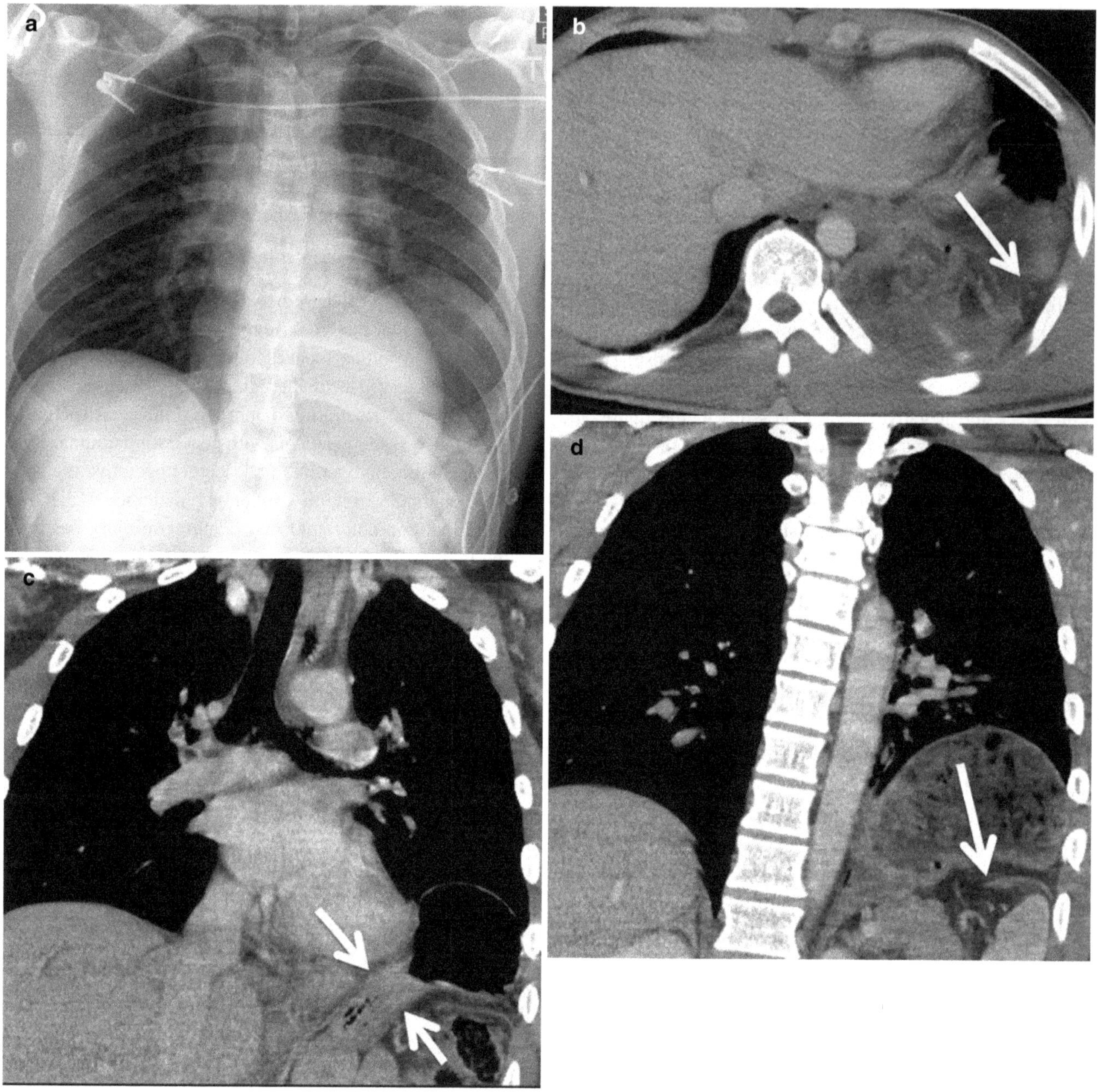

Fig. 12.7 Traumatic diaphragmatic injury with herniation. (**a**) AP chest radiograph shows an elevated left hemidiaphragm with stomach projecting in the lower left hemithorax. (**b**) Axial contrast-enhanced CT demonstrates stomach displaced posteriorly (dependent viscera sign) and suggestion of a waist-like constriction (arrow). (**c**, **d**) Coronal CT images demonstrate herniation of a portion of the stomach into the thorax and depict the collar sign (arrows in (**c**)) and abrupt discontinuity of left hemidiaphragm (arrow in (**d**))

phragm, may mimic traumatic rupture and account for false-positive findings. Intrathoracic herniation has a sensitivity of 55–75% and a specificity of 100% [33]. Waist-like constriction of herniated abdominal contents at the level of diaphragmatic rupture creates the collar sign, best depicted on coronal and sagittal reformations. With thin section helical CT, the collar sign has a sensitivity of 63% and a specificity of 100%. The dependent viscera sign describes the position of the stomach, spleen, or bowel that has herniated into the thorax and lies adjacent the dependent aspect of the chest wall. This sign yields sensitivity of 55–90% for blunt trauma diaphragmatic injuries. Other signs suggestive of diaphragmatic injury include thickening and segmental non-visualization of the diaphragm [33].

Penetrating diaphragm injuries tend to be considerably smaller than blunt diaphragmatic injuries, and accordingly radiologic signs based on the herniation of abdominal viscera are only occasionally helpful. Diagnosis depends on demonstration of a simple breach of the diaphragm. Direct visualization of the diaphragm defect on CT is specific but uncommonly seen. CT demonstration of contiguous injuries on both signs of the diaphragm is the most sensitive CT finding and in many cases and its absence can be used to exclude injury. Unfortunately, its specificity can be diminished if multiple wounds are present. Construction of double oblique CT images along the trajectory of the knife or bullet (trajectography) can improve specificity of diagnosis. Demonstration of a tract extending on both sides of the diaphragm is specific for penetrating diaphragm injury and in many cases is adequate impetus for operative exploration [32].

Key Points

CT Findings in Diaphragmatic Tear

- Blunt
  Injury Findings (Sensitivity of CT – 70–90%)
  - Sharp discontinuity of hemidiaphragm
  - Herniation of omental fat or abdominal viscera
  - Waist-like narrowing of herniated viscera (collar sign)
  - Lack of visualization of hemidiaphragm
  - Dependent viscera sign
- Penetrating
  Injury Findings (Sensitivity of CT – 80–100%)
  - Contiguous injury – single wound
  - Contiguous injury – multiple wounds (decreased specificity)
  - Transdiaphragmatic trajectory

12.13 Thoracic Skeletal or Chest Wall Trauma

Rib fractures have prognostic significance and can by themselves cause physiologic impairment. In general rib fractures are more common in elderly individuals, due to lesser elasticity of the skeleton. In children, on the other hand, rib fractures indicate a significant mechanism of injury and are associated with a higher mortality rate [1].Rib fractures are uncommon in restrained passengers in collisions at speeds of less than 30 miles (<50 km) per hour [1] but overall occur in 60% of patients with blunt thoracic trauma. The most commonly fractured ribs are the fourth through the ninth ribs. Mortality increases slightly in patients with two or more rib fractures visible on CT but increases more sharply when nine or more are visible.

Several patterns of rib fractures are associated with specific injuries. Fractures of the 10th, 11th, and 12th ribs are associated with renal, splenic, and hepatic injuries. First, second, and third ribs are associated with a significant mechanism of injury and are accompanied by aorta or great vessel injury in 14% and tracheobronchial injuries in 2% of cases [34]. Rib fractures accompanied by disruption of chest wall soft tissues can result in lung herniation. In the setting or blunt trauma, this occurs most commonly anteriorly or posteriorly which layers of intercostal muscles are fewest. Patients with greater than four continuous ribs that are fractured in two placed (segmental fractures) are at increased risk for development of a flail chest.... This is a clinical diagnosis in which an unstable portion of the chest wall moves paradoxically during respiration, impairing ventilation.

Sternal fractures are seen predominately in restrained passengers and occur in 8% of individuals with a significant mechanism of injury. The presence of sternal fractures is associated with severity of chest injury, the degree of displacement being the major determinant. Less than 10% of patient with minimally displaced sternal fractures have spine fractures or traumatic pericardial effusions. Patients with completely displaced sternal fractures, however, have >40% chance of having a traumatic pericardial effusion and >30% chance of having a spine fracture. Although associated with cardiac injury, sternal fractures are not associated with ATAI.

Location of fracture within the sternum is also significant, with fractures involving the manubrium having the highest association with spine fractures, usually involving the upper thoracic spine (T5–T6) and the thoracolumbar junction (T12–L1) [35]. Sternomanubrial dislocations share this association with thoracic spine trauma, specifically type 2 dislocations in which the manubrium is displaced posteriorly with respect to the sternal body. This type of dislocation is caused by hyperflexion, the same mechanism often fracturing the thoracic spine. Type-one sternomanubrial dislocations in which the sternal body is displaced posteriorly with respect to the manubrium are usually the result of a direct blow, rather than hyperflexion. Internal mammary arteries can be directly damaged by this posterior displacement of the sternal body.

The sternoclavicular joints and sternum (see above) are important sites to evaluate for fracture or dislocation because injury in these locations can cause adjacent mediastinal hematoma that may raise concern for ATAI if the associated fracture is not identified. Sternoclavicular dislocations are also clinically relevant due to potential direct damage to adjacent structures. These injuries are rare due to extensive ligamentous support, such that forces transmitted along the clavicle are far more likely to fracture the clavicle than dislocate the joint. Anterior sternoclavicular dislocation is the most common type of dislocation, while posterior dislocation is associated with more severe sequelae, such as tracheal, esophageal, and great vessel impingement or injury.

Scapular fractures indicate a significant mechanism of injury and can be seen on 57% of initial chest radiographs [34]. Approximately 50% of patients with a scapular fracture have a pneumothorax. Ipsilateral subclavian, axillary, or brachial artery injury may be present in 11% of patients with scapular fracture [1]. Vascular and neurologic injury are also associated with scapulothoracic disassociations, a more severe injury that separates the scapula and muscular attachments of upper extremity from the thorax without disrupting the overlying skin.

Thoracic spine fractures occur in 3% of blunt trauma patients and are most common in the thoracolumbar region [34]. Wedge compression and burst fractures secondary to hyperflexion and axial load mechanisms are the predominant fracture types [36] and frequently result in significant neurologic impairment. Neurologic impairment is common because the spinal cord occupies a larger percentage of the available space in the canal than in the more spacious cervical and lumbar spine regions. Additionally, thoracic cord blood supply has little collateral reserve, predisposing to ischemic insult.

12.13.1 Radiography and Computed Tomography

CT is more sensitive than chest radiography in the diagnosis of rib and may be used to three-dimensional reformatted images to better visualizing rib trauma. In the setting of a flail chest, this may aid the surgeon in surgical planning. Fixation of rib fractures in the setting of flail segment may decrease the patient duration of mechanical ventilation, but the evidence is not strong, and operative fixation is not commonly performed [37]. Peripheral opacities that parallel the chest wall represent extrapleural hematomas adjacent to rib fractures. Extrapleural hematoma forms superficial to the parietal pleura, arising from bleeding from damaged intercostal vessels, and muscles. These extrapleural hematomas can be identified on CT by the presence of inward displacement of extrapleural fat and are *not* treated by tube thoracostomy. Collections that are biconvex may represent an arterial bleeding source and are more likely to require surgical intervention [38]. The possibility of a flail chest should also be considered whenever a large extrapleural hematoma is seen.

Sternal fractures are rarely seen on frontal radiographs but, similar to rib fractures, are readily seen on CT images, particularly sagittal reconstructions. Diagnosis of sternoclavicular dislocation without CT is also very difficult, even with special radiographic views (e.g., serendipity view).

Radiographic diagnosis of scapulothoracic disassociation relies on detecting scapular displacement via the scapula index, a measurement easily distorted by difference in arm positioning and by rotation. In suspected cases CTA is essential to diagnose occlusion of subclavian and axillary vessels from thrombosis or external compression. MRI is best suited for evaluating associated brachial plexus injuries; the presence of >3 pseudomeningoceles suggests irreversible nerve root damage.

Key Points

- Sternal fracture.
  - Completely displaced—traumatic pericardial effusion (40%) and spine fracture (30%)
  - Minimally displaced—traumatic pericardial effusion/spine fracture (10%)
- Manubrium fracture
  - Thoracic spine (T5–T6) and the thoracolumbar junction (T12–L1)
- Sternomanubrial dislocation
  - Type 2—hyperflexion spinal injury
  - Type 1—internal mammary artery injury
- Posterior sternoclavicular joint dislocation
  - Brachiocephalic vein and aortic arch vessels
- Scapulothoracic disassociation
  - Subclavian/axillary artery, brachial plexus, and pseudomeningoceles

12.14 Concluding Remarks

Over the last two decades, cross-sectional imaging of both blunt and penetrating thoracic traumas has helped clinicians select from among widened options for injury management. Advances in CT imaging and evolution of treatment for ATAI now allow for nonoperative treatment of some injuries and delayed endovascular stent placement for others. Conversely, the presence of signs of penetrating diaphragmatic injury may prompt laparotomy in patients initially triaged to nonoperative management. Despite these improvements in CT imaging, diagnostic uncertainty may still prompt invasive procedures for some injuries (e.g., catheter angiography for supra-aortic vessel injury, bronchoscopy for suspected large airway rupture).

Take-Home Messages

- Patients with minimal ATAI are managed nonoperatively. In the remaining ATAI victims, accurate description of pseudoaneurysm extent may facilitate management with either imaging follow-up or non-emergent endovascular stenting rather than emergent intervention.
- CT demonstration of hemopericardium is a nonspecific finding that can be due to pericardial injury, cardiac contusion, and rarely rupture of right-sided cardiac chambers. Focal constriction of cardiac chambers suggests underlying pericardial rupture, while accompanying IVC distention and periportal edema are indicators of associated tamponade.

- Manubrial fracture and posterior dislocation of the manubrium are strongly associated with spine fractures, while posterior sternal body dislocation, posterior sternoclavicular dislocations, and scapulothoracic disassociation prompt careful evaluation for vascular injuries.
- Blunt diaphragmatic injuries cause large defects that are detectable by direct visualization, displacement of viscera, or deformation of herniated contents (collar sign). Detection of the smaller defects caused by penetrating trauma depends on determining the trajectory of the penetrating object.

References

1. Mayberry J. Imaging in thoracic trauma: the trauma surgeon's perspective. J Thorac Imaging. 2000;15:76–86.
2. Durso A, Caban K, Munera F. Penetrating thoracic injury. Radiol Clin N Am. 2015;53:675–93.
3. Schellenberg M, Inaba K, Bardes JM, Orozco N, Chen J, Park C, et al. The combined utility of extended focused assessment with sonography for trauma and chest x-ray in blunt thoracic trauma. J Trauma Acute Care Surg. 2018;85(1):113–7.
4. Strumwasser A, Chong V, Chu E, Victorino GP. Thoracic computed tomography is an effective screening modality in patients with penetrating injuries to the chest. Inj Int J Care Injured. 2016;47:2000–5.
5. Steenburg SD, Ravenel JG, Ikonomidis JS, Schönholz C, Reeves S. Acute traumatic aortic injury: imaging evaluation and management. Radiology. 2008;248(3):748–62.
6. Kirkham JR, Blackmore CC. Screening for aortic injury with chest radiography clinical factors. Emerg Radiol. 2007;14:211–7.
7. Cowley RA, Turney SZ, Hankins JR, et al. Rupture of thoracic aorta caused by blunt trauma. A fifteen-year experience. J Thorac Cardiovasc Surg. 1990;100:652.
8. Morgan TA, Steenburg SD, Siegel EL, Mirvis SE. Acute traumatic aortic injuries: posttherapy multidetector CT findings. Radiographics. 2010;30:851–67.
9. Costantino M, Gosselin MV, Primack SL. The ABC's of thoracic trauma imaging. Semin Roentgenol. 2006;41:209–25.
10. Raptis C, Hammer M, Raman K, et al. Acute traumatic aortic injury: practical considerations for the diagnostic radiologist. J Thorac Imaging. 2015;30:202–13.
11. Rojas CA, Restrepo CS. Mediastinal hematomas: aortic injury and beyond. J Comput Assist Tomogr. 2009;33:218–24.
12. Gunn ML, Lehnert BE, Lungren RS, et al. Minimal aortic injury of the thoracic aorta: imaging appearances and outcome. Emerg Radiol. 2014;21:227–33.
13. Harris DG, Rabin J, Starnes BW, Khoynezhad A, Conway G, et al. Evolution of lesion-specific management of blunt thoracic aortic injury. J Vasc Surg. 2016;64:500–5.
14. Holly BP, Steenburg SD. Multidetector CT of blunt traumatic venous injuries in the chest, abdomen, and pelvis. Radiographics. 2011;31(5):1415–2.
15. Chen MY, Miller PR, McLaughlin CA, Kortesis BG, Kavanagh PV, Dyer RB. The trend of using computed tomography in the detection of acute thoracic aortic and branch vessel injury after blunt thoracic trauma: single-center experience over 13 years. J Trauma. 2004 Apr;56(4):783–5.
16. Hammer MM, Raptis DA, Cummings KW, et al. Imaging in blunt cardiac injury: computed tomographic findings in cardiac contusion and associated injuries. Injury. 2016;47(5):1025–30.
17. Restrepo CS, Gutierrez FR, Marmol-Velez JA, Ocazionez D, Martinez-Jimenez S. Imaging patients with cardiac trauma. Radiographics. 2012;32:633–49.
18. Plurad DS, Bricker S, Van Natta TL, Neville A, Kim D, et al. Penetrating cardiac injury and the significance of chest computed tomography findings. Emerg Radiol. 2013;20:279–84.
19. Wintermark M, Schnyder P. The Macklin effect: a frequent etiology for pneumomediastinum in severe blunt chest trauma. Chest. 2001;120:543–7.
20. Zylak CM, Standen JR, Barnes GR, Zylak CJ. Pneumomediastinum revisited. Radiographics. 2000;20:1043–57.
21. Conradie JW, Gebremariam FA. Can computed tomography esophagography reliably diagnose traumatic penetrating upper digestive tract injuries? Clin Imaging. 2015;39(6):1039–45.
22. Cassada DC, Munyikwa MP, Monitz MP, et al. Acute injuries of the trachea and major bronchi: importance of early diagnosis. Ann Thorac Surg. 2000;69:1563–7.
23. Kunisch-Hoppe M, Hoppe M, Rauber K, Popella C, Rau WS. Tracheal rupture caused by blunt chest trauma: radiological and clinical features. Eur Radiol. 2000;10:480–3.
24. Scaglione M, Romanoa S, Pinto A, Sparano A, Scialpi MB, Rotondo A. Acute tracheobronchial injuries: impact of imaging on diagnosis and management implications. Eur J Radiol. 2006;59:336–43.
25. Rivas LA, Fishman JE, Múnera F, Bajayo DE. Multislice CT in thoracic trauma. Radiol Clin N Am. 2003;41:599–616.
26. Mille r LA. Chest wall, lung, and pleural space trauma. Radiol Clin N Am. 2006;44:213–24.
27. Rodriguez RM, Friedman B, Langdorf MI, Baumann BM, Nishijima DK, Hendey GW, Medak AJ, Raja AS, Mower WR. Pulmonary contusion in the pan-scan era. Injury. 2016;47(5):1031–4.
28. Huh J, Wall MJ Jr, Estrera AL, Soltero ER, Mattox KL. Surgical management of traumatic pulmonary injury. Am J Surg. 2003;186:620–4.
29. DuBose J, Inaba K, Demetriades D, Scalea TM, O'Connor J, Menaker J, et al. Management of post-traumatic retained hemothorax: a prospective, observational, multicenter AAST study. J Trauma Acute Care Surg. 2012 Jan;72(1):11–22.
30. Moore FO, Goslar PW, Coimbra R, Velmahos G, Brown CV, Coopwood TB Jr, et al. Blunt traumatic occult pneumothorax: is observation safe?–results of a prospective, AAST multicenter study. J Trauma. 2011;70(5):1019–23.
31. Iochum S, Ludig T, Walter F, et al. Imaging of diaphragmatic injury: a diagnostic challenge? Radiographics. 2002;22:S103–18.
32. Dreizin D, Bergquist PJ, Taner AT, Bodanapally UK, Tirada N, Munera F. Evolving concepts in MDCT diagnosis of penetrating diaphragmatic injury. Emerg Radiol. 2015;22:149–56.
33. Nchimi A, Szapiro D, Ghaye B, et al. Helical CT of blunt diaphragmatic rupture. Am J Roentgenol. 2005;184:24–30.
34. Collins J. Chest wall trauma. J Thorac Imaging. 2000;15:112–9.
35. von Garrel T, Ince A, Junge A, Schnabel M, Bahrs C. The sternal fracture: radiographic analysis of 200 fractures with special reference to concomitant injuries. J Trauma. 2004;57:837–44.

36. Kuhlman JE, Pozniak MA, Collins J, Knisely BL. Radiographic and CT findings of blunt chest trauma: aortic injuries and looking beyond them. Radiographics. 1998;18:1085–106.
37. Kasotakis G, Hasenboehler EA, Streib EW, Patel N, Patel MB, Alarcon L, Bosarge PL, Love J, Haut ER, Como JJ. Operative fixation of rib fractures after blunt trauma: a practice management guideline from the Eastern Association for the Surgery of Trauma. J Trauma Acute Care Surg. 2017;82(3):618.
38. Chung JH, Carr RB, Stern EJ. Extrapleural hematomas: imaging appearance, classification, and clinical significance. J Thorac Imaging. 2011;26:218–23.

13

Diagnosis and Staging of Breast Cancer: When and How to Use Mammography, Tomosynthesis, Ultrasound, Contrast-Enhanced Mammography, and Magnetic Resonance Imaging

Fiona J. Gilbert and Katja Pinker-Domenig

Learning Objectives

- To understand when and how to use mammography, digital breast tomosynthesis, ultrasound, contrast-enhanced mammography, and magnetic resonance imaging for the diagnosis and staging of breast cancer.
- To realize the limitations of each imaging modality.
- To understand the information that can be obtained with each imaging modality and their complementary value in this context.

13.1 Mammography

Breast cancer is the most common cause of female cancer deaths in the western world, with early detection of cancer being pivotal for an improved prognosis and survival. Mammography is the mainstay of breast cancer screening and diagnosis [1–3]. Mammography is a two-dimensional image and relies on the identification of morphologic findings that are suspicious for breast cancer (Fig. 13.1). These findings include masses, grouped calcifications, asymmetries, and areas of architectural distortion. A standard screening mammogram consists of mediolateral oblique (MLO) and craniocaudal (CC) views of each breast. The screening exam is intended solely to detect suspicious findings after which the woman would return for additional diagnostic views. Diagnostic mammographic views may include spot compression, magnification, rolled, extended views, and true lateral views among others in order to characterize and localize abnormalities. The Breast Imaging Reporting and Data System (BIRADS) was developed by the American College of Radiology in order to standardize terminology describing mammographic findings [4]. The BIRADS atlas also outlines acceptable performance metrics for screening mammography programs such as a cancer detection rate of ≥2.5 cancers/1000 screens and a recall rate between 5 and 12%. Performance benchmarks are also available for diagnostic mammography, such as a positive predictive value of biopsy of between 20 and 45%. Randomized controlled trials have found that screening mammography has decreased the mortality for breast cancer by 30% [1]. However, with a sensitivity of approximately 70%, mammography has its limitations. Particularly in women with dense breasts, cancers might be occult on mammography [5]. Current recommendations for breast cancer screening in the United States and Europe are somewhat variable. The Society of Breast Imaging, the American College of Radiology, and the National Comprehensive Cancer Network recommend annual screening mammography beginning at the age of 40 years for women at average risk for breast cancer. Due to varying judgments of the benefits and harms of screening, the American College of Obstetricians and Gynecologists guidelines differ from the recommendations issued by the US Preventive Services Task Force, the American Cancer Society, the National Comprehensive Cancer Network, and the American College of Radiology/Society of Breast Imaging (Table 13.1). Women at increased risk for breast cancer (i.e., ≥ 20% lifetime risk) are recommended to undergo supplemental screening in addition to mammography with breast MRI [6, 7]. Women who are BRCA1/2 gene mutation carriers or who are not tested but have an equivalent risk (with TP53 Li Fraumeni syndrome, AT homozygote or supradiaphragmatic radiother-

F. J. Gilbert (✉)
Department of Radiology, School of Clinical Medicine, University of Cambridge, Cambridge, UK
e-mail: fjg28@medschl.cam.ac.uk

K. Pinker-Domenig
Department of Radiology, Breast Imaging Service, Memorial Sloan Kettering Cancer Center, New York, NY, USA
e-mail: pinkerdk@mskcc.org

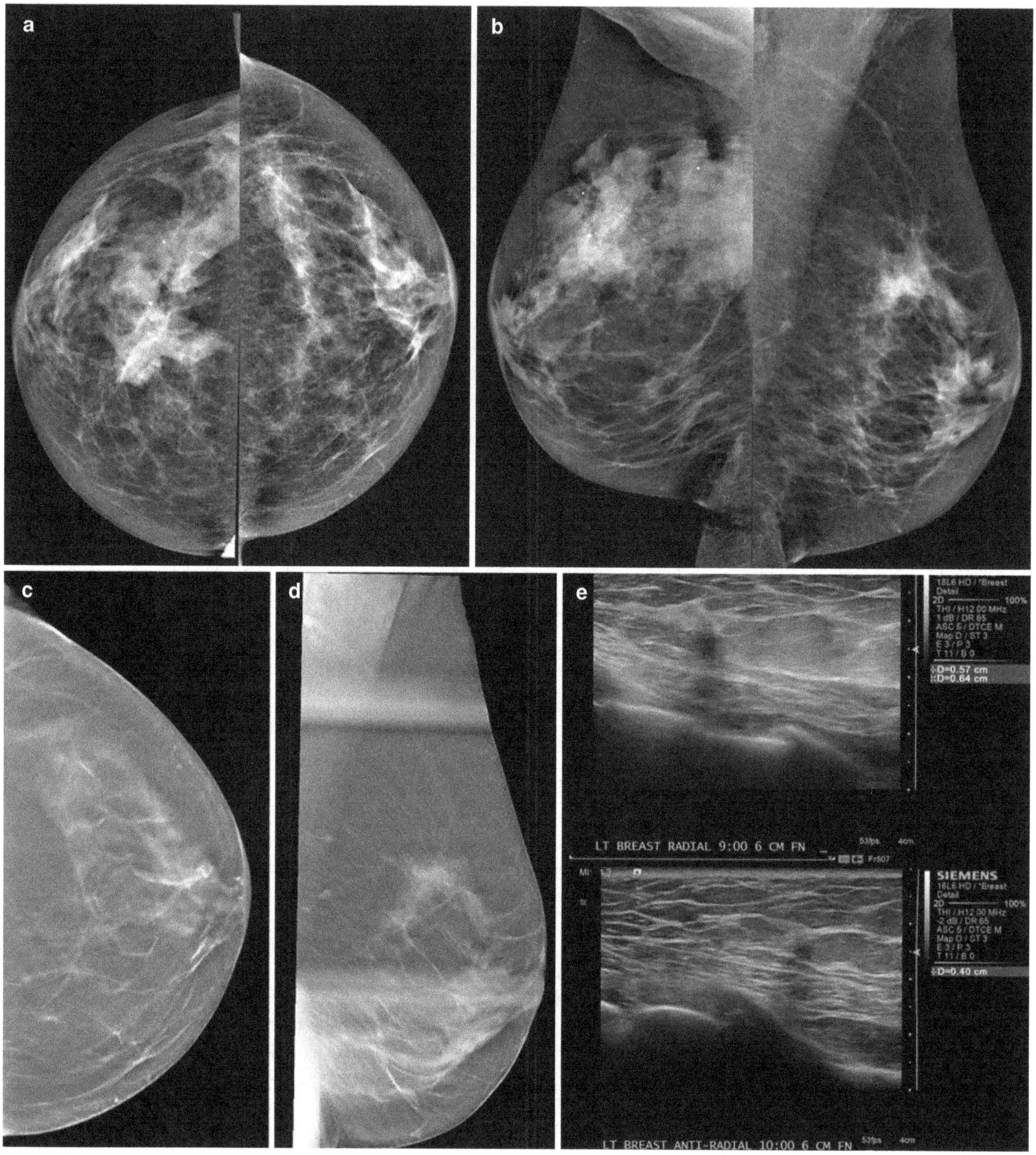

Fig. 13.1 Screen-detected multifocal invasive ductal carcinoma III between the 9 and 10:00 axis of the left breast in a 72-year-old patient with a personal history of right breast cancer, breast conserving therapy and radiation treatment in 1983. (**a**, **b**) CC and MLO views: Post-surgical changes are present in the right breast. There are two new irregular shaped and partially spiculated masses in the 9 and 10:00 axis of the left breast posterior depth which are best appreciated on additional tomosynthesis views CC (**c**) and ML (**d**, spot). On targeted ultrasound (**e**) these correspond to two irregular shaped and marginated hypoechoic masses (9:00 6 cm from the nipple 0.6 × 0.5 cm, 10:00 6 cm from the nipple 0.4 × 0.4 cm)

apy before the age 30 years) are offered annual mammography ± MRI. In addition, recent breast density legislation in the United States requires that women be informed if they have mammographically heterogeneously dense or extremely dense breasts and that supplemental breast cancer screening be considered. This has led to an increased use of mammog-

Table 13.1 Recommendations for breast cancer screening in average-risk women

	UK National Health Service Breast Screening Programme	U.S. Preventive Services Task Force	American Cancer Society	National Comprehensive Cancer Network	American College of Radiology/ Society of Breast Imaging
Clinical breast examination	Not recommended	Insufficient evidence to recommend for or against	Not recommended	Recommend every 1–3 years for women 25–39 years and annually for women 40 years and older	Not recommended
Mammography initiation age	Offer starting at age 50 years	Recommend at age 50 years Age 40–49 years: decision to start screening mammography before age 50 years should be an individual one	Offer at ages 40–45 years Recommend at age 45 years	Recommend at age 40	Recommend at age 40
Mammography screening interval	Three yearly	Biennial	Annual for women aged 40–54 years Biennial with the option to continue annual screening for women 55 years or older	Annual	Annual
Mammography stop age	Continue until age 70 years Beyond age 70 years, women may continue to attend every 3 years	The current evidence is insufficient to assess the balance of benefits and harms of screening mammography women 75 years and older	When life expectancy is less than 10 years	When severe comorbidities limit life expectancy to 10 years or less	When life expectancy is less than 5–7 years

raphy supplemented with whole-breast screening ultrasound in women with dense breast tissue [8].

13.1.1 Staging with Mammography

Mammography, together with ultrasound and MRI as detailed below, is used to detect and characterize lesions found at screening and to evaluate symptomatic women. In patients with breast cancer, diagnostic mammography, often in conjunction with specialized views – latero-medial (LM) and mediolateral (ML), extended CC, magnification, spot compression, and other views – is used to determine lesion size and location as well as to image the surrounding tissue and lymph nodes [9]. Diagnostic mammography is often tailored to the specific problem. For example, in a woman with suspicious mammographic calcifications, magnification views are necessary to evaluate the extent of calcifications (Fig. 13.2). If calcifications are associated with an asymmetry or mass, further evaluation with ultrasound is warranted to search for a solid mass that may indicate an invasive component.

Key Point

- Mammography is a two-dimensional image and relies on the identification of morphologic findings that are suspicious for breast cancer. Mammography is the mainstay of breast cancer screening and diagnosis.

13.2 Digital Breast Tomosynthesis

Digital breast tomosynthesis (DBT) images are created from repeated exposure of the breast tissue from different angles and data processing interpolated into multiple slices typically 0.5 mm thick through the breast tissue. Many retrospective and prospective studies have demonstrated that this technique is acceptable to women, increases the radiation dose by an average of 20%, and increases cancer detection by approximately 15–30% while reducing recall rates by 15–20% by decreasing overlapping shadows mimicking breast cancer [10]. While the technique is excellent for

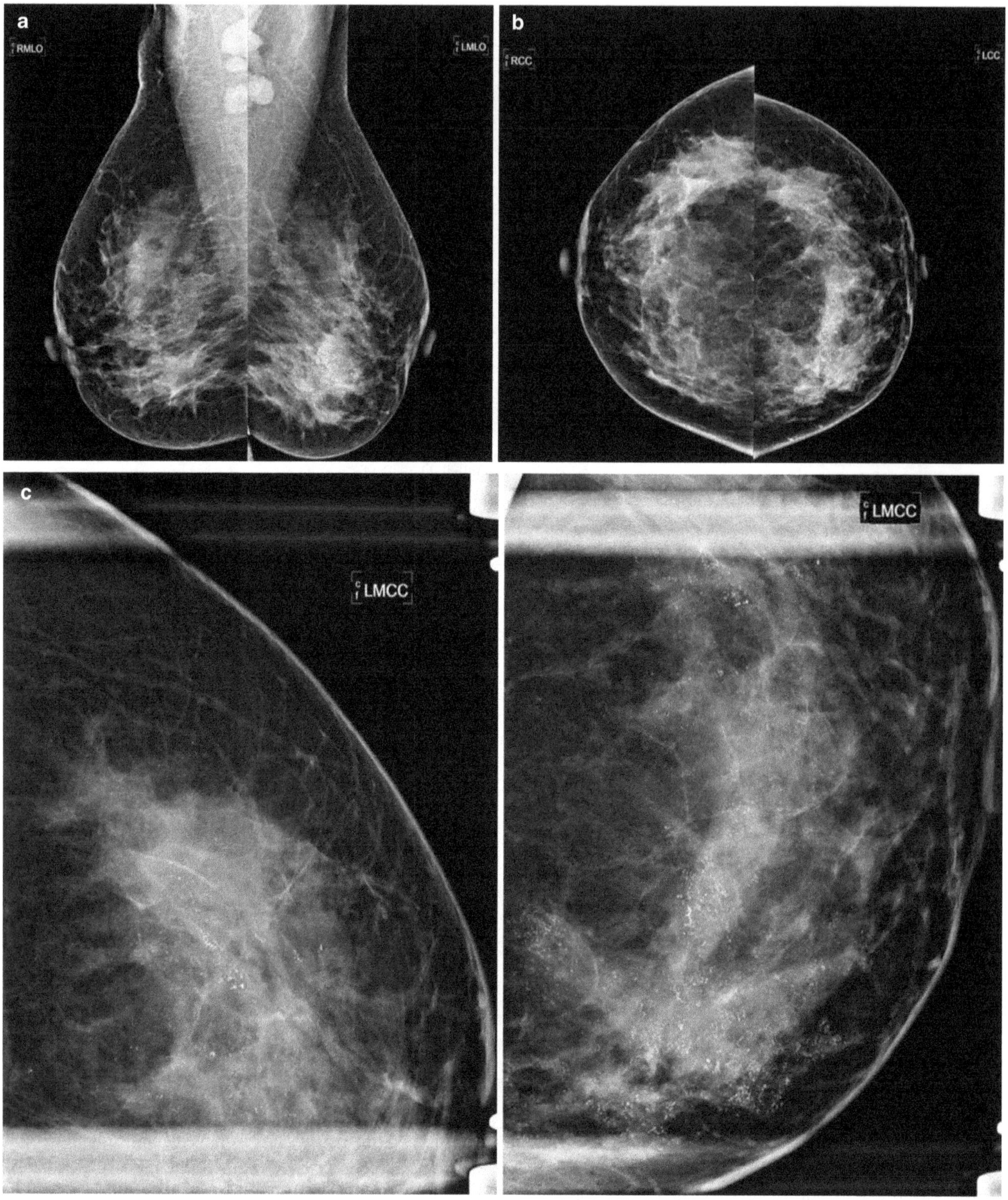

Fig 13.2 Multicentric invasive ductal carcinoma III and ductal carcinoma in situ high grade in a 54-year-old patient presenting with a palpable area of concern in the left breast for diagnostic mammography. CC and MLO views (**a**, **b**) and left magnification views CC (**c**) and ML (**d**). In the right breast there are no suspicious mass or tumor calcifications present. In the left breast there are pleomorphic microcalcifications spanning both the lower inner and outer quadrant. In addition, there is an enlarged axillary lymph node, which was confirmed to be metastatic

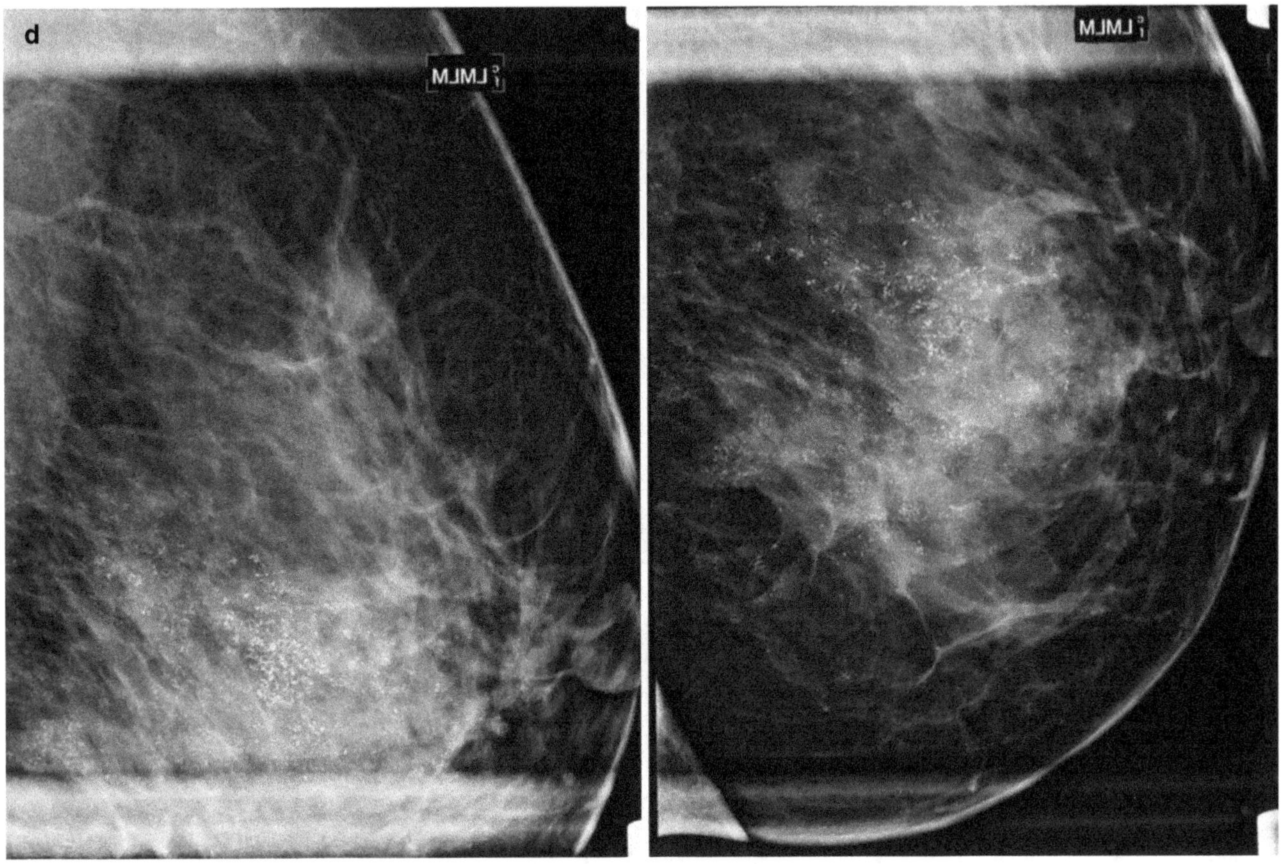

Fig 13.2 (continued)

assessing soft tissue masses, architectural distortion, and asymmetries, the conspicuity and analysis of microcalcification were not improved [11]. However, recently, due to faster processing techniques manufacturers have been able to analyze all pixels instead of "binning" (combining pixels with the effect of reducing resolution) the data to reduce processing time. This means that fine calcification can now be more clearly identified with improved sensitivity and specificity.

DBT has been shown to be particularly useful in women with mixed to dense breast tissue (BIRADS B & C) but is not advantageous in women with very dense breast tissue. DBT is now increasingly used in the clinic either on its own with a 2D composite image or in conjunction with a standard 2D full-field digital mammography (FFDM) image. The advantage of using DBT is that the need for additional views such as the coned view or other supplemental techniques is no longer required [12]. In a recent meta-analysis, 17 studies were found where DBT was compared with 2D mammography in a screening setting. The pooled incremental cancer detection rate was 1.6 cancers/1000 screens compared with 2D FFDM with an overall absolute reduction in recall rates of 2.2%. However, there were differences between European and US-based studies with European studies showing a higher cancer detection rate of 2.4 cancers/1000 screens and a 0.5% increase in recall rates and US studies showing a reduction in the recall rates due the higher recall rates initially [13].

In the symptomatic setting, DBT has been found to have improved diagnostic accuracy compared with 2D mammography and improved reader confidence in distinguishing benign from malignant lesions and is more accurate in assessing tumor size and at identifying multifocal disease [14]. Techniques are also now available for image-guided biopsy using DBT to guide targeting.

Key Point

- DBT has the potential to overcome the primary limitation of standard two-dimensional mammography, a masking effect due to overlapping fibroglandular breast tissue, improving diagnostic accuracy by differentiating benign and malignant features, and increasing lesion conspicuity, particularly in dense breasts.

13.3 Contrast-Enhanced Mammography

Contrast-enhanced mammography (CEM) is an emerging technology in breast imaging. CEM allows both a morphologic evaluation comparable to routine digital mammography and a simultaneous assessment of tumor neovascularity as an indicator of malignancy. Contrast-enhanced spectral mammography (CESM) acquires a low kV image and a high kV image simultaneously before and after the injection of iodinated contrast. Retrospective studies comparing CESM with standard 2D mammography show significant improvement in the sensitivity and specificity for detecting breast carcinomas with CESM; the sensitivity of CESM is 93–100% compared with 71.5–93% for mammography and increases the specificity from 42 to 87.7%. The patient populations in all these studies were either symptomatic patients or patients recalled to assessment after an abnormal screening mammogram [15, 16].

In women with heterogeneously or dense breasts (BIRADS C & D), small occult cancers can be seen with CESM due to increased vascularity from tumor angiogenesis. In women with dense breasts, CESM is one of several supplementary techniques that can be used to avoid overlooking cancer (Fig. 13.3). The low-dose image is virtually as good as a 2D FFDM image and has the same resolution as a conventional image. However, microcalcification due to low-grade DCIS is often not visualized on the subtracted image of CESM.

The disadvantage of this contrast examination is that approximately the same dose of iodinated contrast is injected intravenously, and sensitivity reactions can occur at the same rate as with computed tomography (CT) examinations. This means that CESM must be performed in a center with resuscitation facilities in place, and caution must be exercised in patients with impaired renal function, patients with allergies, and in the elderly.

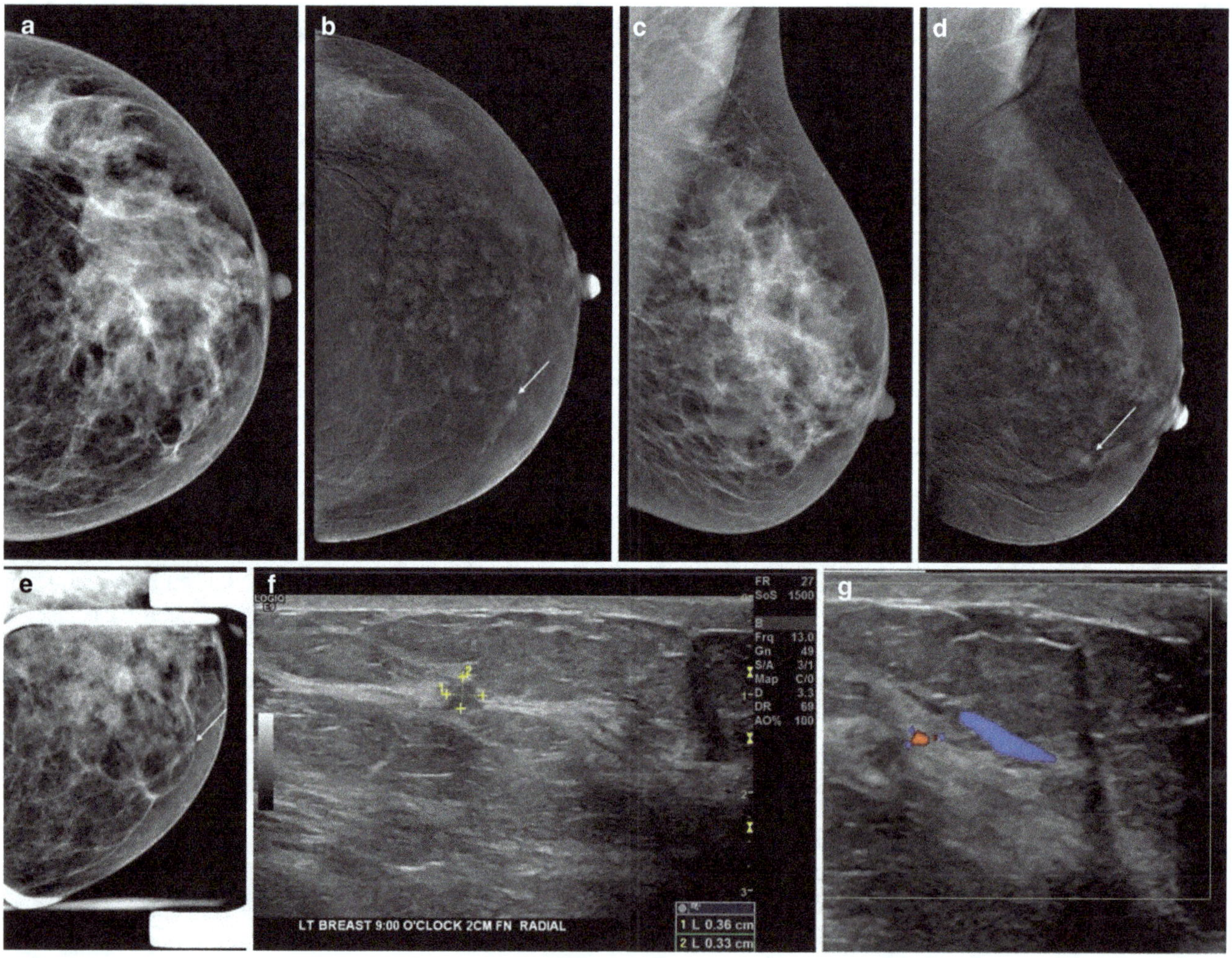

Fig. 13.3 Invasive ductal carcinoma II in a 49-year-old patient who underwent contrast-enhanced mammography with a personal history of right breast cancer and mastectomy and reduction mammoplasty on the left. CC and MLO views (**a**, **c**), contrast-enhanced CC and MLO views (**b**, **d**), left CC spot compression view and diagnostic targeted ultrasound (**f**, **g** with color doppler). On mammography, left lower inner focal asymmetry that does not efface on spot compression correlates to a 0.4 cm enhancing mass on CEM. Targeted ultrasound shows an irregular shaped and marginated hypoechoic mass with vascularization

The diagnostic accuracy in younger women and in those with dense breasts in the symptomatic setting is improved compared with 2D mammography [17].

13.3.1 Staging with CESM

A major advantage of CESM is that the ability to see additional foci of disease is enhanced hugely and, in many studies, it is comparable to MRI. Jochelson et al. found equal sensitivity between MRI and CESM for detecting the index cancer, although MRI was less sensitive for detecting additional tumor foci [18]. Lee-Felker et al. found that MRI had slightly higher sensitivity for the index lesion but equal sensitivity for detecting additional tumor foci [19]. Overall both studies showed that CESM had a significantly improved positive predictive value and specificity compared with MRI, as well as fewer false-positive interpretations. This means that once a cancer is suspected on imaging at the clinic visit, a CESM examination can be performed which has almost comparable sensitivity and specificity to staging breast MRI.

Key Point

- CEM allows both a morphologic evaluation comparable to routine digital mammography and a simultaneous assessment of tumor neovascularity as an indicator of malignancy similar to MRI. CEM has an improved sensitivity and increases the specificity compared with mammography.

13.4 Ultrasound

Handheld ultrasound (US) has improved enormously over the last 20 years with markedly improved resolution and rapid image processing. While it is rarely used as a primary diagnostic tool, US is used in the majority of patients presenting with a clinical symptom as an adjunctive tool to further analyze a mammographic abnormality to determine whether a soft tissue mass is solid or cystic and to differentiate benign from malignant masses. It is also used when there is a negative mammographic examination, but the patient has a clinical symptom or palpable abnormality. The procedure is acceptable to patients, is safe with no ionizing radiation, but is operator dependent. The drawback for conventional US is that in breast tissue with extensive fibrocystic disease and shadowing, small tumors can be overlooked especially if they are invasive lobular disease. Ductal carcinoma in situ (DCIS) can be picked up now due to the improved resolution as microcalcification can produce a speckled pattern but DCIS with no calcification is difficult to detect.

Whole-breast US or Automated Breast US (ABUS) is a technique that is rapidly gaining acceptance. This technique requires the operator to undertake three positions with a flat panel US plate of each breast. The images are reconstructed to produce a 3D examination of the breast. This technique is showing promise in many clinical trials and may become the examination of choice for women with dense breasts in whom a supplemental examination is justified. A third of the United States, France, and Belgium have introduced supplemental imaging techniques such as US for women with BIRADS C & D breast density although in all cases this additional examination is insurance or self-funded. The literature supports the use of the supplemental imaging with studies reporting an additional 4 cancers/1000 screens when used with annual or 2-yearly screening. While the drawback for screening US has traditionally been that it had high recall rates ranging from 10 to 30%, a recent publication from Sweden has shown more promising results with ABUS with recall below 2.5% while good sensitivity is retained [20].

A most valuable aspect of US is the ability to rapidly undertake an image-guided biopsy. This can be done safely, in a timely manner at the first visit to the clinic and has a degree of accuracy without any precautions save checking for a bleeding diathesis.

13.4.1 Staging with US

US is widely used to confirm a diagnosis of cancer and to look for additional disease in the breast which is found in up to 20% cases. Additional disease is more often found toward the nipple and in the same quadrant as the index tumor.

Assessment of the axilla to look for abnormal lymph nodes is a very popular approach. The short axis diameter of axillary nodes is less than 5 mm in size, but in reality there is a large variation in normal lymph node size. Hence, the more reliable indicators of disease are abnormal shape (rounded), loss of echogenicity of the hilum, thickened cortex by more than 3 mm, or irregular lobulated cortex. When proving malignancy prior to surgery, US-guided core biopsies are undertaken.

US is also used extensively as a second-look tool in patients with abnormalities found on MRI particularly when the features are not diagnostic.

Lastly, US is used in localization techniques prior to surgery including the placing of a guide wire into the cancer to aid surgical procedure. This can be done accurately and efficiently under US guidance.

Key Point

- US is widely used to confirm a diagnosis of cancer, to look for additional disease in the breast, for image-guided breast biopsy and localization, assessment of the axilla, and as a second-look tool in patients with abnormalities found on MRI.

13.5 Magnetic Resonance Imaging

Magnetic resonance imaging (MRI) is established valuable technique in breast imaging with multiple clinical indications, such as preoperative staging, response assessment to neoadjuvant therapy, scar vs. recurrence, assessment of breast implant integrity, evaluation of patients with cancer of unknown primary, and screening of high-risk patients [21, 22]. Dynamic contrast-enhanced magnetic resonance imaging (DCE-MRI) provides high-resolution breast morphology and enhancement kinetics to depict angiogenesis as a tumor-specific feature. Undisputedly DCE-MRI is the most sensitive modality for breast cancer detection with a pooled sensitivity of 93%; in terms of specificity, it has good pooled specificity of 71% [23]. In women who are at high risk for breast cancer, several studies have demonstrated that DCE-MRI is the superior screening modality compared with conventional imaging techniques [6, 7]

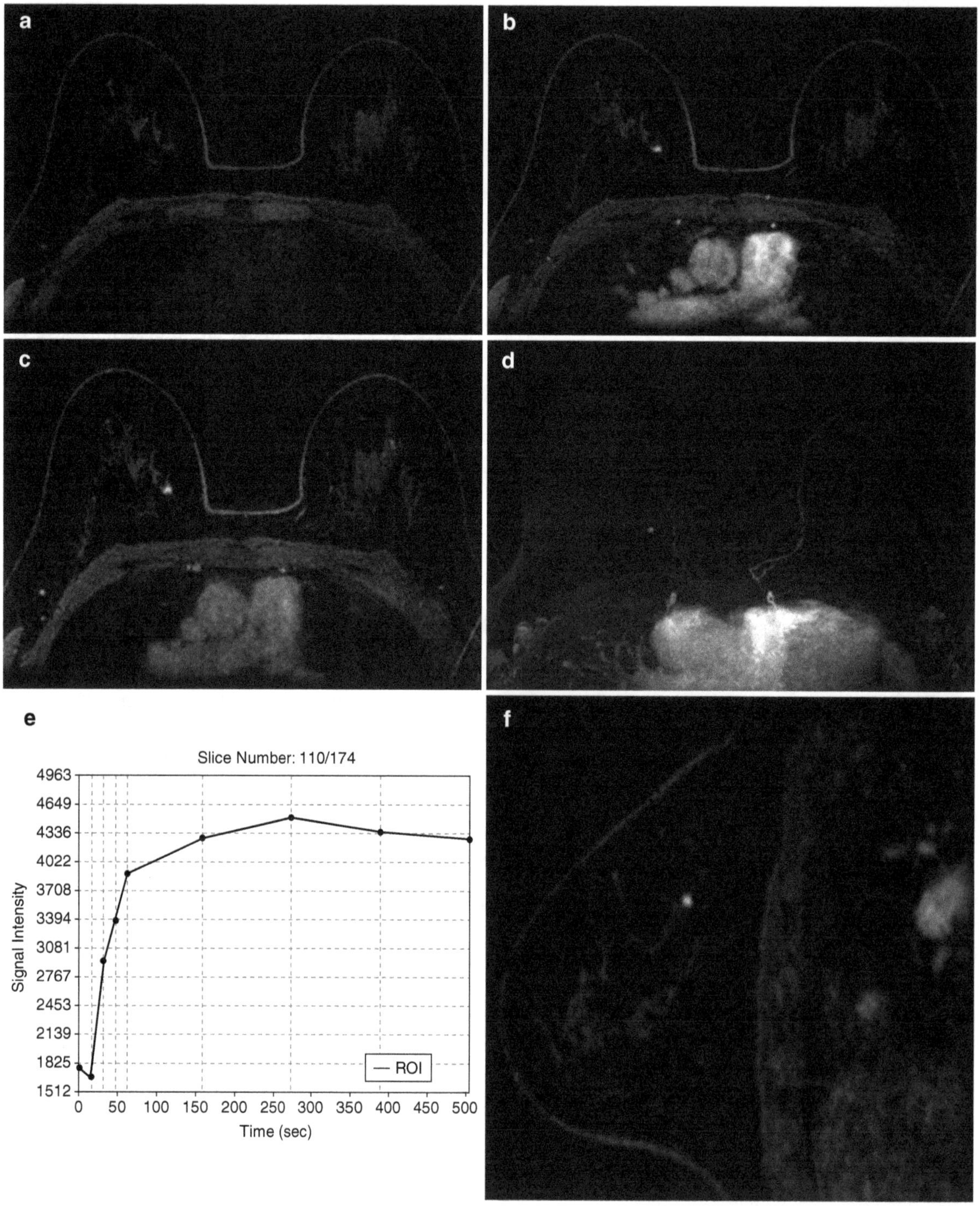

Fig. 13.4 0.4 cm invasive ductal carcinoma III medially in the right breast of a high-risk 51-year-old patient undergoing screening MRI. DCE-MRI (**a**, **b**, **c**) and MIP (**d**) shows round circumscribed mass with initial fast (**b**)/delayed plateau (**c**) enhancement signal intensity graph (**e**) sagittal view (**f**). Screening mammography and ultrasound were negative

(Fig. 13.4). Therefore, adjunct screening with DCE-MRI is recommended for women with a high (>20%) lifetime risk of breast cancer [21, 22, 24], facilitating earlier cancer detection and reducing interval cancers [25–27] in this population. This has also prompted a most recent similar recommendation for its use in women with an intermediate (>15%) lifetime risk of breast cancer [28]. To overcome limitations in DCE-MRI specificity and assess more functional data, additional MRI parameters can be combined with DCE-MRI; this approach is known as multiparametric MRI (MP MRI). In this context, diffusion-weighted imaging (DWI) with apparent diffusion coefficient (ADC) mapping has emerged as the most robust and valuable parameter with a reported sensitivity of up to 96% for breast cancer detection and a specificity of up to 100% for breast tumor characterization [29, 30] and is therefore increasingly implemented in clinical routine.

13.5.1 Staging with MRI

In patients with a biopsy-proven breast cancer, MRI may be used for the assessment of disease extent and detection of additional lesions in the same (multifocal) or different quadrants (multicentric) or in the contralateral breast potentially impacting patient management (Figs. 13.5 and 13.6). In this context DCE-MRI is more useful than mammography and US when staging multifocal and multicentric disease or when DCIS is present (Fig. 13.5) [31]. In addition, numerous studies have shown that DCE-MRI is superior to mammography and US for assessment of tumor size, yet there is still over- and underestimation in up to 15% of patients [31, 32]. Although an improved preoperative disease assessment can be expected to improve surgical outcomes, currently the evidence is controversial [33, 34] with respect to breast cancer histopathology and other studies. There is a good body of

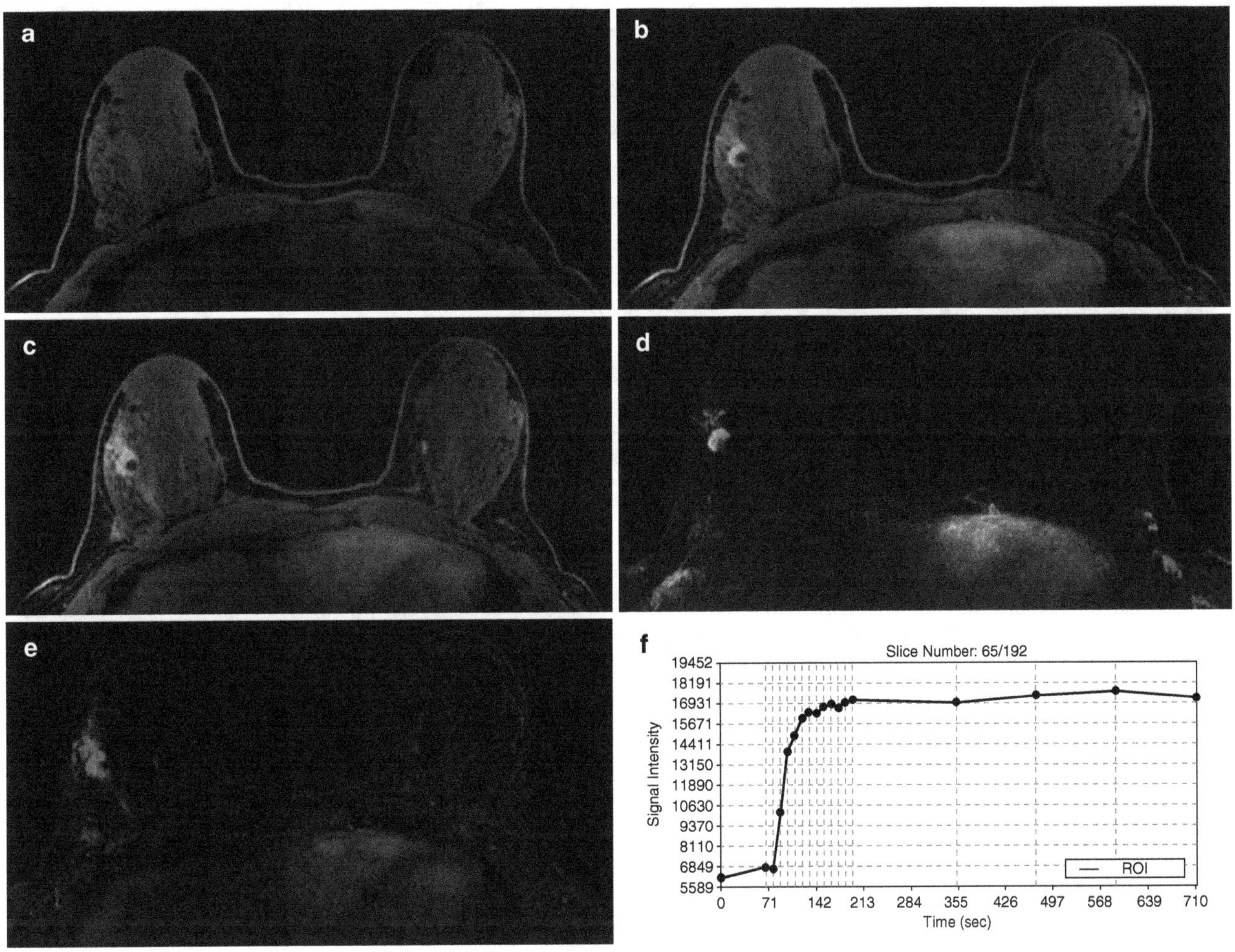

Fig. 13.5 MRI for staging of extent of disease in a 50-year-old patient with an invasive ductal carcinoma III with extensive intraductal component (EIC). On DCE-MRI (**a**, **b**), subtractions (**d**) and MIP (**e**). In the 9:00 axis mid depth there is a round irregular marginated mass with initial fast (**b**, **f**)/delayed plateau (**c**, **f**) enhancement measuring 1.4 × 1.4 × 1.1 cm with susceptibility artifact from clip marker. Extending from the index cancer into the anterior third of the breast there is a heterogeneous segmental non-mass enhancement representing the EIC. The index cancer and the contiguous non-mass enhancement span an area of approximately 3.8 × 1.6 × 1.5 cm. The non-mass enhancement engulfs a biopsy marker from a prior benign breast biopsy

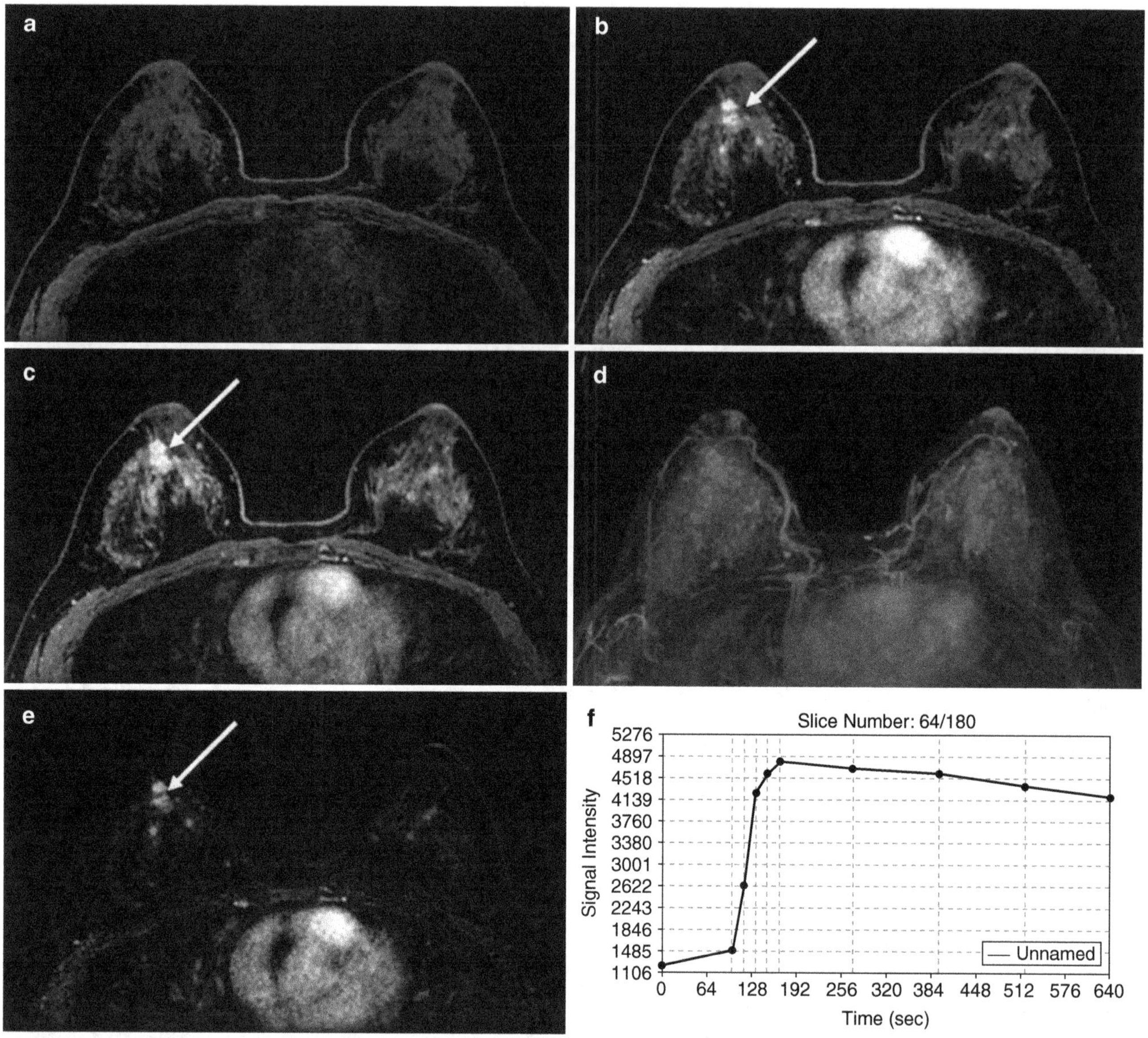

Fig. 13.6 Ductal carcinoma in situ (DCIS) intermediate grade, atypical ductal hyperplasia (ADH) and lobular carcinoma in situ classic type in 46-year-old patient with a history of right breast ADH and status post excisional biopsy undergoing screening MRI. Screening mammography and targeted second look sonography were negative. MRI-guided biopsy of the non-mass enhancement in the right breast retroareolar area shows right DCIS, ADH and LCIS. High resolution DCE-MRI (**a–c**), subtractions (**e**) and MIP (**d**) show in the early phase unique areas of non-mass enhancement with initial fast/delayed persistent enhancement (**f**)

evidence that staging MRI has a value in invasive lobular cancer (ILC), a histopathological breast cancer subtype that is typically underestimated by mammography and US, and reduces re-excision rates in ILC, ranging from 11 to 18% [35, 36]. It has to be noted that presurgical MRI often detects additional suspicious lesions that are occult on mammography and US, thus potentially leading to more extensive surgery. Histopathological verification is therefore mandatory before changes of treatment strategies are recommended based on these additional findings. The primary goal of surgery is to reduce tumor burden and is usually part of a sophisticated treatment strategy that includes radiation therapy, chemotherapy, and hormonal therapy. Although additional cancerous lesions detected by DCE-MRI might be effectively treated with these therapies, to date, there is a lack of evidence that preoperative DCE-MRI improves overall or disease-free survival [37].

DCE-MRI may also detect cancers that were occult on mammography and/or sonography in the contralateral breast in approximately 3% of women with unilateral cancer detected by mammography or US [38]. The detection of these initially unsuspected tumors may have a greater impact on patient outcomes than the detection of additional ipsilateral tumor foci as these would not be treated with concomitant radiation therapy. Although patient prognosis is determined by the size and grade of the index cancer, early detection of second cancers may be associated with a slight increase in survival, especially in patients younger than 50 years old [22]. Another indication of pretreatment breast MRI is as a problem-solving tool when tumor size differs significantly among imaging modalities or clinical examination and to evaluate eligibility for partial breast radiation therapy [21].

Key Point

- DCE-MRI is the most sensitive modality for breast cancer detection with excellent sensitivity and good specificity. MRI is used for the assessment of disease extent and detection of additional lesions. DCE-MRI is more useful than mammography and US when staging multifocal and multicentric disease or when DCIS is present.

13.6 Concluding Remarks

In conclusion, imaging plays a pivotal role in breast cancer detection and staging and helps in guiding treatment decisions. Imaging modalities for diagnosis and staging of breast cancer comprise mammography, DBT, ultrasound, CEM, and MRI. Whereas mammography is the mainstay of breast cancer screening and diagnosis, other imaging modalities such as DBT and CEM have emerged with the potential to overcome limitations in sensitivity and specificity adding valuable information in breast cancer staging. US is widely used to confirm a breast cancer diagnosis, to look for additional disease and for image-guided breast biopsy and localization, staging of the axilla, and as a second-look tool in patients with suspicious findings on MRI. DCE-MRI remains the most sensitive modality for breast cancer detection with excellent sensitivity and good specificity and is more useful than mammography and US for the assessment of disease extent and detection of additional disease. Each imaging modality has its limitations and advantages and therefore may be used in conjunction to facilitate an optimal breast cancer staging and treatment.

Take-Home Messages

- Mammography is the mainstay of breast cancer screening and diagnosis.
- Breast US is widely used to confirm a diagnosis of breast cancer, to look for additional disease in the breast and for image-guided breast interventions.
- DBT, CEM, and MRI increase cancer detection, especially in women with dense breasts at increased risk of cancer.
- MRI of the breast is superior to other imaging modalities for the assessment of disease extent and detection of additional disease.

References

1. Tabar L, Vitak B, Chen TH, Yen AM, Cohen A, Tot T, et al. Swedish two-county trial: impact of mammographic screening on breast cancer mortality during 3 decades. Radiology. 2011;260(3):658–63.
2. Hellquist BN, Duffy SW, Abdsaleh S, Bjorneld L, Bordas P, Tabar L, et al. Effectiveness of population-based service screening with mammography for women ages 40 to 49 years: evaluation of the Swedish Mammography Screening in Young Women (SCRY) cohort. Cancer. 2011;117(4):714–22.
3. Moss SM, Wale C, Smith R, Evans A, Cuckle H, Duffy SW. Effect of mammographic screening from age 40 years on breast cancer mortality in the UK Age trial at 17 years' follow-up: a randomised controlled trial. Lancet Oncol. 2015;16(9):1123–32.
4. D'Orsi CJ, Sickles EA, Mendelson EB, Morris EA, et al. ACR BI-RADS® atlas, breast imaging reporting and data system. 5th ed. Reston, VA: American College of Radiology; 2013.
5. Pisano ED, Gatsonis C, Hendrick E, Yaffe M, Baum JK, Acharyya S, et al. Diagnostic performance of digital versus film mammography for breast-cancer screening. N Engl J Med. 2005;353(17):1773–83.
6. Riedl CC, Luft N, Bernhart C, Weber M, Bernathova M, Tea MK, et al. Triple-modality screening trial for familial breast cancer underlines the importance of magnetic resonance imaging and questions the role of mammography and ultrasound regardless of patient mutation status, age, and breast density. J Clin Oncol. 2015;33(10):1128–35.
7. Krammer J, Pinker-Domenig K, Robson ME, Gonen M, Bernard-Davila B, Morris EA, et al. Breast cancer detection and tumor characteristics in BRCA1 and BRCA2 mutation carriers. Breast Cancer Res Treat. 2017;163(3):565–71.
8. Tagliafico AS, Calabrese M, Mariscotti G, Durando M, Tosto S, Monetti F, et al. Adjunct screening with tomosynthesis or ultrasound in women with mammography-negative dense breasts: interim report of a prospective comparative trial. J Clin Oncol. 2016;
9. Lee SC, Jain PA, Jethwa SC, Tripathy D, Yamashita MW. Radiologist's role in breast cancer staging: providing key information for clinicians. Radiographics. 2014;34(2):330–42.
10. Gilbert FJ, Tucker L, Young KC. Digital breast tomosynthesis (DBT): a review of the evidence for use as a screening tool. Clin Radiol. 2016;71(2):141–50.
11. Gilbert FJ, Tucker L, Gillan MG, Willsher P, Cooke J, Duncan KA, et al. Accuracy of digital breast tomosynthesis for depicting breast cancer subgroups in a UK retrospective reading study (TOMMY Trial). Radiology. 2015;277(3):697–706.
12. Gilbert FJ, Selamoglu A. Personalised screening: is this the way forward? Clin Radiol. 2018;73(4):327–33.
13. Marinovich ML, Hunter KE, Macaskill P, Houssami N. Breast cancer screening using tomosynthesis or mammography: a meta-analysis of cancer detection and recall. J Natl Cancer Inst. 2018;110(9):942–9.
14. Michell MJ, Batohi B. Role of tomosynthesis in breast imaging going forward. Clin Radiol. 2018;73(4):358–71.

15. Lobbes MB, Lalji U, Houwers J, Nijssen EC, Nelemans PJ, van Roozendaal L, et al. Contrast-enhanced spectral mammography in patients referred from the breast cancer screening programme. Eur Radiol. 2014;24(7):1668–76.
16. Lalji UC, Houben IP, Prevos R, Gommers S, van Goethem M, Vanwetswinkel S, et al. Contrast-enhanced spectral mammography in recalls from the Dutch breast cancer screening program: validation of results in a large multireader, multicase study. Eur Radiol. 2016;26(12):4371–9.
17. Tennant SL, James JJ, Cornford EJ, Chen Y, Burrell HC, Hamilton LJ, et al. Contrast-enhanced spectral mammography improves diagnostic accuracy in the symptomatic setting. Clin Radiol. 2016;71(11):1148–55.
18. Jochelson MS, Dershaw DD, Sung JS, Heerdt AS, Thornton C, Moskowitz CS, et al. Bilateral contrast-enhanced dual-energy digital mammography: feasibility and comparison with conventional digital mammography and MR imaging in women with known breast carcinoma. Radiology. 2013;266(3):743–51.
19. Lee-Felker SA, Tekchandani L, Thomas M, Gupta E, Andrews-Tang D, Roth A, et al. Newly diagnosed breast cancer: comparison of contrast-enhanced spectral mammography and breast MR imaging in the evaluation of extent of disease. Radiology. 2017;285(2):389–400.
20. Wilczek B, Wilczek HE, Rasouliyan L, Leifland K. Adding 3D automated breast ultrasound to mammography screening in women with heterogeneously and extremely dense breasts: Report from a hospital-based, high-volume, single-center breast cancer screening program. Eur J Radiol. 2016;85(9):1554–63.
21. Sardanelli F, Boetes C, Borisch B, Decker T, Federico M, Gilbert FJ, et al. Magnetic resonance imaging of the breast: recommendations from the EUSOMA working group. Eur J Cancer. 2010;46(8):1296–316.
22. Mann RM, Balleyguier C, Baltzer PA, Bick U, Colin C, Cornford E, et al. Breast MRI: EUSOBI recommendations for women's information. Eur Radiol. 2015;25(12):3669–78. https://doi.org/10.1007/s00330-015-3807-z.
23. Zhang L, Tang M, Min Z, Lu J, Lei X, Zhang X. Accuracy of combined dynamic contrast-enhanced magnetic resonance imaging and diffusion-weighted imaging for breast cancer detection: a meta-analysis. Acta Radiol. 2016;57(6):651–60.
24. Saslow D, Boetes C, Burke W, Harms S, Leach MO, Lehman CD, et al. American Cancer Society guidelines for breast screening with MRI as an adjunct to mammography. CA Cancer J Clin. 2007;57(2):75–89.
25. Sardanelli F, Podo F, Santoro F, Manoukian S, Bergonzi S, Trecate G, et al. Multicenter surveillance of women at high genetic breast cancer risk using mammography, ultrasonography, and contrast-enhanced magnetic resonance imaging (the high breast cancer risk Italian 1 study): final results. Investig Radiol. 2011;46(2):94–105.
26. Kuhl CK, Schrading S, Leutner CC, Morakkabati-Spitz N, Wardelmann E, Fimmers R, et al. Mammography, breast ultrasound, and magnetic resonance imaging for surveillance of women at high familial risk for breast cancer. J Clin Oncol. 2005;23(33):8469–76.
27. Passaperuma K, Warner E, Causer PA, Hill KA, Messner S, Wong JW, et al. Long-term results of screening with magnetic resonance imaging in women with BRCA mutations. Br J Cancer. 2012;107(1):24–30.
28. Monticciolo DL, Newell MS, Moy L, Niell B, Monsees B, Sickles EA. Breast cancer screening in women at higher-than-average risk: recommendations from the ACR. J Am Coll Radiol. 2018;15(3. Pt A):408–14.
29. Dorrius MD, Dijkstra H, Oudkerk M, Sijens PE. Effect of b value and pre-admission of contrast on diagnostic accuracy of 1.5-T breast DWI: a systematic review and meta-analysis. Eur Radiol. 2014;24(11):2835–47.
30. Chen X, Li WL, Zhang YL, Wu Q, Guo YM, Bai ZL. Meta-analysis of quantitative diffusion-weighted MR imaging in the differential diagnosis of breast lesions. BMC Cancer. 2010;10:693.
31. Esserman L, Hylton N, Yassa L, Barclay J, Frankel S, Sickles E. Utility of magnetic resonance imaging in the management of breast cancer: evidence for improved preoperative staging. J Clin Oncol. 1999;17(1):110–9.
32. Boetes C, Mus RD, Holland R, Barentsz JO, Strijk SP, Wobbes T, et al. Breast tumors: comparative accuracy of MR imaging relative to mammography and US for demonstrating extent. Radiology. 1995;197(3):743–7.
33. Turnbull L, Brown S, Harvey I, Olivier C, Drew P, Napp V, et al. Comparative effectiveness of MRI in breast cancer (COMICE) trial: a randomised controlled trial. Lancet. 2010;375(9714):563–71.
34. Gonzalez V, Sandelin K, Karlsson A, Aberg W, Lofgren L, Iliescu G, et al. Preoperative MRI of the breast (POMB) influences primary treatment in breast cancer: a prospective, randomized, multicenter study. World J Surg. 2014;38(7):1685–93.
35. Mann RM, Loo CE, Wobbes T, Bult P, Barentsz JO, Gilhuijs KG, et al. The impact of preoperative breast MRI on the re-excision rate in invasive lobular carcinoma of the breast. Breast Cancer Res Treat. 2010;119(2):415–22.
36. Houssami N, Turner R, Morrow M. Preoperative magnetic resonance imaging in breast cancer: meta-analysis of surgical outcomes. Ann Surg. 2013;257(2):249–55.
37. Ryu J, Park HS, Kim S, Kim JY, Park S, Kim SI. Preoperative magnetic resonance imaging and survival outcomes in T1-2 breast cancer patients who receive breast-conserving therapy. J Breast Cancer. 2016;19(4):423–8.
38. Pediconi F, Catalano C, Roselli A, Padula S, Altomari F, Moriconi E, et al. Contrast-enhanced MR mammography for evaluation of the contralateral breast in patients with diagnosed unilateral breast cancer or high-risk lesions. Radiology. 2007;243(3):670–80.

14

Follow-Up of Patients with Breast Cancer: Imaging of Local Recurrence and Distant Metastases

Ulrich Bick and Thomas H. Helbich

Learning Objectives

- To learn about the strengths and weaknesses of the different imaging modalities for local surveillance of patients with a personal history of breast cancer.
- To understand that mammography is the only routinely recommended imaging modality with which to detect local recurrence or contralateral breast cancer.
- To discuss the role and effectiveness of imaging modalities in the staging and surveillance of patients with breast cancer after primary therapy.
- To show that there is little justification for imaging to detect metastasis in asymptomatic breast cancer patients.

14.1 Introduction

Breast cancer is the leading cause of cancer-related death among women worldwide, with variable incidence and mortality rates. Fortunately, mortality has decreased because of advances in screening and treatment [1, 2]. The 10-year survival rate of breast cancer ranges from 70 to 80%, with up to 90% for local and 60% for regional disease [3]. The annual hazard of recurrent disease (local and or metastases) ranges between 2 and 5% in years 5–20 after diagnosis. The yield for recurrent disease is likely to be higher in patients with advanced stages of disease [4]. Recent studies have demonstrated that the onset of local recurrence is an independent predictor for survival [5]. Thus management of patients with breast cancer during surveillance plays an important role. The aims of any follow-up are to detect early local recurrence or contralateral breast cancer and to diagnose and treat cancer and/or therapy-related diseases such as metastases and osteoporosis [3]. Considering these facts a well-defined, evidence-based surveillance protocol is needed to manage patients with breast cancer after the initial diagnosis, including staging and follow-up. Currently mammography every 1–2 years is the only recommended evidence-based imaging modality. In asymptomatic patients, there are no data to indicate that any imaging or laboratory test leads to a survival benefit. In symptomatic patients or in case of clinical findings appropriate tests should be performed immediately [3–8].

The purpose of this chapter is to address the role and effectiveness of imaging modalities in the staging and surveillance of patients with breast cancer after primary therapy.

14.2 Surveillance Recommendations for Local Recurrence

Local recurrence in breast cancer can be defined as recurrent disease to the ipsilateral breast, chest wall, or regional lymph nodes. Most local recurrences in breast cancer can be treated with curative intent and early detection of local recurrence will improve the overall prognosis of the patients [9]. Overall, the incidence of an ipsilateral breast recurrence (including ipsilateral new primary cancers) in women with spontaneous early-stage breast cancer treated with breast-conserving therapy will be around 0.5–1% per year and may especially in estrogen-receptor-positive tumors remain elevated well beyond 10 years after diagnosis [9, 10]. However, a variety

U. Bick (✉)
Department of Radiology, Charité - Universitätsmedizin Berlin, Berlin, Germany
e-mail: ulrich.bick@charite.de

T. H. Helbich (✉)
Department of Biomedical Imaging and Image-guided Therapy, Division of Molecular and Gender Imaging, Medical University of Vienna, Vienna, Austria
e-mail: thomas.helbich@meduniwien.ac.at

of factors will influence the likelihood and timing of local recurrence. In particular, involved surgical margins, nonadherence to adjuvant therapy guidelines, large size, and aggressive biology of the primary tumor, young patient age at diagnosis, and presence of familial or genetic risk factors may substantially increase recurrence rates.

14.2.1 Surveillance After Breast-Conserving Surgery

The backbone of surveillance of the ipsilateral breast in asymptomatic women with a personal history of breast cancer and who were treated with breast-conserving surgery is mammography [11–13]. However, specific recommendations vary substantially between countries and institutions regarding the optimal time to begin of mammographic surveillance after local treatment (e.g., 6–24 months after surgery) and the frequency (from semiannual mammography of the ipsilateral breast during the first 2 or 3 years after surgery to mammography only every 2–3 years) [9]. As sensitivity of mammography in the treated breast may be lower due to posttreatment changes [9], mammography is usually accompanied by a clinical exam and in many European countries by breast ultrasound [3]. This has the advantage that the axilla and regional lymph nodes can be evaluated at the same time. Digital breast tomosynthesis (DBT) has the potential to improve screening accuracy compared to 2D mammography; however data regarding DBT in the follow-up of patients with breast cancer is limited [14]. Contrast-enhanced magnetic resonance imaging (MRI) has the highest sensitivity regarding ipsilateral breast cancer recurrence. MRI is therefore an excellent tool for surveillance of asymptomatic high-risk women with a personal history of breast cancer as well as for problem-solving in otherwise indeterminate cases. However, the available evidence is currently insufficient to recommend for or against MRI as routine surveillance method in all normal-risk women with a personal history of breast cancer [15].

14.2.2 Follow-Up After Mastectomy

Most women treated with mastectomy with or without reconstruction can safely be followed by clinical exam alone or in conjunction with ultrasound. As long as the breast parenchyma has been completely removed during mastectomy, routine mammography on the affected side will not be necessary [16]. However it should be noted that some centers will ignore this advice and perform regular mammography in asymptomatic women after mastectomy with or without reconstruction [17]. If there is suspicion of significant residual breast parenchyma after mastectomy, breast MRI can reliably confirm or exclude residual parenchyma. Ipsilateral remaining breast tissue after mastectomy in women who have not received radiation therapy substantially increases the risk for local recurrence and may require re-excision or careful imaging surveillance [18]. In patients with mastectomy and implant reconstruction, MRI is superior to mammography and palpation regarding detection of recurrent disease [19]. MRI will be especially valuable in cases with prepectoral positioning of the implant to exclude pectoral recurrence behind the implant, as this area will not be accessible to clinical exam and ultrasound.

14.2.3 Imaging Patients with Local Symptoms

Any locoregional symptom such as a palpable lump, new pain, changes in breast configuration, or skin changes in a patient with a personal history of breast cancer should be carefully evaluated by a thorough clinical exam and tailored imaging. Many palpable abnormalities are readily accessible to targeted ultrasound. Additional imaging such as mammography and/or MRI can be added as needed. Positron emission tomography-computed tomography (PET/CT) can be very helpful in cases with suspected axillary recurrence, especially if the findings are not accessible to percutaneous biopsy.

14.2.4 Strengths and Weaknesses of Different Surveillance Methods

14.2.4.1 Clinical Exam

The value of a thorough clinical exam that consists of history-taking, inspection, and palpation of the breast and regional lymph nodes for the detection of local breast cancer recurrences should not be underestimated. Skin changes detected during clinical inspection may be the only sign of a local recurrence around the surgical scar or even for the existence of skin metastases. Palpation of the regional lymph nodes is also an important part of the clinical exam, especially if mammography only (no accompanying ultrasound) surveillance regimes are employed. About half of all ipsilateral breast recurrences will have a positive finding on clinical exam, and about a one-third of ipsilateral breast recurrences will be detected by the clinical exam with negative mammography [9]. This proportion is substantially higher than for healthy women undergoing routine mammography screening. Most guidelines therefore recommend clinical follow-up visits for breast cancer patients in the first 5 years after diagnosis at shorter intervals than the imaging surveillance (e.g., every 3–6 months) [3]. These visits also provide psychological support, motivate to follow adjuvant treatments recommendations, and help to detect treatment related problems early.

14.2.4.2 Mammography

Regular, usually annual mammography is the foundation of every surveillance regime in women after breast-conserving therapy. Ultrasound (US) and/or MRI can be used to supplement, but not to replace mammography in this situation. Between 50 and 80% of ipsilateral breast recurrences will be detectable by mammography. Key to this is the detection of suspicious microcalcifications by mammography, often an early sign of residual or recurrent disease (Fig. 14.1). High breast density as well as postoperative changes such as hematoma, seroma, fat necrosis, or scarring may reduce the sensitivity of mammography. There is hope that DBT will be able to overcome these limitations at least in part, by reducing problems due to superposition.

> **Key Point**
> - The detection of suspicious microcalcifications by mammography plays a crucial role in the early detection of not only in situ but also invasive ipsilateral breast cancer recurrence.

14.2.4.3 Ultrasound

Breast US is an ideal complementary technique to the clinical exam and mammography. It enables direct correlation with and work-up of clinical as well as mammographic findings. In addition, US is able to evaluate the chest wall or the reconstructed breast after mastectomy. Breast ultrasound is also an excellent tool to evaluate the regional lymph nodes. In contrast to mammography, the detection performance of US is not affected by dense breast tissue. The main limitation of US is the high number of non-specific or false-positive findings, although this is less of a problem if US is performed on a regular basis during follow-up.

14.2.4.4 MRI of the Breast

MRI of the breast has by far the highest sensitivity for invasive breast cancer of all available imaging modalities. This translates into a very high negative predictive value approaching 100% and makes MRI the ideal problem-solving tool. If no relevant contrast enhancement is found on MRI in the area of an equivocal clinical, mammographic, or sonographic finding, clinically relevant changes can be excluded with sufficient certainty, and the patient can safely be placed on short-term follow-up. With the exception of the immediate postoperative phase, MRI can also reliably differentiate between postoperative changes/scarring and recurrence. However, it is important to realize that local recurrence may lack typical malignant features at imaging such as irregular borders or rapid contrast uptake on MRI. Therefore histological confirmation, if necessary by open excisional biopsy, is advisable for all new solid lesions with enhancement on MRI (Fig. 14.2). The disadvantage of MRI is that many otherwise occult benign breast changes (including high-risk lesions) will also show enhancement on MRI. For MRI to have the highest benefit in routine surveillance/screening, the underlying incidence of malignant changes has to be high enough, or the positive predictive value of an abnormal MRI finding will be too low. This is the reason why routine surveillance with MRI is currently recommended only in the high-risk setting [15].

> **Key Point**
> - Any new solid enhancing lesion in the ipsilateral breast or chest wall should be considered suspicious for recurrence regardless of size, morphology, or enhancement characteristics.

14.2.4.5 Other Imaging

Contrast-enhanced mammography is an emerging technology, which may serve as an alternative if MRI cannot be performed (e.g., due to claustrophobia). Positron emission technologies such as PET/PEM are not recommended for routine surveillance of the breast due to the relatively high associated radiation dose associated with these modalities. However, PET/CT may be helpful in the evaluation of a possible regional lymph node recurrence or if there is the possibility of additional distant metastasis.

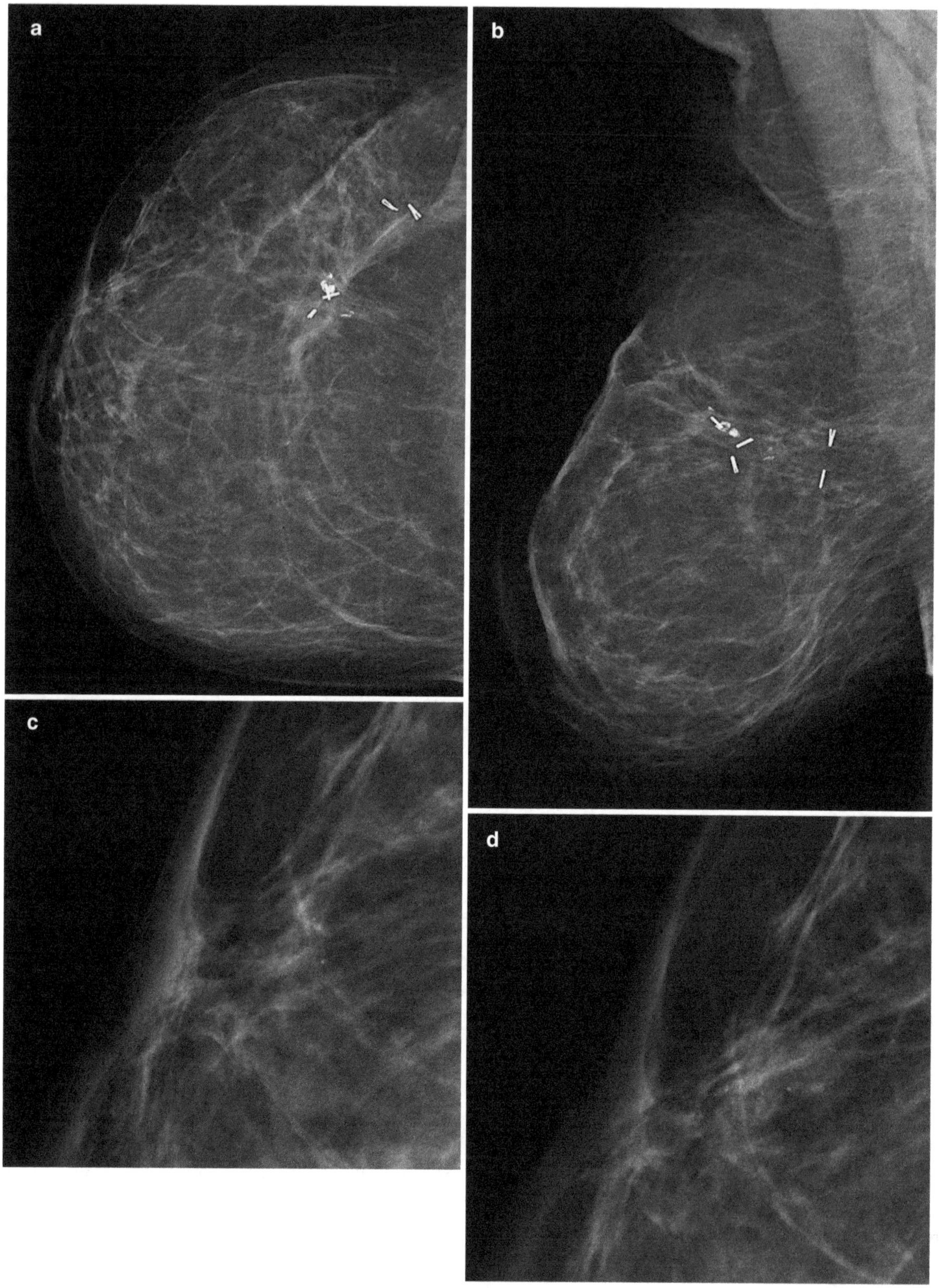

Fig. 14.1 A 48-year-old asymptomatic female, 11 years after breast-conserving treatment for right breast cancer (invasive NST with associated DCIS high-grade, pN2, pN1a, G2, ER/PR positive, Her2 negative) treated with adjuvant chemotherapy and endocrine therapy under routine surveillance. CC (**a**) and MLO (**b**) views of the right breast. Enlarged views of the retroareolar region of the prior CC 1 year ago (**c**) and the current CC (**d**) demonstrate a slight increase in the number of subtle calcifications in this area. Clinical exam and tailored ultrasound were normal. Stereotactic vacuum-assisted biopsy with specimen radiography of the obtained cores (**e**) and post-biopsy views (**f**) to confirm correct clip placement was performed and revealed a poorly differentiated invasive breast cancer (NST). Mastectomy confirmed a 13-mm invasive breast cancer (rpT1c, rpN0, G3, ER 100%, PR 100%, Her2 negative, MIB-1 proliferation index 10%). The patient was placed on tamoxifen and is currently healthy at age 53

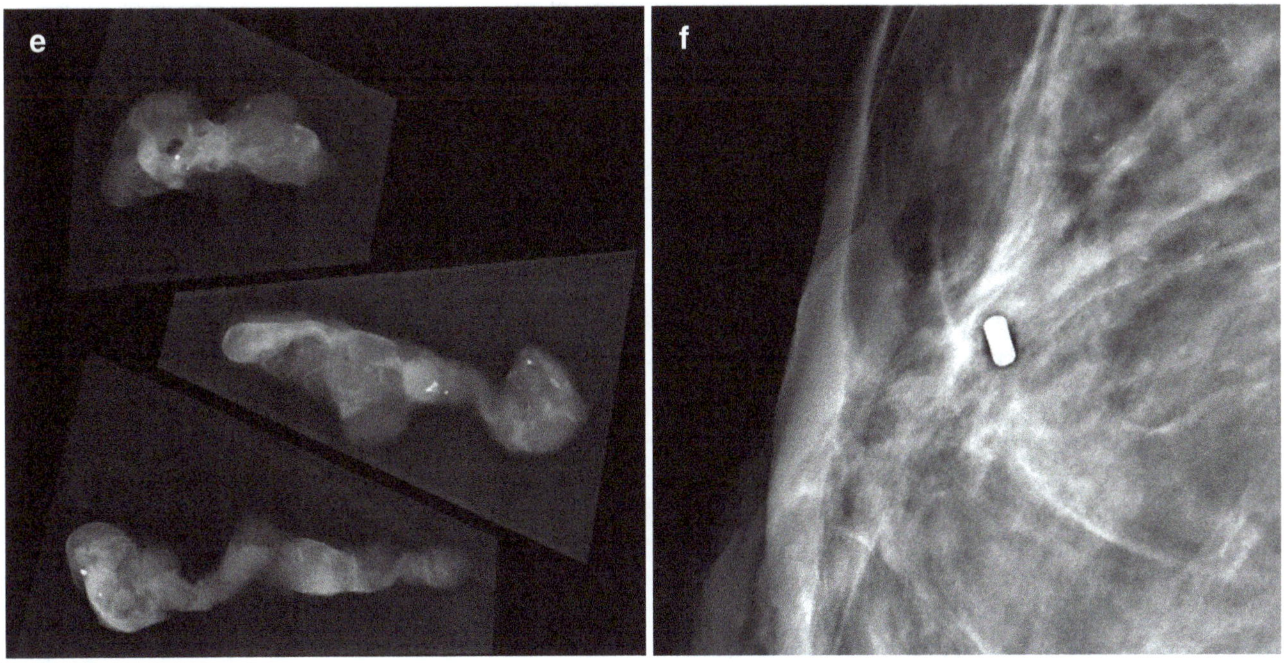

Fig. 14.1 (continued)

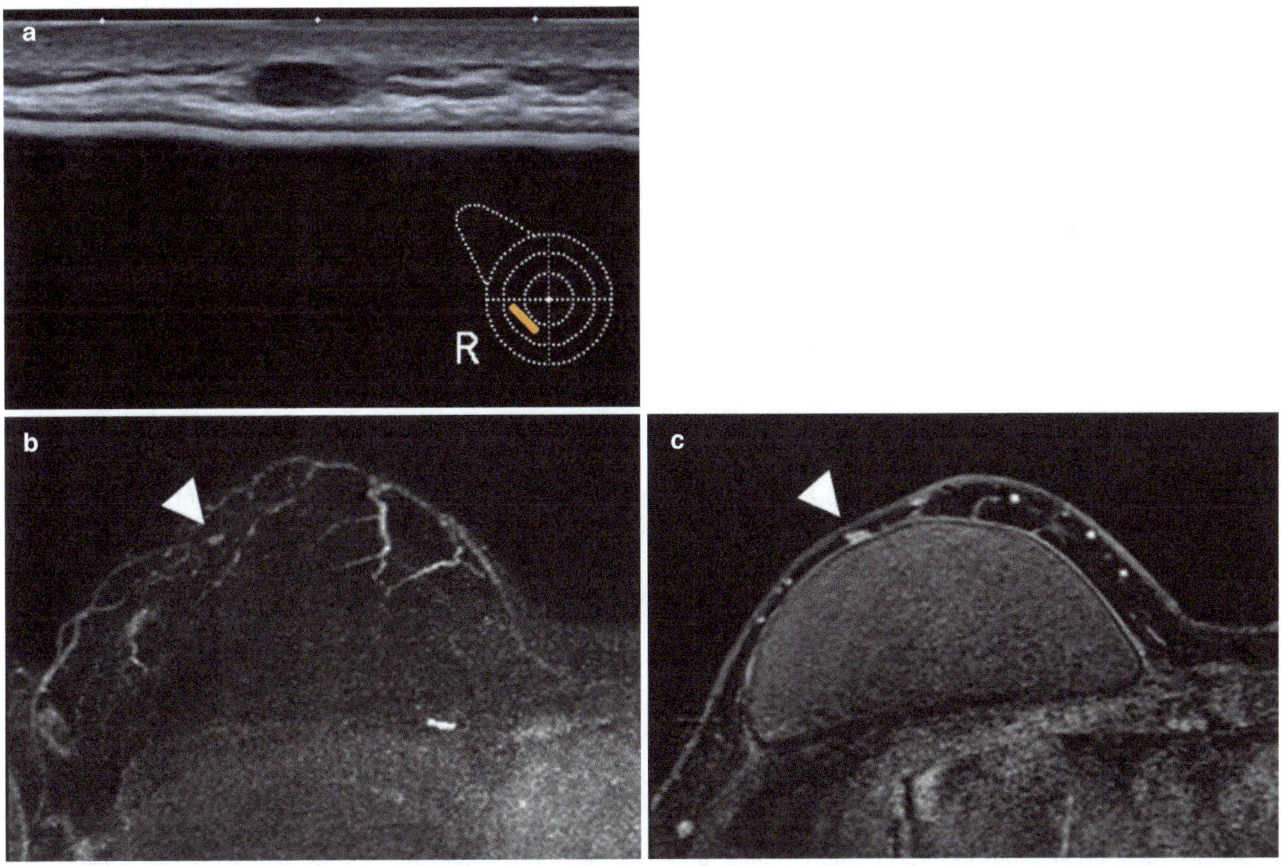

Fig. 14.2 A 37-year-old asymptomatic female, 6 years after right nipple-sparing mastectomy and implant reconstruction for extensive DCIS. Routine surveillance ultrasound (**a**) shows a new, small, oval, circumscribed, hypoechoic mass with parallel orientation in the remaining subcutaneous tissue surrounding the implant on the right. Contrast-enhanced MRI for further evaluation was performed. MIP images in the second minute after contrast enhancement (**b**) and delayed images with fat saturation (**c**) confirm a small, oval, circumscribed enhancing mass with persistent enhancement in the delayed phase. On surgical excision an invasive breast cancer (NST) with a maximum size of 6 mm was found (pT1b, pN0, G2, ER 100%, PR 0%, Her2 positive, MIB-1 proliferation index 30%). The patient was treated with chemotherapy in combination with trastuzumab as well as tamoxifen and is currently healthy at age 40

14.3 Imaging of Distant Metastases

14.3.1 Initial Staging

Once breast cancer is diagnosed, staging of the axilla must be performed. Currently, sentinel lymph node biopsy is recommended because imaging is not accurate enough [7]. Several guidelines recommend against the routine use of imaging modalities to stage asymptomatic metastases in newly diagnosed breast cancer [4]. Modern imaging technologies have improved the detection capability; thus the current NCCN guidelines [8] recommend against routine staging of patients with stage I and II disease but recommend CT (lung plus abdomen) or MRI (abdomen/liver) in addition to bone scintigraphy for stage III and IV disease. The use of FDG-PET/CT is viewed with caution though several studies demonstrate more accurate breast cancer staging with PET/CT. The use of FDG-PET/CT changed the clinical stage in 30% and found unsuspected metastases in 21% of patients with stage IIA and IIIC disease. Particular in younger patients (<40 years of age), an upstaging of 17% was seen in stage IIB disease [20]. Even more in bone metastases FDG-PET/CT outperforms CT or bone scintigraphy, with accuracies of up to 90%. The role of PET/CT may be less clinically relevant in extensive metastatic disease; however there are cases where a single metastasis is detected which affects the prognosis and the therapy (Fig. 14.3). The results of FDG-PET/CT are excellent; however it should be noted that its utility depends on cancer type being less sensitive in lobular breast cancer disease. Nevertheless it can be expected that PET/CT with more specific tracers than FDG will enhance the ability to stage breast cancer more accurately and will allow better prediction and assessment of treatment response during targeted therapy [7].

Key Point

- NCCN guidelines recommend against routine staging of patients with stage I and II disease but recommend CT or MRI in addition to bone scintigraphy for stage III and IV disease [8].

14.3.2 Distant Metastases

Distant recurrence (metastasis) is the main cause of breast cancer death. Mastectomy or lumpectomy followed by radiation therapy does not influence this risk [21]. The most common sites for breast cancer metastases are the skeleton, lung, liver, and brain [22]. In a Cochrane review by Rojas et al., which included 3055 women, there was no difference in overall or disease-free survival rates for patients who underwent intensive laboratory and imaging testing compared to those managed with clinical visits and mammography were seen [22]. Similar results were observed in two multicentric randomized surveillance studies performed in Italy in asymptomatic breast cancer patients. In both studies patients were randomized in two groups. One group had intensive follow-up, including bone scintigraphy, chest x-ray, and ultrasound of the liver, whereas the control group was examined only with imaging and laboratory test when clinical symptoms were present. In both studies intensive testing found more metastases; however, there was no significant difference seen in the overall survival between the two groups [23, 24]. As a consequence [3, 5, 6], several guidelines (Table 14.1) do not recommend intensive surveillance that would include routine blood tests, blood tests for tumor markers, chest x-ray, ultrasound of the liver, CT, MRI, or even PET/CT [5]. Nevertheless, surveillance programs vary among countries, organizations, and physicians. Physicians and patients favor intensive surveillance. In addition patients overestimate the role of laboratory and imaging tests and often incorrectly perceive the significance of a normal test [25, 26]. Keating et al. showed that patients who received care from oncologists had higher rates of testing than patients who were followed by their primary care physicians [25]. Grunfeld et al. [27] saw similar results were seen be in a retrospective study of 11,219 asymptomatic breast cancer survivors. Twenty-five percent of all patients had fewer than the recommended surveillance mammograms, and 50% had more than the recommended surveillance for metastatic disease (including bone scans, chest x-ray, CT, or MRI). Higher morbidity (more mastectomies) and seeing both an oncologist and primary care physicians increased the odds of having more intense imaging testing. Other studies found similar results, with the overuse of blood tests although rising tumor markers (i.e., CA 15-3 and CEA) suggest recurrence in asymptomatic patients [28]. Recently several studies demonstrated that in breast cancer patients with rising CA 15-3 and CEA levels the use of FDG-PET/CT would be of high diagnostic value, reporting an accuracy of up to 92% [29, 30]. Although FDG-PET/CT is not recommended for follow-up, suspected cases of recurrence that have equivocal conventional studies would be the best candidate for PET/CT [29]. In a recent study, Parmar et al. [5] assessed the role of imaging modalities in follow-up programs. Surprisingly, only 55% of patients showed strict adherence to the surveillance program. During the study period (2011–2007), the use of bone scans and mammograms decreased (21% to 13% and 81% to 75%, respectively), whereas use of MRI and FDG-PET/CT increased significantly (0.5% to 7% and 2% to 9%, respectively).

Overall, when imaging and laboratory tests are ordered in asymptomatic patients during follow-up surveillance, the cost-effectiveness and accuracy of applying supplemental testing must be considered. In addition efforts should be made to a more intensively educate of physicians to reduce to use of non-guideline conforming surveillance testing. Nevertheless, it has been evidentially seen that physicians

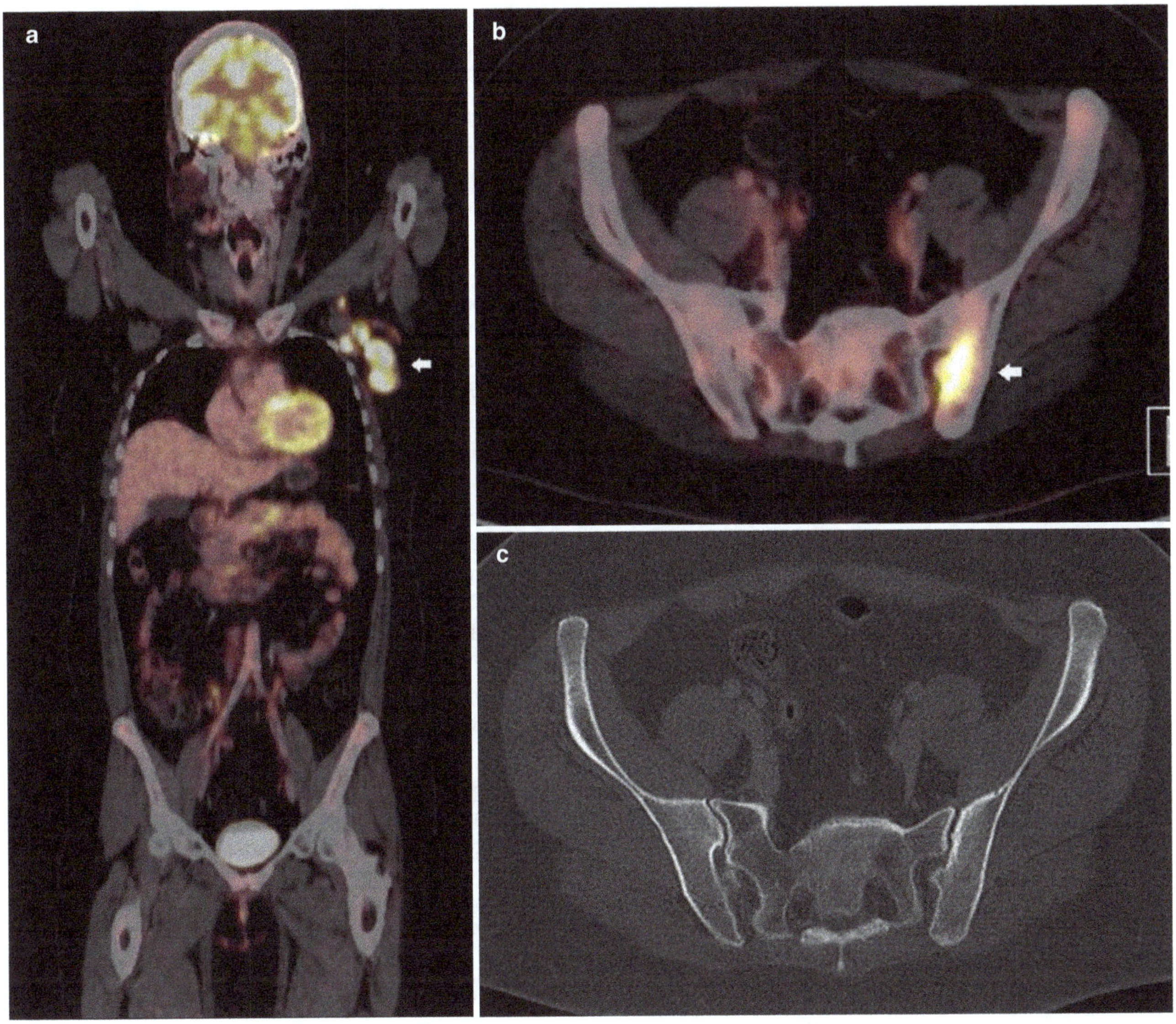

Fig. 14.3 A 41-year-old female with multicentric biopsy proven left breast cancer measuring 8 cm in dimensions and suspicious ipsilateral axillary nodes (stage T3 N1). Patient underwent 18F-FDG PET/CT for staging (histology: invasive ductal carcinoma NOS, G3, ER weakly positive, PR negative, HER2 positive, p53 weakly positive (10%), MIB-1 positive). (**a**) Coronal fused PET/CT image shows bulky FDG avid left axillary nodes (arrow). (**b**) Axial fused PET/CT image shows a FDG avid lesion in the left ilium (arrow) and biopsy proven osseous metastases. This was occult on the CT component (**c**). PET/CT correctly upstaged the disease to stage IV thus illustrating the value of PET/CT in distant staging

and patients are not confident in the current surveillance programs with mammography as the only imaging modality considering the development of new and promising imaging technologies [29, 30]. Currently there is no evidence that early detection of metastases during follow-up improves survival. However, early detection may allow more accurate and curative intervention, and this may be the cause for the current trends, in which advanced imaging modalities other than mammography are used [5, 29].

Key Point

- Breast cancer patients who receive intensive screening and surveillance with imaging and laboratory studies have no survival benefit compared to those who undergo testing after clinical symptoms are evident.

14.3.3 Imaging for Bone, Lung, and Liver Metastases

Current guidelines (Table 14.1) recommend against the routine use of laboratory or imaging tests to detect asymptomatic metastases during staging or follow-up after breast cancer diagnosis. This paragraph describes briefly which imaging modalities should be used to detect distant metastases if clinical symptoms are present [6]. To detect skeletal metastases, bone scintigraphy is more effective than conventional radiography. Several recent studies suggest that FDG-PET/CT, PET/MRI, or whole-body MRI is significantly more accurate than bone scintigraphy, but both can still miss some metastases, particularly sclerotic ones. It is expected that these new imaging techniques will replace current technologies (Fig. 14.4). To detect lung metastases chest x-ray and CT are recommended. Chest x-ray is considered the most reasonable approach because of the low costs. In case of any questionable findings, CT is recommended as a baseline for monitoring and for follow-up. Liver metastases are not as common as lung or bone metastases; however, their appearance is associated with the worst prognosis. In symptomatic patients CT or MRI is recommended as more lesions can be diagnosed with a higher accuracy compared to US. Particularly for follow-up during therapy MRI should be advantageously used. Breast cancer is second only to lung carcinoma as a cause of brain metastases. Contrast-enhanced MRI has largely replaced CT for the detection and evaluation of brain lesions because of its high sensitivity (Fig. 14.5) [6].

14.3.4 Assessing Treatment Response of Distant Metastases

Once a breast cancer patient has been diagnosed with metastases, accurate assessment of treatment response is of the uppermost importance. Currently follow-up assessment is based on anatomic imaging (CT or MRI) (Fig. 14.6). Treatment response, particularly in clinical trials, is evaluated by the RECIST (Response Evaluation Criteria in Solid Tumors) 1.1 criteria. A change in the size of a given metastasis during treatment is a measure of response. In soft tissue metastases (e.g., liver, lung, and brain), this approach is currently acceptable. However, in bone metastases – the most common site of metastatic disease – this approach is problematic unless there is an extra-osseous soft tissue mass associated with the bone lesion. If FDG-PET/CT is used metabolic activity can be assessed and thus determine the response to treatment [7, 29, 30]. By comparing FDG-PET/CT with conventional anatomic CT, Vranjesevic et al. showed that the PPV (93% vs. 85%) and NPV (84% vs. 59%) of FDG-PET/CT were higher than with conventional imaging [7]. Other PET tracers (e.g., 18F-fluorothymidine) predict response at an early time point, and thus treatment change can be determined earlier which may lead to a better outcome with respect to disease burden and morbidity. Such approaches have been seen in lymphoma patients and should be implemented for breast cancer as well [7]. In addition PET/CT shows great promise in the assessment of patients who have various responses in different sites of metastases

Table 14.1 Surveillance recommendations for women treated for primary breast cancer

	Year	History and physical examinations	Mammography (MG)	Other tests
American Society of Clinical Oncology	2012	Every 3–6 month for first 3 years Every 6–12 months for years 4–5 Annual follow-up thereafter	Posttreatment MG 1 year after initial mammogram At least 6 months after completion of radiation therapy Annual MG	Chest radiography, bone scans, liver US, CT, PET, MRI, or other laboratory tests: NOT recommended in asymptomatic patients with no specific findings on clinical examinations
National Comprehensive Cancer Network	2018	Every 4–6 months for 5 years Annual follow-up thereafter	MG every 12 months	MRI considered in women with lifetime risk of second primary breast cancer greater than 20% Imaging and laboratory tests not recommended in asymptomatic patients
European Society of Medical Oncology	2013	Every 3–4 months for first 2 years Every 6 months from year 3–5 Annual follow-up thereafter	Ipsilateral (after BCS) and contralateral MG every 1–2 years	MRI may be indicated for young women with dense breasts, genetic of familial predispositions Laboratory or imaging tests not recommended in asymptomatic patients
National Institute for Clinical Excellence	2011	Regular check-up, determined by physician or patient	Annual MG	Laboratory or imaging tests not recommended routinely

Note: Modified from [5]

BCS breast-conserving surgery, *CT* computed tomography, *MRI* magnetic resonance imaging, *PET* positron emission tomography, *US* ultrasonography

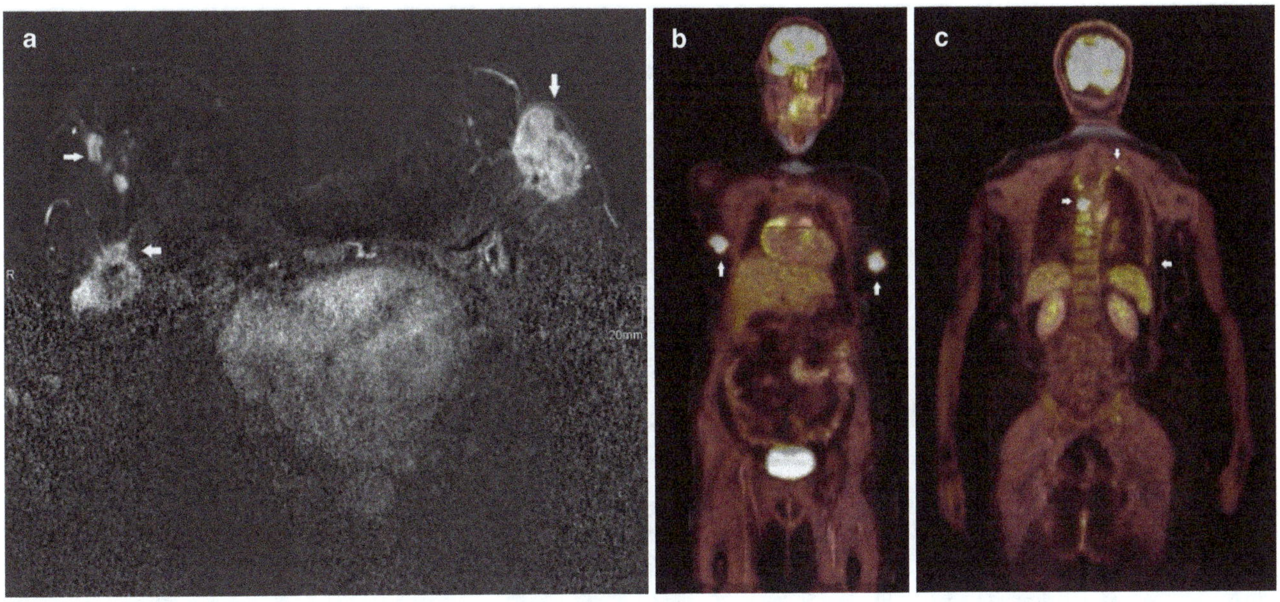

Fig. 14.4 A 66-year-old female with bilateral biopsy proven multicentric breast cancers underwent whole-body 18F-FDG PET/MRI which enables "one stop" staging of both locoregional and distant disease (histology: right invasive ductal carcinoma NOS, G2, ER/PR positive, HER2 negative, p53 weakly positive (10%), MIB-1 20% positive; left invasive ductal carcinoma NOS G2, ER/PR positive, HER2 weakly positive (20%), p53 weakly positive (10%), MIB-1 10% positive). (**a**) Contrast-enhanced axial T1 subtracted breast MRI image shows multicentric disease on the right (arrows) involving the skin, nipple, and chest wall and a dominant left breast mass (arrow) involving the nipple; bilateral T4 tumors (**b, c**) Coronal fused whole-body PET/MRI images show bilateral FDG avid breast tumors (arrows) (**b**) and multiple FDG avid osseous metastases (arrows) (**c**). PET/MRI also revealed bilateral FDG avid axillary and supraclavicular nodes (not shown). Overall stage T4, N3, M1

due to tumor heterogeneity. Several studies have reported discordant responses between bone and non-bone metastases in 30–43% [7]. Further FDG-PET/CT demonstrated response in patients who had no change at anatomic CT and predicted progression-free survival and disease-specific survival significantly better than CT [7].

14.4 Concluding Remarks

A well-defined evidence-based surveillance protocol is needed to manage patients with breast cancer after the initial diagnosis, as well as during staging and follow-up. The aims of any follow-up are to detect early local recurrence and to diagnose and treat cancer and/or therapy-related diseases such as metastases. Currently, mammography every 1–2 years is the only recommended evidence-based imaging modality. In asymptomatic patients, there are no data to indicate that any imaging or laboratory test leads to a survival benefit; thus these tests are not recommended during surveillance. Recent guidelines recommend CT or MRI in addition to bone scintigraphy for stage III and IV disease at the time of diagnosis. In the near future, it can be expected that sensitive imaging tests (whole-body MRI or PET/CT/MRI) will enhance the ability to stage breast cancer more accurately and will allow better prediction and assessment of treatment response during targeted therapy.

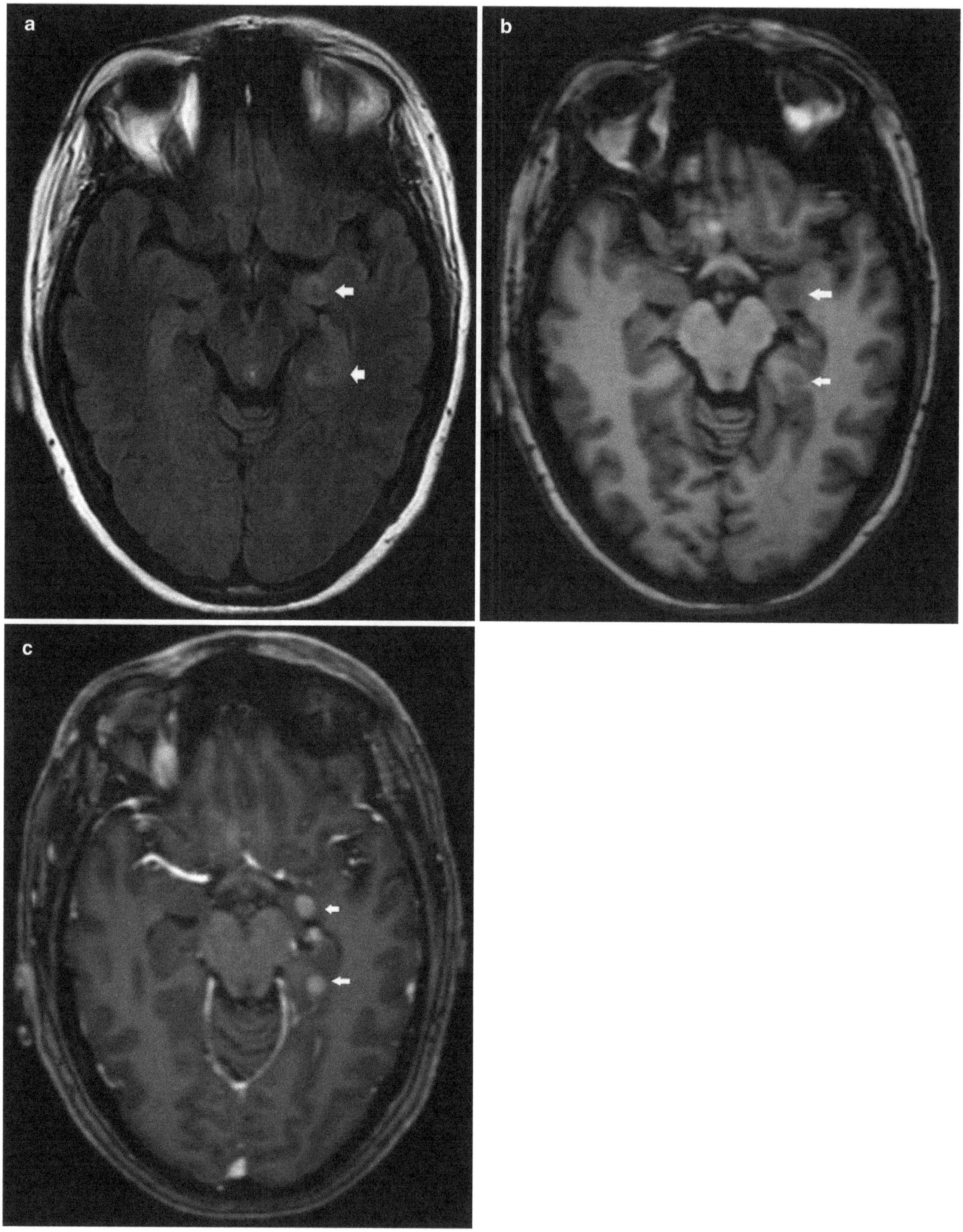

Fig. 14.5 A 40-year-old female with biopsy proven left breast cancer underwent contrast-enhanced brain MRI for further evaluation of headache (histology: invasive ductal carcinoma NOS, G2, ER positive, PR negative, HER2 positive, p53 negative, MIB-1 positive). Axial FLAIR (**a**), T1(**b**) and post-contrast T1 (**c**) images show enhancing left temporal lesions in keeping with brain metastases which are heterogeneous predominantly hypointense on FLAIR and hypointense on T1 (arrows)

Fig. 14.6 A 76-year-old female with biopsy proven right breast cancer and ipsilateral nodal disease (histology: invasive lobular carcinoma, G3, ER/PR negative, HER-2 positive, p53 positive, MIB-1 positive) with multiple mixed lytic and sclerotic osseous metastases in the spine and sternum on the sagittal CT bone window image (arrows) (**a**). Post chemotherapy the breast and nodal lesions regressed (not shown). On the post-chemotherapy sagittal CT image (**b**), the osseous metastases (arrows) show interval increased sclerosis in keeping with posttreatment changes

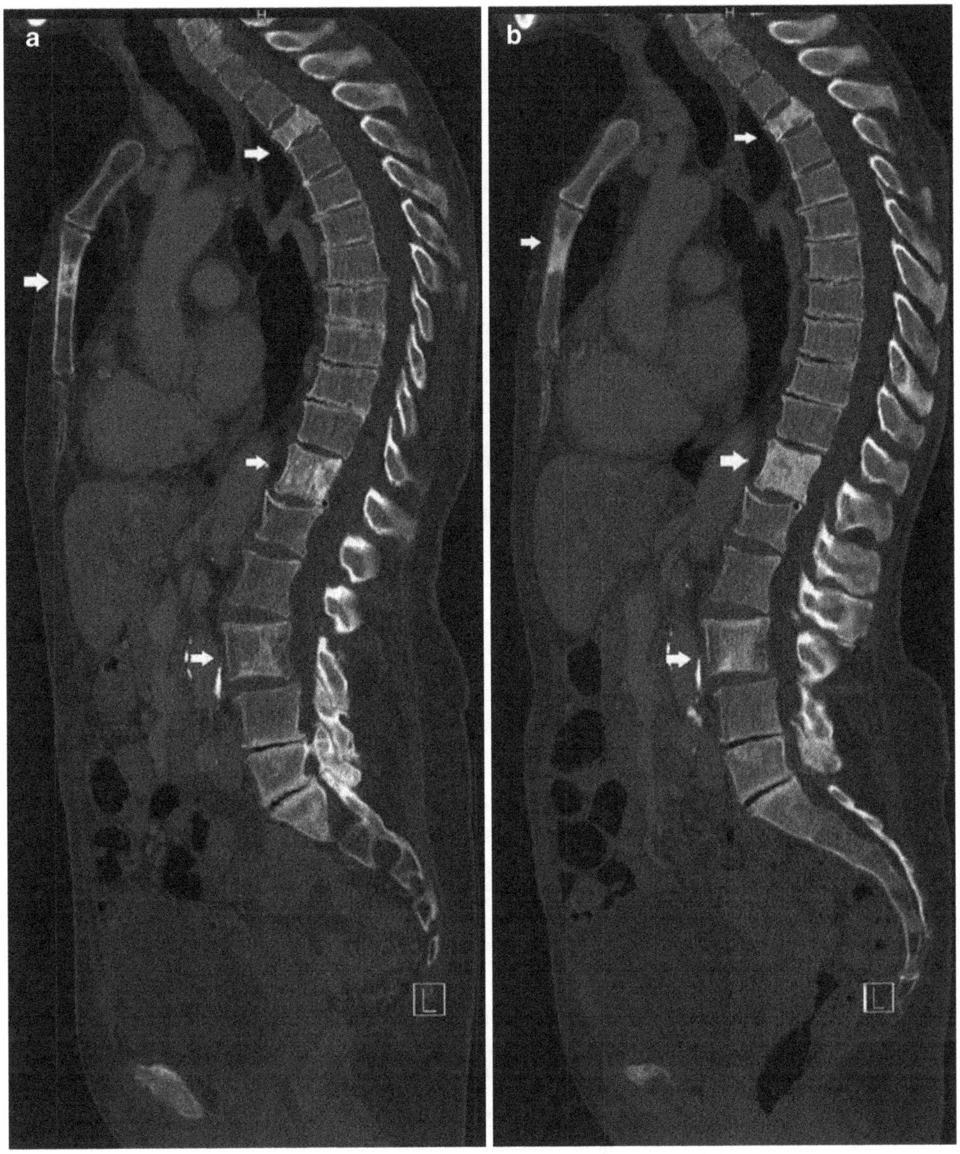

Take-Home Messages

- Regular, usually annual mammography is the cornerstone of surveillance of the ipsilateral breast in patients with a personal history of breast cancer who were treated with breast-conserving therapy.
- Local breast cancer recurrence may lack the typical imaging features of primary breast cancer, and reliable diagnosis is often based on the combination of a thorough clinical exam and tailored multimodality imaging.
- Current guidelines do not recommend intensive surveillance in asymptomatic breast cancer patients, which includes routine blood tests, chest x-ray, ultrasound of the liver, CT, MRI, or even PET/CT. At time of diagnosis, CT or MRI in addition to bone scintigraphy is recommended in stage III and IV disease.
- More sensitive imaging tests (e.g., whole-body MRI or PET/CT/MRI) will enhance the ability to stage breast cancer more accurately and may change current guidelines.

References

1. Siegel R, Naishadham D, Jemal A. Cancer statistics. CA Cancer J Clin. 2013;63:11–30.
2. Berry DA, Cronin KA, Plevritis SK, et al. Effect of screening and adjuvant therapy on mortality from breast cancer. N Engl J Med. 2005;353:1784–92.
3. Senkus E, Kyriakides S, Penault-Llorca F, et al. Primary breast cancer: ESMO Clinical Practice Guidelines for diagnosis, treatment and follow-up. Ann Oncol. 2013;24:vi7–vi23.
4. Brennan ME, Houssami N. Evaluation of the evidence on staging imaging for detection of asymptomatic distant metastases in newly diagnosed breast cancer. Breast. 2012;21:112–23.
5. Yoon JH, Kim MJ, Kim EK, Moon HJ. Imaging surveillance of patients with breast cancer after primary treatment: current recommendations. KJR. 2015;16:219–28.
6. Moy L, Bailey L, D'Orsi C, et al. ACR appropriateness criteria stage I breast cancer: initial workup and surveillance for local recurrence and distant metastases in asymptomatic women. J Am Coll Radiol. 2017;14:S282–92.
7. Jochelson M. Breast Cancer Staging. Physiology trumps anatomy. https://www.sbi-online.org/RESOURCES/WhitePapers/TabId/595/ArtMID/1617/ArticleID/597/Breast-Cancer-Staging-Physiology-Trumps-Anatomy.aspx
8. National Comprehensive Cancer Network, Inc. 2018. The NCCN Evidence BlocksTM, NCCN Guidelines. Version 1.2018.
9. Houssami N, Ciatto S. Mammographic surveillance in women with a persona history of breast cancer: how accurate? How effective? Breast. 2010;19:439–45.
10. Spronk I, Schellevis FG, Burgers JS, et al. Incidence of isolated local breast cancer recurrence and contralateral breast cancer: a systematic review. Breast. 2018;39:70–9.
11. Lam DL, Houssami N, Lee JM. Imaging surveillance after primary breast cancer treatment. AJR. 2017;208:676–86.
12. Muradali D, Kennedy EB, Eisen A, et al. Breast screening for survivors of breast cancer: a systematic review. Prev Med. 2017;103:70–5.
13. Robertson C, Ragupathy SK, Boachie C, et al. Surveillance mammography for detecting ipsilateral breast tumour recurrence and metachronous contralateral breast cancer: a systematic review. Eur Radiol. 2011;21:2484–91.
14. Sia J, Moodie K, Bressel M, et al. A prospective study comparing digital breast tomosynthesis with digital mammography in surveillance after breast cancer treatment. Eur J Cancer. 2016;61:122–7.
15. Saslow D, Boetes C, Burke W, et al. American Cancer Society guidelines for breast screening with MRI as an adjunct to mammography. CA Cancer J Clin. 2007;57:75–89.
16. Khatcheressian JL, Hurley P, Bantug E, et al. Breast cancer follow-up and management after primary treatment: American Society of Clinical Oncology clinical practice guideline update. J Clin Oncol. 2013;31:961–5.
17. Noroozian M, Carlson LW, Savage JL, et al. Use of screening mammography to detect occult malignancy in autologous breast reconstructions: a 15-year experience. Radiology. 2018;289:39–48.
18. Margolis NE, Morley C, Lotfi P, et al. Update on imaging of the postsurgical breast. Radiographics. 2014;34:642–60.
19. Bone B, Aspelin P, Isberg B, et al. Contrast-enhanced MR imaging of the breast in patients with breast implants after cancer surgery. Acta Radiol. 1995;36:111–6.
20. Riedl CC, Slobod E, Jochelson M, et al. Retrospective analysis of 18F-FDG PET/CT for staging asymptomatic breast cancer patients younger than 40 years. J Nucl Med. 2014;55:1578–83.
21. Buchholz TA, Hunt KK. Breast-conserving therapy: conventional whole breast irradiation. In: Harris JR, Lippman ME, Morrow M, Osborne CK, editors. Disease of the breast. Philadelphia, PA: Lippincott Williams & Wilkins; 2010.
22. Rojas MP, Telaro E, Russo A, et al. Follow-up strategies for women treated for early breast cancer. Cochrane Database Syst Rev. 2005;1:CD001768.
23. Rosselli Del Turco M, Palli D, Cariddi A, Ciatto S, Pacini P, Distante V. Intensive diagnostic follow-up after treatment of primary breast cancer. A randomized trial. National Research Council Project on Breast Cancer follow-up. JAMA. 1994;271:1593–7.
24. The GIVIO Investigators. Impact of follow-up testing on survival and health-related quality of life in breast cancer patients. A multicentre randomized controlled trial. JAMA. 1994;271:1587–92.
25. Keating NL, Landrum MB, Guadagnoli E, Winer EP, Ayanian JZ. Surveillance testing among survivors of early-stage breast cancer. J Clin Oncol. 2007;25:1074–81.
26. Loomer L, Brockschmidt JK, Muss HB, Saylor G. Postoperative follow-up of patients with early breast cancer. Patterns of care among clinical oncologists and a review of the literature. Cancer. 1991;67:55–60.
27. Grunfeld E, Hodgson DC, Del Giudice ME, Moineddin R. Population- based longitudinal study of follow-up care for breast cancer survivors. J Oncol Pract. 2010;6:174–81.
28. Chang HT, Hu C, Chiu YL, Peng NJ, Liu RS. Role of 2-[18F] fluoro-2-deoxy-D-glucose-positron emission tomography/computed tomography in the post-therapy surveillance of breast cancer. PLoS One. 2014;9:e115127.
29. Paydary K, Seraj SM, Zadeh MZ, et al. The evolving role of FDG-PET/CT in the diagnosis, staging, and treatment of breast cancer. Mol Imaging Biol. 2018; https://doi.org/10.1007/s11307-018-1181-3.
30. Champion L, Brain E, Giraudet AL, et al. Breast cancer recurrence diagnosis suspected on tumor marker rising: value of whole-body 18FDG-PET/CT imaging and impact on patient management. Cancer. 2011;117:1621–162.

15

CT and MRI in Suspected Ischemic Heart Disease

Albert de Roos and Konstantin Nikolaou

Learning Objectives

- To understand basic approaches of CT and MRI in ischemic heart disease.
- To learn systematic approach to diagnose ischemic heart disease.
- To learn about differential diagnoses shown by CT and MRI.

15.1 Introduction

CT and MRI have made enormous strides over the past decades becoming established imaging techniques in patients with suspected ischemic heart disease. The impact of these imaging techniques cannot be overestimated in the diagnosis and prognostication of patients with ischemic heart disease. As ischemic heart disease is highly prevalent, any contribution to improving the diagnosis and work-up of these patients by noninvasive imaging techniques has direct implications to more cost-effective diagnosis and therapy. For a long time, the mainstay in the diagnosis and treatment of ischemic heart disease was conventional x-ray angiography and echocardiography. The recognition of limitations inherent to these well-established diagnostic methods has led to a surge of interest in cardiovascular imaging by CT and MRI. In addition, nuclear medicine imaging is a well-established imaging technology for myocardial perfusion assessment in patients with suspected ischemic heart disease. The strength of this imaging technology is the wealth of outcome data for patient management, but CT and MRI have also made big strides to pose as an alternative for myocardial perfusion imaging as well as other approaches to assess the functional significance of coronary artery disease.

CT and MRI have their own strengths and weaknesses to provide diagnostic information in the work-up of patients with suspected ischemic heart disease. The main breakthrough was coronary CT angiography providing unparalleled high-quality noninvasive visualization of coronary artery disease, now firmly established as the preferred tool to exclude coronary artery disease in patients with intermediate likelihood for coronary disease based on their clinical risk profile. The main limitation of CT was the lack of functional information to estimate the significance of a stenosis as a flow-limiting lesion that may cause myocardial ischemia. Nowadays CT may provide this crucial information for patient management by rest/stress CT perfusion and noninvasive estimation of the fractional flow reserve (CT-FFR). The integration of diagnosing coronary artery anatomy (stenosis) in conjunction with functional assessment (ischemia) provides a complete tool for clinical decision-making (indication for percutaneous coronary intervention or bypass surgery). In contrast, MRI has lacked behind to CT as a robust imaging tool for noninvasive coronary artery imaging. The main strengths of cardiac MRI are the unsurpassed high-quality images of cardiac anatomy and global left ventricular function and a wide armamentarium for myocardial tissue characterization. For example, MRI late gadolinium enhancement (LGE) started over 30 years ago and took a relative long time before becoming established as a unique noninvasive tool to assess the transmural extent of a myocardial scar with great clinical implications. The combined use of cine MRI and LGE is clinically highly relevant to characterize ischemic heart disease and to differentiate ischemic from nonischemic heart disease. Cine MRI is unsurpassed in accuracy for precisely measuring structure (wall thickness) and function (ejection fraction). Next to LGE, a number of other

A. de Roos (✉)
Department of Radiology, Leiden University Medical Center, Leiden, South Holland, The Netherlands
e-mail: a.de_roos@lumc.nl

K. Nikolaou
Department of Diagnostic and Interventional Radiology, University Hospitals Tubingen, Tubingen, Germany
e-mail: Konstantin.Nikolaou@med.uni-tuebingen.de

MRI techniques have been established for myocardial tissue characterization that provide additional information on acute versus chronic scar (T2 mapping, STIR) and diffuse myocardial fibrosis (T1 mapping, extracellular volume or ECV). Combining these MRI techniques for tissue characterization has some similarity with how a pathologist may combine different staining techniques for tissue characterization to come to a final diagnosis. MRI myocardial tissue "staining" has been established as an invaluable tool for characterizing myocardial disease in patients with suspected ischemic heart disease as well as in patients with unexplained heart failure to differentiate ischemic heart disease from the large number of nonischemic cardiomyopathies (nonischemic dilated cardiomyopathy, hypertrophic cardiomyopathy, amyloid, other storage diseases, and alike).

Patients are referred to cardiac or chest CT and MRI by various medical disciplines (e.g., cardiology, internal medicine, emergency department) with different clinical questions and scenarios. For example, many referrals for evaluating acute chest pain come from the emergency department ("rule out pulmonary embolism"). The current high volume of pulmonary embolism referrals may lead to a number of unexpected findings on chest CT, as the yield of this referral for a positive diagnosis of pulmonary embolism is quite low and the clinical work-up of these patients may be suboptimal. The high-quality CT images of today, even if ungated, provide good diagnostic information on cardiac anatomy and coronary disease. So, coronary artery disease is becoming an "incidental finding" on routine chest CT requested for other indications. Radiologists are now in a central and responsible position to diagnose or rule out not only pulmonary embolism in acute chest pain evaluation but also be prepared to diagnose the extensive differential diagnosis (over 30 differential diagnoses) of a patient presenting with acute chest pain (main causes are life-threatening acute coronary occlusion, aortic dissection, and pulmonary embolism).

In this course we will discuss the role of CT and MRI in patients with suspected ischemic heart disease. First, the basic aspects of the pathophysiology (ischemic cascade) and technology will be shortly summarized. Secondly, the specific utility of CT and MRI in suspected ischemic heart disease will be illustrated using patient examples. The patient presentations will also consider a stepwise approach on how to differentiate ischemic from nonischemic cardiomyopathies and the differential diagnosis of acute chest pain.

Key Point

- LGE is helpful MRI technique to differentiate ischemic from nonischemic cardiomyopathy.

15.2 Cardiac MRI

15.2.1 MRI Techniques

Myocardial function is typically evaluated using cine balanced steady-state free precession (bSSFP) imaging, providing optimal contrast between the blood pool (bright signal) and myocardium (intermediate-low signal). Cine MRI is used to assess ventricular function and valvular function in various orientations (transverse, angulated). As a starting point, the transverse cine images provide a global impression on left ventricular function, regional function (scar, aneurysm), and valvular function (stenosis jet, regurgitation jet, valve morphology). Short-axis cine images are routinely applied for calculation of ventricular volumes (ejection fraction is very important for clinical decision-making and prognostication). LGE-MRI is the reference standard for imaging myocardial scar. Based on inversion recovery methods, contrast is created between normal (dark, gadolinium excluded from intact cells) myocardium and scar (white due to gadolinium accumulation). Both acute and chronic infarct may display LGE. Acute infarcts show LGE due to cell membrane breakdown, whereas chronic collagen scar has little cellular volume and larger volume of distribution and therefore accumulates gadolinium. A particular strength of LGE is visualization of very small scars as well as the transmural extent of necrosis (starts at the subendocardium and may progress through the ventricular wall as a wave front with longer durations of coronary occlusion). Myocardial signal intensity depends on the T1, T2, T2*, and proton density of the tissue. All these parameters are actively explored for better characterizing the severity of myocardial injury. Quantitative maps of myocardial T1, T2, T2*, and extracellular volume (ECV) are attractive alternative methods for better tissue characterization. Quantitative methods for characterizing myocardial tissue based on parametric mapping of T1 and T2 have been explored as an objective tool of detecting and quantifying focal as well as global myocardial tissue alterations. In combination with extracellular contrast agent (gadolinium) injection, T1 mapping can also estimate the extracellular volume (ECV) fraction. Non-contrast enhanced, native T1 mapping and ECV mapping are explored as a diagnostic tool in both acute and chronic myocardial infarction and may be used to assess the area at risk (edema). Many other disease processes in the myocardium may result in elevated (e.g., myocarditis, amyloidosis) or decreased (e.g., Fabry disease, high iron content) native T1 values. Native T2 mapping can detect edema in myocarditis, area at risk, and acute myocardial infarction. Technical details of pulse sequences, acquisition protocols, scanner adjustments, artifacts, image processing (windowing) and other confounders are affecting and complicating reliable determination of parametric maps. Well-controlled and optimized techniques are crucial to improve accuracy (saturation methods), precision (inversion methods), and reproducibility of the use of parametric imaging. The acquisition technique combines an inversion or saturation pulse to pertubate T1, sampling of the relaxation curve, and a model to fit the sampled curve and extract the myocardial T1 value. Initial methods for pixel-wise parametric T1 mapping are MOLLI and shMOLLI (modified Look-Locker inversion and shortened breath-hold modified Look-Locker inversion, respectively) sequences. Inversion methods (e.g., MOLLI, shMOLLI), saturation methods (e.g., SASHA, saturation recovery single-shot acquisition), and combined inversion and saturation methods (e.g., SAPPHIRE, saturation pulse prepared heart-rate-independent inversion recovery) are explored to optimize the reliability of acquisition schemes. Motion artifacts have been reduced by schemes that allow high-resolution imaging at the same cardiac and respiratory phase. The ECV in the myocardium is estimated from the concentration of extracellular contrast agent in the myocardium relative to the blood in a dynamic state. The formula for calculation of ECV incorporates hematocrit (determined for each individual from blood sample or synthetic Ht, reflecting blood volume of distribution) and change in relaxation rate between precontrast and postcontrast (proportional to gadolinium concentration, 15 min after bolus injection). Quantitative T2 mapping is commonly performed using single-shot T2-prepared SSFP approach, although other approaches are available. For example, images may be acquired at three echo times, and after monoexponential curve fitting, a pixel-wise T2 map is produced.

The initial area at risk after coronary occlusion (before necrosis develops) may be visualized as a bright region by using T2-weighted MRI techniques. Multiple MRI techniques are available to provide optimal T2 contrast. T2-weighted imaging is also helpful to differentiate acute (white) from chronic scar (dark), as both may show similar LGE. Shortly after coronary occlusion edema may develop in the area at risk (the myocardium dependent on that coronary artery) and may be shown as a bright region on T2-weighted imaging. Initially dark-blood T2-weighted sequences were used for defining the presumed edema in the area at risk. However, when limitations and artifacts of these techniques raised some controversy on their utility, T2 mapping, T1 mapping, early gadolinium enhancement, and contrast-enhanced bSSFP cine MRI were proposed as alternative methods to visualize the area at risk. The area at risk appears bright on T2-weighted imaging (long T2) or dark on T1-weighted imaging (long T1) and in the bright range of the color scale on quantitative T1 and T2 maps due to long T1 and long T2. The endocardial surface area (approximation of the wave front) method of acute infarction has also been used to estimate the area at risk. The ischemic cascade may further progress with necrosis starting at the subendocardial level and depending on duration of occlusion may progress throughout the entire wall (transmural, full thickness infarct). LGE MRI may show the transmural extent of the infarct to best advantage. In large infarcts with extensive necrosis, a central area of no enhancement may be seen (microvascular obstruction). T2* imaging is useful to detect intramyocardial hemorrhage due to susceptibility for breakdown products of hemoglobin. Intramyocardial hemorrhage is considered as an additional marker of more severe myocardial injury, like microvascular obstruction. A number of other complications may be observed on cardiac MRI in ischemic heart disease (aneurysm, thrombus, contained rupture).

Key Point

- Acute as well as chronic myocardial infarction show LGE. T2-weighted MRI is helpful to differentiate acute from chronic myocardial injury.

15.3 Myocardial Infarction

Acute coronary occlusion leads to myocardial necrosis in the distribution area of the culprit coronary artery. Occlusion of the left anterior descending area will cause necrosis in the anterolateral wall, occlusion of the right coronary artery most commonly involves the inferoseptal wall, and occlusion of the circumflex coronary artery will involve the lateral wall. Inversely, recognizing scar in these locations may help to suspect the culprit artery. Ischemic heart disease can be suspected by regional abnormalities in the distribution area of individual coronary arteries. LGE is currently the highest-resolution method for detecting acute myocardial infarction with very high sensitivity, even to demonstrate microinfarcts (e.g., embolic infarction in patients undergoing percutaneous coronary intervention). The size of the region of hyperenhancement is a clinically validated measurement of infarct size, correlating with the degree of elevations of cardiac enzymes and other markers of necrosis. Acute myocardial infarcts will show LGE with variable transmurality and sometimes central microvascular obstruction (larger infarcts, worse prognosis). Microvascular obstruction and related no-reflow phenomenon can prevent reperfusion of the core of the infarct after reperfusion therapy and indicates more severe ischemia. Note the transmural extent of the infarct (grading more or less than 50% of wall thickness, indicating residual viability if less than 50%). Viability assessment based on grading transmurality of the infarct may help to guide revascularization options (percutaneous intervention or bypass surgery). When analyzing patients with heart failure, the first step is to suspect regional abnormalities in the myocardium (e.g., a scar or wall thinning in the anterior wall is likely due to occlusion of the left anterior descending (LAD) artery). Wall thinning indicates the presence of long-standing scar (i.e., chronic infarct). For example, coronary CT angiography may show occlusion of the LAD and MRI may show LGE of chronic scar in the anterior wall. However, recanalization of a coronary artery may occur after myocardial infarction; therefore not all patients with a previous infarct will reveal occlusive coronary artery disease. Complications of previous infarcts include a left ventricular aneurysm (wide connection, involving all wall layers, true aneurysm), pseudoaneurysm (narrow neck, pericardial enhancement due to contained rupture in pericardial sack, predilection for inferior wall, large size), and thrombus adjacent to scar (best shown on LGE imaging). Thrombus is a common complication after myocardial infarction and may be missed by echocardiography, especially in apical location. LGE imaging is helpful to detect both acute and chronic infarction. T2-weighted imaging is used to differentiate acute versus chronic infarction. CT may also show the infarct as a perfusion defect and sometimes late iodine enhancement may reveal the infarct, although LGE MRI is better suited to demonstrate late enhancement with greater conspicuity. It is important to be aware of "incidental perfusion defects" in the myocardium when evaluating chest CT in patients with unexplained chest pain. In the scenario of acute chest pain, look for the presence and extent of coronary calcifications as a marker of coronary atherosclerosis (visual grading minor, moderate or severe works well as compared to the Agatston score). Coronary anomalies may be noted in young patients (coronary aneurysm in Kawasaki disease) or "malignant" course between the pulmonary artery and aorta (cause for ischemia and sudden death in young people). There are a number of anatomic variants of coronary anatomy that may have limited clinical significance (e.g., anomalous course of circumflex posterior to aorta, bridging of LAD).

15.4 Heart Failure

In patients presenting with heart failure the first question is whether coronary artery disease (previous infarcts) is the underlying problem. Coronary CT angiography and cardiac MRI are well suited to assess comprehensively the presence and extent of ischemic cardiomyopathy (see above). However, many patients with unexplained heart failure may suffer from a large number of other disease entities that may lead to heart failure. A common cause for heart failure is idiopathic, nonischemic dilated cardiomyopathy. The systematic analysis of CT and MRI images may help to clarify the diagnosis of nonischemic dilating cardiomyopathy. Coronary CT angiography will most commonly show normal coronary anatomy, although sometimes coexisting coronary disease may be noted. The overall appearance of the left ventricle indicates global dilation and diffuse wall thinning in patients with nonischemic dilating cardiomyopathy (in contrast to ischemic cardiomyopathy where we expect regional scar or wall thinning), although sometimes three-vessel coronary artery disease may also result in this phenotype (hibernating left ventricle where bypass surgery can be advantageous to reverse global ischemia). Cardiac MRI using cine imaging will show the same appearance in a dynamic format. Cine MRI is very accurate to estimate the volumes and ejection fraction. The ejection fraction is a crucial parameter to decide for ICD placement. LGE will most commonly show no scar or LGE in patients with nonischemic dilating cardiomyopathy. In a minority of these patients, a scar in the middle of the ventricular wall can be shown (midwall scar is a trigger point for arrhythmias and may be an indication for preventive ICD placement).

Another common cause for heart failure is characterized by the hypertrophic phenotype. The hypertrophic phenotype has a number of underlying causes for myocardial thickening. The wall thickening can be local ("humps and bumps") in any location, most common in the septum in patients with genetically determined hypertrophic cardiomyopathy (the most common cause for sudden death in young people), but can also present as diffuse wall thickening. Simple explanations for left ventricular hypertrophy may be the presence of long-standing high blood pressure and outflow obstruction (e.g., aortic valve stenosis, bicuspid aortic valve). Sometimes physiological hypertrophy may occur in endurance athletes that may be reversible after stopping heavy exercise. After excluding these obvious causes for left ventricular hypertrophy, it is important to analyze cine MRI images and LGE images to narrow the differential diagnosis of the hypertrophic phenotype. Cardiac MRI is now playing a crucial role in systematically analyzing the potential underlying cause in unexplained heart failure presenting with the hypertrophic phenotype. The genetic hypertrophic phenotype is an important first consideration. Most commonly local hypertrophy will be recognized in the septum, but it may occur in any location and may even present with diffuse, global hypertrophy. There are a number of secondary helpful clues for this diagnosis on imaging. On cine imaging there may be a jet phenomenon in the outflow tract to the aorta (hypertrophic obstructive cardiomyopathy, exaggerated by the elongated anterior leaflet of the mitral valve, systolic anterior motion (SAM)), secondary mitral regurgitation with enlargement of the left atrium is frequent, supernormal ejection fraction (hypercontractile left ventricle), and clefts in the myocardium. LGE is helpful to assess scar distributed in the myocardium in genetic hypertrophy (nonischemic pattern) and is a marker for arrhythmia risk. Cardiac amyloidosis is another disease that may present with the hypertrophic phenotype and is characterized by diffuse subendocardial LGE (not confined to a coronary artery distribution area). A number of other storage diseases may present with the hypertrophic phenotype (e.g., Fabry disease, typical LGE in posterolateral wall, sometimes focal hypertrophy, dilated aorta). Fabry disease is characterized by sphingolipid accumulation intracellularly (shown by native T1 mapping, ECV unchanged), sometimes complicated by diffuse or focal scar. Therapy is available for Fabry disease, so important to recognize and diagnose early. Inflammatory diseases (SLE, myocarditis, sarcoid) may present also with heart failure and the hypertrophic phenotype. Myocarditis may be recognized by subepicardial LGE in typical locations. A number of drugs may accumulate in the heart and present with heart failure and hypertrophy (e.g., amiodarone, hydroxychloroquine used in rheumatology, simulating Fabry disease).

Key Point

- MRI is a first-line modality to diagnose the underlying cause in patients with heart failure.

15.5 Cardiac CT

15.5.1 CT Technique and Low-Dose CT Coronary Angiography

Technical developments such as wide detectors, dual source configuration, low kV scanning and high-pitch acquisitions have allowed to establish coronary CT angiography (CCTA) as an imaging modality that provides high temporal and spatial resolution, for motion-free cardiac imaging and detailed visualization of coronary or myocardial pathology. With increasing utilization of coronary CT angiography, especially low-dose CCTA acquisitions are constantly improving, in order to combine CT's high anatomical resolution with short examination times while still maintaining very low radiation exposure. Specifically, high-pitch CT (pitch >3), low kV (as low as 70 kV), and iterative reconstruction algorithms have resulted in cardiovascular exams with radiation exposure of <1 mSv [1]. For a detailed visualization of the cardiac and coronary anatomy, ECG-triggered protocols are recommended, although it has also been demonstrated, that the detection of the coronary arteries is possible even in a non-ECG-triggered spiral mode with high temporal resolution [2]. Most CCTA cases today will be scanned in a prospective ECG-triggered sequential scan ("step-and-shoot mode") or, if a dual-source CT scanner is available, in high-pitch scan mode, whereas retrospective ECG-gating should be avoided or reserved to special cases (high heart rates, arrhythmia) due to potentially high radiation exposure.

15.5.2 Stable Angina

Consequently, CCTA has emerged as a noninvasive, robust, and well-established diagnostic tool for the assessment and evaluation of patients with known or suspected CAD and in stable angina pectoris. There is a large body of evidence for these indications, demonstrating a high diagnostic accuracy with a sensitivity ranging from 94 to 99% and a specificity of 64–83% for the detection of significant coronary stenoses (i.e., diameter stenoses >50% in a morphological assessment) [3]. Clinically, with its high negative predictive value ranging from 97 to 99%, CCTA represents a reliable diagnostic imaging tool to rule out obstructive CAD, especially in low- to intermediate-risk settings [3–6]. As such, large-scale registries and prospective trials have shown that CCTA serves as a valuable alternative to invasive diagnostic testing in patients with stable angina [7–9] and low to intermediate pretest likelihood of CAD (e.g., asymptomatic, younger patients) and in those with less extensive coronary artery calcification, especially in patients who are unable to undergo stress testing for functional testing [6, 9]. An example of a negative coronary CT angiography in a relatively young female patient with suspected CAD is provided in Fig. 15.1. Furthermore, due to the ability of CCTA for visualization and assessment of coronary atherosclerotic plaque, three-dimensional vessel trajectories and anatomical features of the coronary vessel segments as well as detection of pathological coronary artery alterations such as calcifications or occlusions, CCTA is gaining recognition as a useful imaging tool in pre-procedural planning of cardiovascular interventions, providing improved success rates for revascularization and post-procedural outcome after percutaneous techniques [10]. Besides its diagnostic value, there is also an increasing role of CCTA to predict cardiovascular risk over time, as several follow-up studies report an excellent prognosis for patients negative at CCTA for any CAD or coronary atherosclerosis, whereas outcome in patients with obstructive and also nonobstructive CAD is substantially worse [11, 12].

15.5.3 Acute Chest Pain

The work-up of patients in the emergency room is complex and sometimes suboptimal, leading to a high number of unnecessary hospital admissions. Both CT and MRI have been successfully used as a gatekeeper to diagnose life-threatening causes of acute chest pain (i.e., acute myocardial infarction, aortic dissection, and pulmonary embolism). In the setting of acute chest pain potentially caused by an acute coronary syndrome (ACS) or non-ST-elevation myocardial infarction (NSTEMI), there is strong evidence that CCTA improves the efficiency of clinical decision-making in the

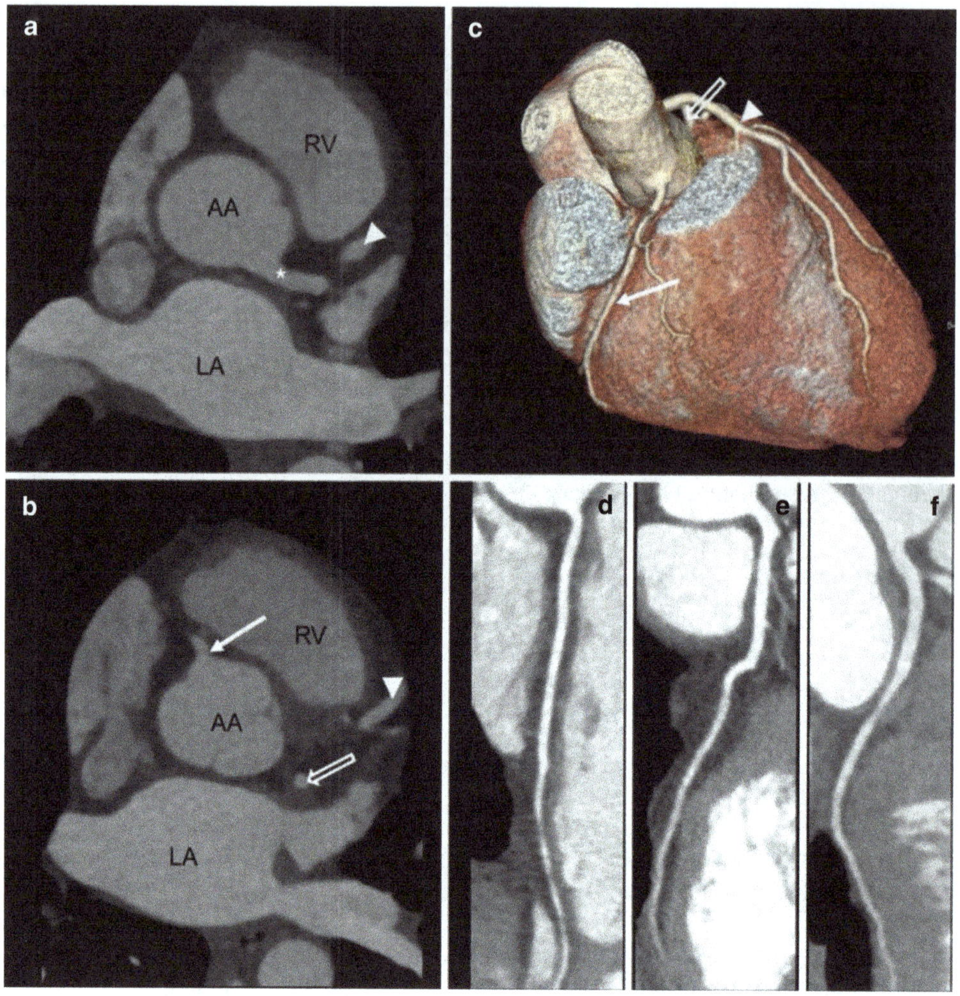

Fig. 15.1 Coronary CT of a 48-year-old female with exertional atypical chest pain. The CT reveals the absence of coronary atherosclerotic plaque or stenosis. (**a**) Axial slice demonstrating the left main coronary artery (asterisk) and the left anterior descending coronary artery (arrow head). (**b**) Origin of the right coronary artery (white arrow) and proximal segment of the left anterior descending coronary artery (arrow head) and left circumflex coronary artery (open arrow). (**c**) Volume rendered three-dimensional reconstruction showing the left anterior descending coronary artery as well as the branch of the right coronary artery and the circumflex coronary artery. (**d–f**) Multiplanar curved reconstructions of the right coronary artery (**d**), the left anterior descending coronary artery (**e**), and the circumflex coronary artery (**f**) demonstrating the absence of coronary atherosclerotic plaque or coronary artery stenosis. *AA* ascending aorta, *LA* left atrium, *RV* right ventricle

emergency department, resulting in a shorter length of hospitalization and reduced costs [13]. Several large randomized trials (CT-STAT, ACRIN-PA, ROMICAT II, and CT-COMPARE) compared coronary CT angiography to the current standard of care in patients with acute chest pain [13–16]. Their clinical implementations illustrated the reliability of a negative coronary CT angiography in identifying patients for discharge from the emergency department [17]. Here, coronary CT angiography allows for fast and safe triage of patients. In clinical practice, individuals demonstrating severe coronary stenosis are often directly referred to invasive catheter angiography, and patients with intermediate stenosis, high overall plaque burden, or equivocal findings typically undergo functional testing [18, 19].

Key Point

- Coronary CT angiography is a first-line modality for excluding coronary artery disease in patients with intermediate likelihood of disease.

15.6 Functional Assessment of Coronary Artery Disease

15.6.1 CT-Based Fractional Flow Reserve (CT-FFR) and Imaging of Myocardial Perfusion

Given its established value in morphologic imaging of CAD, research efforts over the last years have focused on providing information beyond the assessment of coronary stenosis and atherosclerotic vessel wall changes. To date, CT offers two different approaches to assess the functional relevance of a given stenosis: (A) myocardial perfusion imaging (which can be performed in a dynamic or static fashion) and (B) the calculation of a CT-based fractional flow reserve (CT-FFR). CT myocardial perfusion is based on the first-pass effect of iodinated contrast media through the myocardium during vasodilator stress (pharmacologically induced using regadenoson, adenosine, or dipyridamole). The study can either be performed by obtaining one single scan during maximum enhancement (also referred to as "static" or "snapshot/

single-shot" perfusion imaging) or by acquiring multiple scans during contrast passage (i.e., a "dynamic," time-resolved imaging of myocardial perfusion). The benefit of the "snapshot" protocol is the reduction of radiation exposure, whereas the "dynamic" protocol enables the absolute quantification of myocardial blood flow and volume. Perfusion defects as obtained by these techniques are identified as areas of hypo-attenuated myocardium compared to perfusion at baseline. While reversible malperfusion indicates ischemic myocardium, persistent perfusion defects are considered to represent myocardial scar tissue [20, 21]. The calculation of the CT-FFR using flow dynamics from coronary computed tomography angiography images is another noninvasive method for the assessment of flow dynamics [22]. This novel approach allows lesion-specific flow analysis throughout the coronary tree without additional imaging or vasodilator stress, i.e., this calculation is based on the original CCTA examination. The currently most widely used technique (known as FFRCT) uses a complex reconstruction algorithm to create a three-dimensional (3D) model of the coronary arteries and assess the left ventricular mass which is directly proportional to the total blood flow at rest. By combining the information of branch diameter from the 3D model and resting blood flow, it is possible to specifically calculate the blood flow for each coronary segment (see an example in Figs. 15.2 and 15.3). Recently, freely available and simplified approaches using a one-dimensional (1D) analysis (cFFR) are under investigation [23].

Key Point

- The presence or absence of flow limitation caused by a coronary artery stenosis can be estimated by computational fluid dynamics using the coronary CT dataset noninvasively on-site.

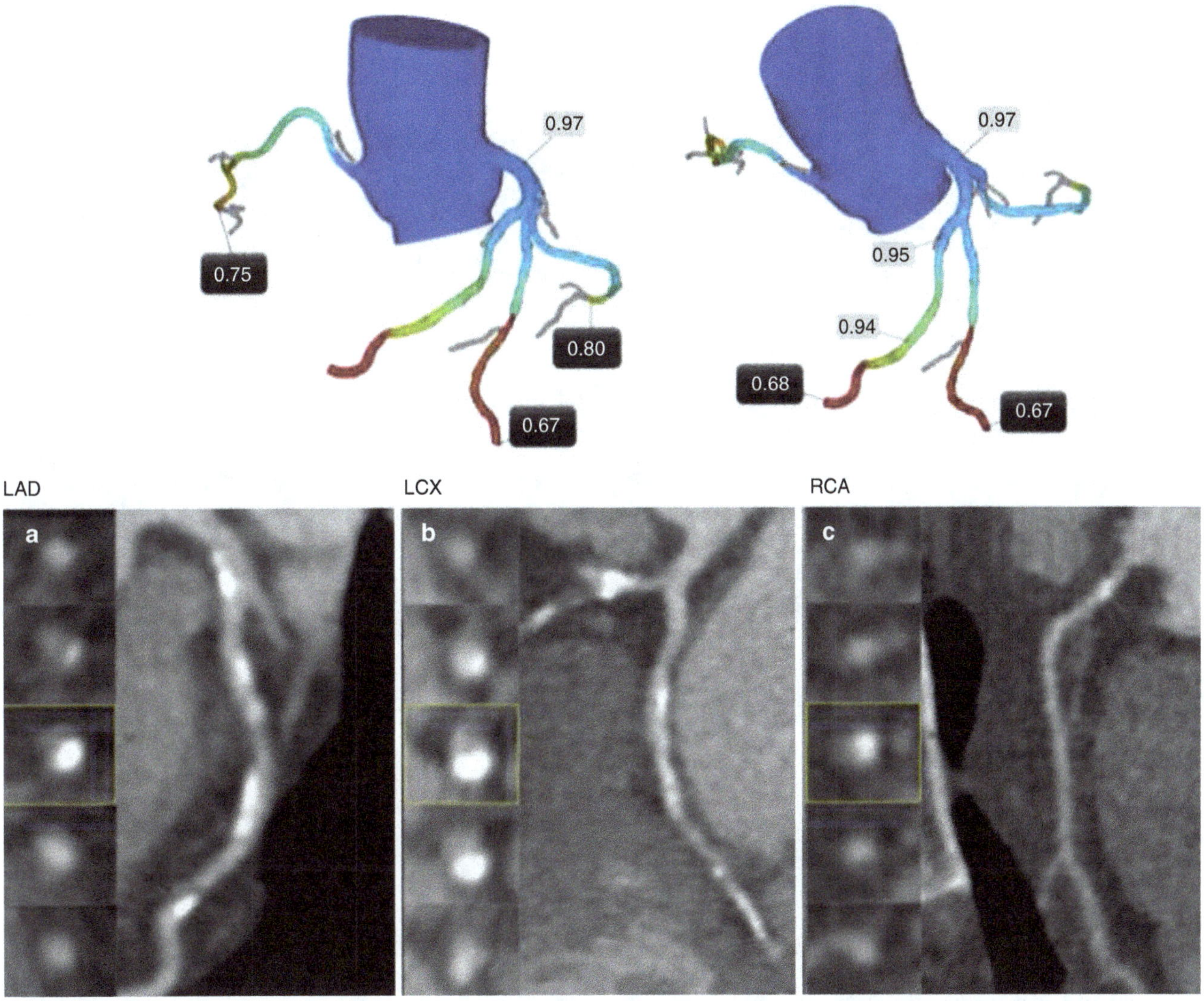

Fig. 15.2 Example of a CT-based derivation of fractional flow reserve model (CT-FFR, upper bar) and source coronary CT datasets demonstrating diffuse calcified and non-calcified plaques with hemodynamically relevant coronary stenosis present in the distal left anterior descending coronary artery (also A) and a large diagonal branch (red color-coding in the FFR model), whereas the right coronary artery and the left circumflex coronary artery (C and B, respectively) have diffuse coronary artery disease without hemodynamically relevant coronary lesions

15.7 Assessment of Atherosclerotic Plaque

Given its high spatial resolution, CCTA offers the unique potential to noninvasively visualize, characterize, and quantify atherosclerotic plaque [24]. The notion of vulnerable plaques is a rather complex concept; however, specific high-risk plaque features can be identified on standard CCTA datasets. Several adverse features associated with vulnerable plaques have already been identified with CCTA; these include the presence of positive remodeling, low-attenuation plaque, spotty calcifications, and the napkin ring sign (see a typical low-attenuation plaque in Fig. 15.3) [25–28]. In contrast, larger calcification is more likely to be found in stable coronary lesions. Although the evidence is still very limited, detailed assessment of plaque morphology for detection of high-risk plaque features in patients presenting to the ED with acute chest pain but negative initial electrocardiogram and troponin may provide incremental diagnostic value, as the presence of high-risk plaque increases the likelihood of ACS, independent of significant CAD and clinical risk assessment, including age, sex, and number of cardiovascular risk factors [29]. Thus, identification of such high-risk plaques may thus improve risk estimates for the individual patient and may be of use in the selection of patients who benefit from revascularization.

15.8 Summary

Cardiac MR and CT imaging have seen an incredible speed of development over the past years. Today, both technique are readily and widely available and have reached a point of robustness while providing complex and complementary information at the same time, making both ever more important in clinical routine management of CAD patients.

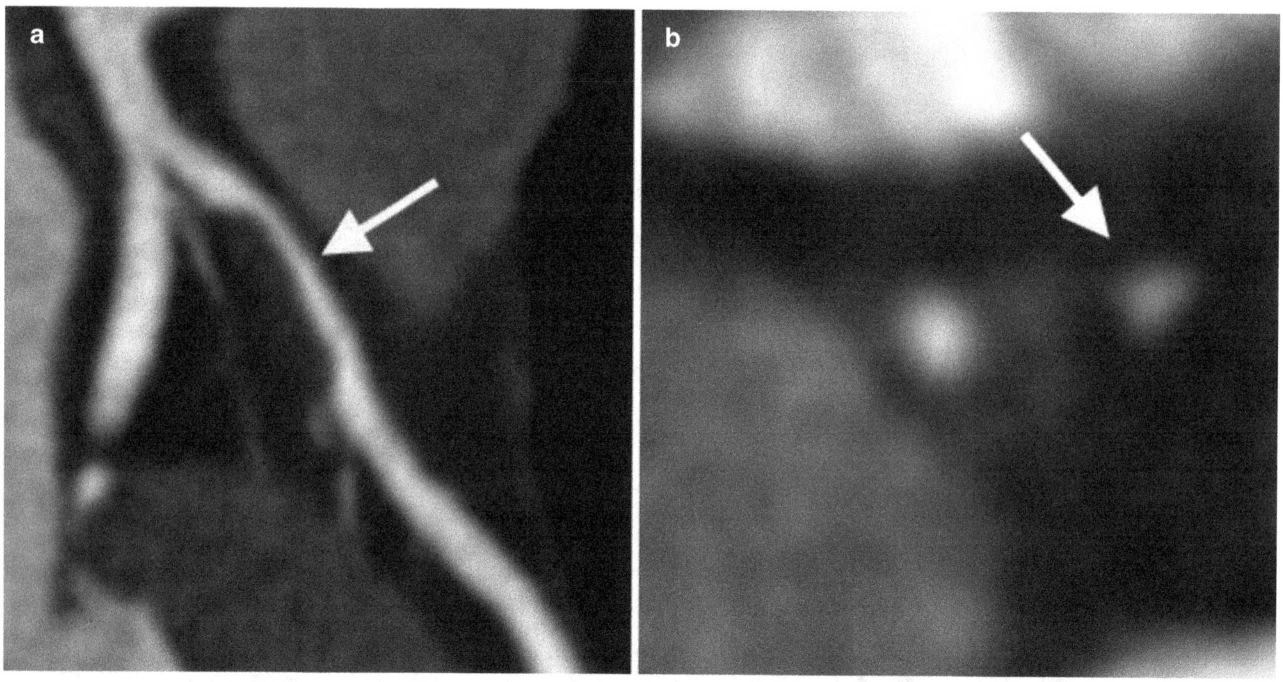

Fig. 15.3 Coronary CT of an atherosclerotic plaque in the LAD, demonstrating high-risk plaque features, including low-attenuation and positive remodeling in the proximal segment of the left anterior descending coronary artery. (**a**) curved multiplanar reformat and corresponding cross section of the vessel (**b**)

Take-Home Messages

- Parametric T1 mapping of the myocardium may provide an objective method to diagnose acute infarction, area at risk, and diffuse fibrosis unseen by LGE.
- Late gadolinium enhancement by MRI has the unique feature to demonstrate the transmural extent of scar. Transmural extent of scar is very important for diagnosis of remaining myocardial viability and therefore for clinical decision-making in patients with ischemic heart disease.
- Coronary CT angiography is highly reliable for excluding coronary artery disease in patients with intermediate likelihood of disease.
- Functional assessment of an intermediate coronary stenosis requires ischemia testing by using myocardial perfusion or estimating fractional flow reserve by state-of-the-art CT techniques to guide treatment options.

References

1. Rompel O, Glockler M, Janka R, et al. Third-generation dual-source 70-kVp chest CT angiography with advanced iterative reconstruction in young children: image quality and radiation dose reduction. Pediatr Radiol. 2016;46:462–72.
2. Bridoux A, Hutt A, Faivre JB, et al. Coronary artery visibility in free-breathing young children on non-gated chest CT: impact of temporal resolution. Pediatr Radiol. 2015;45:1761–70.
3. Budoff MJ, Dowe D, Jollis JG, et al. Diagnostic performance of 64-multidetector row coronary computed tomographic angiography for evaluation of coronary artery stenosis in individuals without known coronary artery disease: results from the prospective multicenter ACCURACY (Assessment by Coronary Computed Tomographic Angiography of Individuals Undergoing Invasive Coronary Angiography) trial. J Am Coll Cardiol. 2008;52:1724–32.
4. Hadamitzky M, Taubert S, Deseive S, et al. Prognostic value of coronary computed tomography angiography during 5 years of follow-up in patients with suspected coronary artery disease. Eur Heart J. 2013;34:3277–85.
5. Marwan M, Hausleiter J, Abbara S, et al. Multicenter evaluation of coronary dual-source CT angiography in patients with intermediate Risk of Coronary Artery Stenoses (MEDIC): study design and rationale. J Cardiovasc Comput Tomogr. 2014;8:183–8.
6. Meijboom WB, Meijs MF, Schuijf JD, et al. Diagnostic accuracy of 64-slice computed tomography coronary angiography: a prospective, multicenter, multivendor study. J Am Coll Cardiol. 2008;52:2135–44.
7. Douglas PS, Hoffmann U, Patel MR, et al. Outcomes of anatomical versus functional testing for coronary artery disease. N Engl J Med. 2015;372:1291–300.
8. Otaki Y, Arsanjani R, Gransar H, et al. What have we learned from CONFIRM? Prognostic implications from a prospective multicenter international observational cohort study of consecutive patients undergoing coronary computed tomographic angiography. J Nucl Cardiol. 2012;19:787–95.
9. Task Force M, Montalescot G, Sechtem U, et al. 2013 ESC guidelines on the management of stable coronary artery disease: the Task Force on the management of stable coronary artery disease of the European Society of Cardiology. Eur Heart J. 2013;34:2949–3003.
10. Opolski MP, Achenbach S. CT angiography for revascularization of CTO: crossing the borders of diagnosis and treatment. JACC Cardiovasc Imaging. 2015;8:846–58.
11. Hadamitzky M, Achenbach S, Al-Mallah M, et al. Optimized prognostic score for coronary computed tomographic angiography: results from the CONFIRM registry (COronary CT Angiography EvaluatioN For Clinical Outcomes: An InteRnational Multicenter Registry). J Am Coll Cardiol. 2013;62:468–76.
12. Dougoud S, Fuchs TA, Stehli J, et al. Prognostic value of coronary CT angiography on long-term follow-up of 6.9 years. Int J Cardiovasc Imaging. 2014;30:969–76.
13. Hoffmann U, Truong QA, Schoenfeld DA, et al. Coronary CT angiography versus standard evaluation in acute chest pain. N Engl J Med. 2012;367:299–308.
14. Goldstein JA, Chinnaiyan KM, Abidov A, et al. The CT-STAT (Coronary Computed Tomographic Angiography for Systematic Triage of Acute Chest Pain Patients to Treatment) trial. J Am Coll Cardiol. 2011;58:1414–22.
15. Litt HI, Gatsonis C, Snyder B, et al. CT angiography for safe discharge of patients with possible acute coronary syndromes. N Engl J Med. 2012;366:1393–403.
16. Hamilton-Craig C, Fifoot A, Hansen M, et al. Diagnostic performance and cost of CT angiography versus stress ECG—a randomized prospective study of suspected acute coronary syndrome chest pain in the emergency department (CT-COMPARE). Int J Cardiol. 2014;177:867–73.
17. Cury RC, Abbara S, Achenbach S, et al. Coronary Artery Disease - Reporting and Data System (CAD-RADS): An Expert Consensus Document of SCCT, ACR and NASCI: Endorsed by the ACC. JACC Cardiovasc Imaging. 2016;9:1099–113.
18. Meinel FG, Bayer RR 2nd, Zwerner PL, De Cecco CN, Schoepf UJ, Bamberg F. Coronary computed tomographic angiography in clinical practice: state of the art. Radiol Clin N Am. 2015;53:287–96.
19. Taylor AJ, Cerqueira M, Hodgson JM, et al. ACCF/SCCT/ACR/AHA/ASE/ASNC/NASCI/SCAI/SCMR 2010 appropriate use criteria for cardiac computed tomography. A report of the American College of Cardiology Foundation Appropriate Use Criteria Task Force, the Society of Cardiovascular Computed Tomography, the American College of Radiology, the American Heart Association, the American Society of Echocardiography, the American Society of Nuclear Cardiology, the North American Society for Cardiovascular Imaging, the Society for Cardiovascular Angiography and Interventions, and the Society for Cardiovascular Magnetic Resonance. J Am Coll Cardiol 2010;56:1864-94.
20. George RT, Jerosch-Herold M, Silva C, et al. Quantification of myocardial perfusion using dynamic 64-detector computed tomography. Investig Radiol. 2007;42:815–22.
21. Dweck MR, Williams MC, Moss AJ, Newby DE, Fayad ZA. Computed tomography and cardiac magnetic resonance in ischemic heart disease. J Am Coll Cardiol. 2016;68:2201–16.
22. Pijls NH, De Bruyne B, Peels K, et al. Measurement of fractional flow reserve to assess the functional severity of coronary-artery stenoses. N Engl J Med. 1996;334:1703–8.
23. Nakanishi R, Budoff MJ. Noninvasive FFR derived from coronary CT angiography in the management of coronary artery disease: technology and clinical update. Vasc Health Risk Manag. 2016;12:269–78.
24. Nance JW Jr, Bamberg F, Schoepf UJ, et al. Coronary atherosclerosis in African American and white patients with acute chest pain: characterization with coronary CT angiography. Radiology. 2011;260:373–80.
25. Motoyama S, Kondo T, Sarai M, et al. Multislice computed tomographic characteristics of coronary lesions in acute coronary syndromes. J Am Coll Cardiol. 2007;50:319–26.
26. Maurovich-Horvat P, Schlett CL, Alkadhi H, et al. The napkin-ring sign indicates advanced atherosclerotic lesions in coronary CT angiography. J Am Coll Cardiol Img. 2012;5:1243–52.
27. Otsuka K, Fukuda S, Tanaka A, et al. Napkin-ring sign on coronary CT angiography for the prediction of acute coronary syndrome. J Am Coll Cardiol Img. 2013;6:448–57.
28. Motoyama S, Sarai M, Harigaya H, et al. Computed tomographic angiography characteristics of atherosclerotic plaques subsequently resulting in acute coronary syndrome. J Am Coll Cardiol. 2009;54:49–57.
29. Puchner SB, Liu T, Mayrhofer T, et al. High-risk plaque detected on coronary CT angiography predicts acute coronary syndromes independent of significant stenosis in acute chest pain: results from the ROMICAT-II trial. J Am Coll Cardiol. 2014;64:684–92.

16

Imaging of Nonischemic Cardiomyopathy

David A. Bluemke and Shawn D. Teague

Learning Objectives

- Identify nonischemic pattern of delayed enhancement.
- Develop a differential diagnosis for dilated cardiomyopathy.
- Evaluate the functional impact of nonischemic cardiomyopathy.

16.1 Introduction

Symptomatic myocardial disease not the result of flow-limiting coronary artery disease or prior myocardial infarction is commonly known as nonischemic cardiomyopathy. Clinical manifestations include arrhythmia, palpitations, heart failure, shortness of breath, lower extremity edema, syncope, and chest pain. Nonischemic cardiomyopathy is more common in women and younger patients. In general, the prognosis for nonischemic cardiomyopathy is better than for ischemic disease. There may be either systolic, diastolic, or combined heart failure. Infiltrative cardiomyopathies in particular tend to result in diastolic dysfunction.

In most patients, ischemic cardiomyopathy should be considered and excluded prior to further work-up of nonischemic cardiomyopathy. Echocardiography is the primary modality for evaluating left ventricular function as well as valvular and diastolic function. Advanced techniques including pulsed tissue Doppler and 3-D imaging have added diagnostic and prognostic information when evaluating nonischemic cardiomyopathy. Stress tests either exercise or chemical with or without imaging are commonly used to exclude underlying ischemia. If these studies are inconclusive, the patient may require cardiac catheterization with ventriculography. However, if the patient is low to intermediate likelihood for coronary artery disease, coronary computed tomography angiography can be performed to differentiate between ischemic and nonischemic cardiomyopathy. Positron emission tomography may be utilized for the evaluation of cardiac sarcoidosis.

Cardiac MRI (CMR) is considered the reference standard to assess myocardial anatomy, function, and viability and often reveals the underlying etiology of heart failure [1]. Delayed enhancement in nonischemic cardiomyopathy usually occurs in a mid-myocardial or subepicardial location rather than subendocardial or transmural as seen in ischemic disease. The location of delayed enhancement can also help to guide myocardial biopsy thus increasing yield of a diagnosis. It can also be utilized to screen in genetically positive but phenotypically negative patients to better help with risk stratification. Finally, there has been significant prognostic value shown related to the location and extent of delayed enhancement.

16.2 Hypertrophic

Hypertrophic cardiomyopathy is the most common genetic cardiac disorder with heterogeneous phenotypic expression. Patients present clinically most commonly with sudden death from ventricular fibrillation, atrial fibrillation, or heart failure but may be asymptomatic. MRI is utilized not only to make the diagnosis of hypertrophic cardiomyopathy but also to characterize the morphologic types related to the distribution of the hypertrophied muscle. Different types include apical, mid-ventricular, concentric, and mass-like although the most common is asymmetric septal hypertrophy. Ventricular wall thickness of >30 mm (normal <15 mm) has

D. A. Bluemke
Department of Radiology, University of Wisconsin School of Medicine and Public Health, Madison, WI, USA
e-mail: dbluemke@wisc.edu

S. D. Teague (✉)
Department of Radiology, National Jewish Health, University of Colorado School of Medicine, Denver, CO, USA
e-mail: teagues@njhealth.org

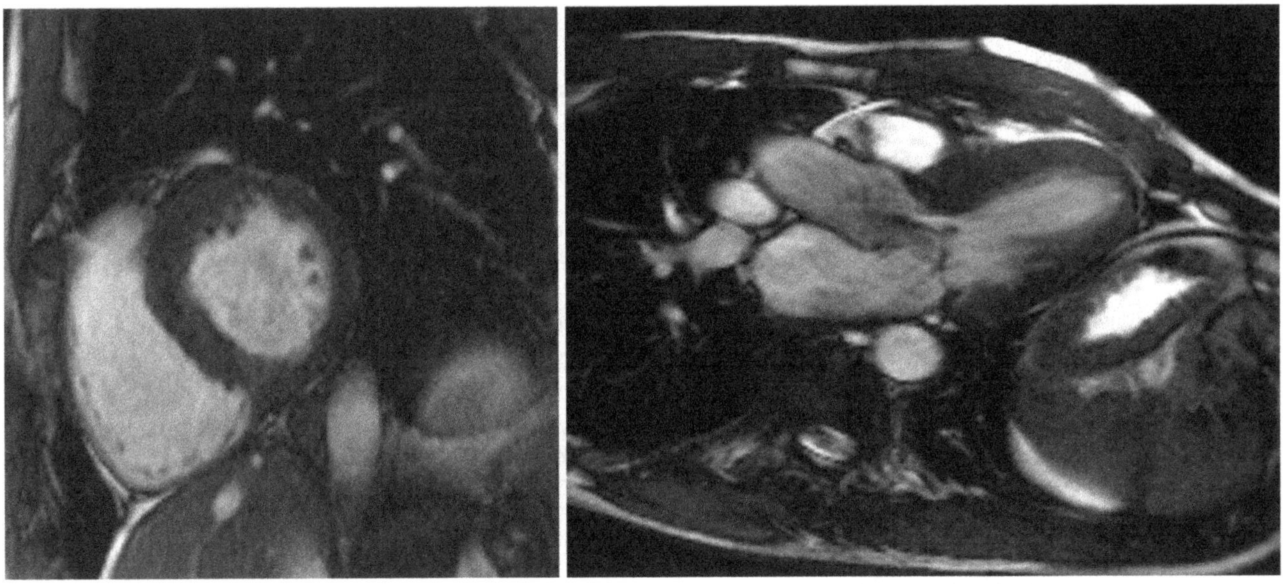

Fig. 16.1 Septal hypertrophic cardiomyopathy. Short axis steady-state free precession image demonstrates thickening of the myocardium involving the anteroseptal segment of the basal left ventricle. Three-chamber image from a cine steady-state free precession series demonstrates septal hypertrophy with anterior motion of the anterior leaflet of the mitral valve and associated flow jet in the left ventricular outflow tract below the level of the aortic valve

been shown to be an independent risk factor for sudden cardiac death [2]. MRI is the procedure of choice for monitoring left ventricular mass over time and in response to treatment.

The area of hypertrophy in asymmetric septal type is commonly located at the basal aspect of the interventricular septum which can result in left ventricular outflow tract obstruction as shown in Fig. 16.1. Using phase-contrast imaging on MRI, the degree of obstruction can be evaluated based on the velocity in the left ventricular outflow tract using the modified Bernoulli equation (gradient = 4 V^2) to calculate the gradient (severe >50 mm Hg). If conservative treatments are not effective, septal ablation or surgical procedures may be required for LVOT obstruction. The accelerated flow in the left ventricular outflow tract can result in systolic anterior motion of the mitral valve which can result in mitral regurgitation. Not only can these two findings be identified during MRI examinations, but the severity of mitral regurgitation can also be quantified. MRI can also be utilized to assess cardiac function and regional wall motion.

Delayed enhancement imaging is performed in all hypertrophic cardiomyopathy patients in order to evaluate for interstitial fibrosis, microfibrillar disarray, or microvascular obstruction. The delayed enhancement images are positive in 60% of these patients [3]. While the delayed enhancement is most commonly seen in a patchy distribution in the mid-myocardium at the right ventricular insertion point, it can be seen throughout the hypertrophied myocardium and sometimes even in the non-hypertrophied muscle. Delayed enhancement has demonstrated prognostic information in several studies of cardiac outcomes including worsening heart failure symptoms, ventricular arrhythmias, ICD discharge, and sudden cardiac death [4]. The absence of delayed enhancement has prognostic information as well with overall lower risk for adverse cardiac outcomes although the risk is still not absent [5]. Not only is the presence or absence of delayed enhancement important, but the extent of late delayed enhancement is a significant predictor of adverse cardiac outcomes [5]. The largest study to date in this patient cohort demonstrated that only the extent of delayed enhancement was a strong predictor of adverse cardiac events and mortality [6]. Limited studies are available regarding the utilization of MRI to monitor treatment for hypertrophic cardiomyopathy.

Key Point

- In hypertrophic cardiomyopathy, MRI is used not only to make the diagnosis but also to characterize the morphology and evaluate for outflow obstruction.

16.3 Dilated Cardiomyopathy

16.3.1 Idiopathic

Idiopathic dilated cardiomyopathy represents an end-stage pump failure of the heart; the disease is considered to be idiopathic when no immediate cause is discerned. However, it is believed that this end-stage condition of the heart may be produced by a variety of toxic, metabolic, or infectious agents. Idiopathic dilated cardiomyopathy may be the late sequela of infection such as viral myocarditis. In some cases, genetic abnormalities are also associated with this condition. In this condition, there is gradual increased left ventricular end-systolic and end-diastolic volumes with continuously declining ejection fraction. The walls of the ventricle are thinned.

On CMR, decreased function, ventricular dilatation, and wall thinning are readily demonstrated. However, the primary advantage of CMR compared to other imaging modalities is the use of late gadolinium enhancement. Late gadolinium is not seen in all patients. However, in some patients, there is characteristic enhancement if the mid-myocardium in a non-coronary artery distribution. This pattern of late gadolinium enhancement has also been recognized in postmortem hearts as a hallmark of this condition. Right ventricular dilatation is also characteristic of idiopathic dilated cardiomyopathy. Furthermore, the presence and extent of myocardial late enhancement have been shown to predict the clinical outcome [7]. After adjustment for LVEF and other conventional prognostic factors, both the presence of fibrosis and the extent of midwall enhancement on CMR were independently and incrementally associated with all-cause mortality.

16.3.2 Viral Myocarditis

The use of CMR for the evaluation of viral myocarditis is increasingly accepted. The diagnosis of viral myocarditis is challenging, as no single test may be used alone for diagnosis. Patient presentation is with chest pain in the setting of a recent or ongoing viral syndrome. The primary differential diagnoses include acute coronary artery syndrome and pericarditis. Other inflammatory myocarditis may also be considered. Troponin values are typically only mildly elevated.

CMR is used for assessment of inflammatory changes such as edema, hyperemia, and myocyte necrosis. No single pathognomonic finding is present. Rather, the Lake Louise criteria are applied. This requires abnormalities in two of the three tissue characterization techniques: T2-weighted images for edema, T1 early gadolinium enhancement imaging for hyperemia, and late gadolinium enhancement for myocyte necrosis and fibrosis. T1 and T2 mapping techniques can help reduce uncertainty that is otherwise associated with qualitative assessment of signal intensity change. A recent multicenter study showed that LV function may be normal or mildly depressed [8]. Overall sensitivity of CMR was 82%. Late gadolinium enhancement may be present in a nonischemic pattern in 80% of cases. The distribution of LGE is typically either subepicardial or midwall. Pericardial effusions are not common.

16.3.3 Takotsubo Myocarditis

Takotsubo is a transient condition involving a distinctive pattern of left ventricular dysfunction. The unusual aspect of the LV dysfunction is its temporal relationship with stressful events, either emotional (e.g., death of a loved one) or physical (e.g., major neurological or abdominal surgery). Patients with this condition recover normal function either days to weeks of the clinical presentation. The underlying etiology is an excess of catecholamines precipitated by a stressful event. The primary differential diagnosis is an acute coronary artery syndrome or possibly viral myocarditis.

The term *takotsubo* derives from the original Japanese description of the syndrome; there is distinct apical ballooning of the left ventricle that resembles an octopus pot. The ventricular dilation involves multiple coronary territories, beginning in the mid-ventricle but extending into the apex. Ventricular hypokinesis is present, particularly in these dilated myocardial regions. One of the primary CMR features is myocardial edema seen on T2-weighted images. Perfusion images are normal. Typically, LGE images do not show focal lesions that my otherwise be associated with acute myocardial infarction. However, LGE is infrequently reported in less than 10% of cases [9].

16.3.4 Alcoholic Cardiomyopathy

Alcoholic cardiomyopathy is an acquired cardiomyopathy. For diagnosis, documentation of long-term consumption of alcohol at high quantities (>80 g per day over 5 years or more) is required. For many patients, successful clinical history over this period is not available. Like other dilated cardiomyopathies, alcoholic cardiomyopathy is characterized by global ventricular dilatation, decreased myocardial function, and myocardial thinning in its end-stage presentation. Women may be more susceptible than men given equivalent quantities of ingested alcohol. Pathologic changes are similar to idiopathic dilated cardiomyopathy.

No specific CMR findings are present, other than that of abnormal ventricular size and shape. Scar patterns may be assumed to be nonischemic in nature, so that CMR can exclude myocardial scar associated with prior infarction [10]. As opposed to echocardiography, CMR may be useful to exclude other etiologies of cardiomyopathy such ischemic heart disease, iron overload, or amyloidosis.

16.3.5 Left Ventricular Noncompaction

Left ventricular noncompaction cardiomyopathy (LVNC) is a rare primary genetic cardiomyopathy characterized by excess myocardial trabeculation more than twice as thick as the underlying myocardial wall (Fig. 16.2) [11]. The trabeculae carneae consist of slim columns of myocardial cells at the luminal ventricular surfaces. The function of the trabecula is to increase cardiac output and enable oxygen supply prior to coronary vascularization. During myocardial development, trabeculae compact leading to an increase in thickness of the compact myocardium.

LVNC is associated with heart failure, regional wall motion abnormalities, and myocardial fibrosis. The ratio of the thickness of noncompacted (NC) versus compacted (C) myocardium (NC/C) is a simple and fast method to quantify trabeculation [12]; a ratio greater than 2.3 to 1 is commonly used as an MRI index of noncompacted myocardium. Although the NC/C ratio is easy to measure, the specificity is low; 33% of the subjects in the MESA cohort had a NC/C ratio greater than 2.3 [13]. Improved specificity of the NC/C ratio is obtained when several segments show high NC/C ratios and LV dysfunction is present. In a study by Wan et al., the mean number of compacted segments was 7.4; noncompaction was present in the apical segments in all patients. Forty percent of patients demonstrated a nonischemic pattern of late gadolinium enhancement, most commonly midmyocardial in location [14].

16.3.6 Collagen Vascular Disease/Connective Tissue Disorders

Connective tissue disease consists of a heterogeneous group of disorders including systemic lupus erythematosus, systemic sclerosis, and Sjogren's syndrome, as well as overlap

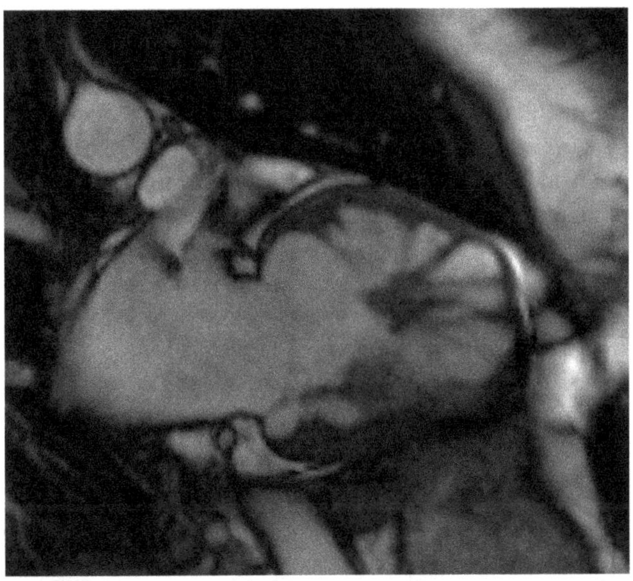

Fig. 16.2 Noncompaction cardiomyopathy. Vertical long axis view of the left ventricle shows a stellate pattern of prominent trabeculation. The left ventricle is dilated, and the myocardium at the apical anterior wall is thinned

between these conditions. Cardiac involvement includes abnormalities of valves, myocardium, and pericardium. The underlying common pathologic features are abnormal activation of the immune system, often targeted toward small blood vessels and internal organs.

Myocardial involvement is often subclinical, with diffuse myocardial fibrosis. Ejection fraction is preserved in early stages of disease in the majority of cases. Reports of focal late gadolinium enhancement are highly variable, from 0 (in our own experience) to 60% of patients [15]; likely this variability depends on the particular subset of patients evaluated. As a result, T1 mapping techniques, including evaluation of extracellular volume fraction, have been evaluated. The primary T1 mapping findings are (a) increased native T1, (b) increased extracellular volume fraction, and (c) decreased T1 times after gadolinium administration [16]. However, these findings are not specific, and changes in myocardial T1 mapping parameters are not distinct from other nonischemic cardiomyopathies.

Key Point

- Clinical history, ventricular structure and function, and pattern of late gadolinium enhancement are used to identify subtypes of dilated cardiomyopathy by CMR.

16.4 Restrictive

16.4.1 Amyloid

Cardiac involvement in amyloidosis is common with deposition of insoluble glycoproteins in the extracellular spaces of myocardial tissue, valve leaflets, and vessels. It can result in restrictive cardiomyopathy which is the leading cause of death in approximately half of amyloid patients.

On cine imaging, there is biventricular myocardial thickening with normal ventricular chamber size, atrial enlargement, and preserved systolic function. Diastolic dysfunction can be demonstrated on mitral inflowing imaging with cine phase-contrast pulse sequence imaging. In the late fibrotic stage, cine images can demonstrate mitral and tricuspid insufficiency.

There is rapid redistribution of gadolinium from the blood pool resulting in altered T1 kinetics in which the myocardium nulls before the blood pool on inversion time (TI) scout images. The altered kinetics can make selection of an appropriate TI time difficult. Phase-sensitive inversion recovery (PSIR) sequence images can be helpful given that they are independent of the TI value. The prognostic value of delayed enhancement imaging has not shown consistent

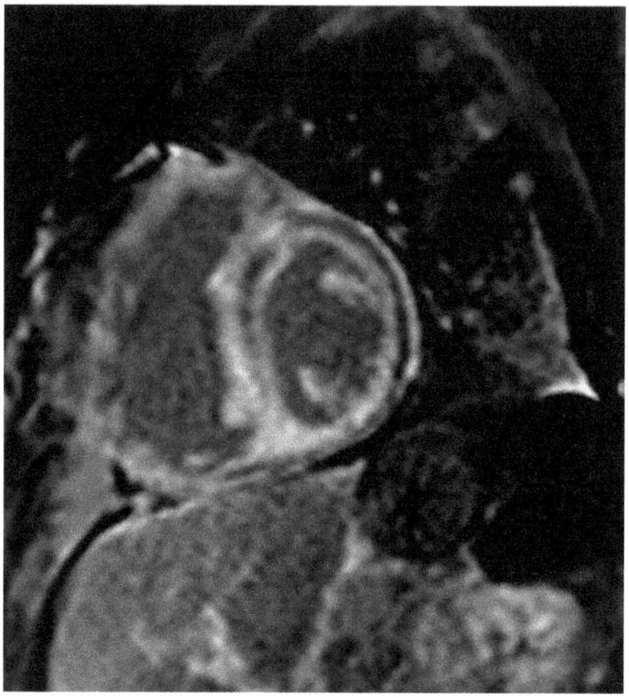

Fig. 16.3 Cardiac amyloid. Short axis delayed enhancement image demonstrates diffuse subendocardial delayed enhancement with more extensive diffuse delayed enhancement in the septum. Note the blood pool is also dark on these images when there is appropriate nulling of the myocardium in the lateral wall which is very characteristic for myocardial amyloidosis

value. The emerging T1 mapping and ECV estimation techniques have shown promise in correlating with cardiac function and risk stratification [17]. The delayed enhancement pattern is quite variable but most often diffuse and irregular in a noncoronary distribution as shown in Fig. 16.3.

CMR has shown promise in differentiating subtypes of cardiac amyloidosis primarily between light chain amyloid and transthyretin-related amyloidosis based on LV mass as well as location and extent of delayed enhancement. The determination of subtype is important given differences in treatment as well as determining prognosis with survival worse for light chain amyloid.

16.4.2 Sarcoid

The hallmark of cardiac sarcoidosis is the presence of necrotizing granulomas in the myocardium. In the acute phase, there can be myocardial thickening and edema with delayed enhancement of the mid-myocardium and/or subepicardium. Perfusion or early post contrast T1-weighted images may demonstrate increased contrast enhancement suggesting inflammation with hyperemia. In the chronic phase, edema is absent, but wall thickening and delayed enhancement may be seen. In the burnt-out phase, transmural delayed enhancement may be seen [18] with wall thinning. The imaging appearance alone can be difficult to distinguish from myocarditis.

Delayed enhancement has prognostic value as a predictor of death as well as other adverse events such as aborted sudden death, appropriate ICD discharge, and ventricular arrhythmias [19]. It is a stronger predictor than other measures such as LVEF and symptoms. The lack of delayed enhancement also appears to have high negative predicative value with respect to adverse outcomes.

CMR also appears to have value in monitoring disease status during treatment with steroids [20]. Steroid treatment has been associated with decrease in delayed enhancement as well as overall improvement in functional parameters.

The AHA consensus guidelines reserve the recommended use of CMR for diagnosis and differentiation from other cardiomyopathies as well as for functional assessment rather than specifically for risk stratification and prognosis [21].

Key Point

- Midwall myocardial delayed enhancement is suggestive of an infiltrative process rather than ischemia and raises concern for a restrictive cardiomyopathy.

16.5 Storage Disease

16.5.1 Hemochromatosis

Systemic iron overload due to hemosiderosis or transfusion-dependent anemias can result in dilated or restrictive cardiomyopathy with progressive diastolic and systolic dysfunction. Dysrhythmias are also commonly present.

Myocardial iron deposition, in the form of ferritin and hemosiderin, is demonstrated on gradient-echo images. Utilizing multiple different TE values, the absolute T2* value can be determined which is the best indicator of myocardial iron content [22]. A T2* <20 ms is considered diagnostic of significant iron overload. T2* values have been shown to detect iron overload earlier than changes of LVEF and have also been shown to be a strong independent predictor of adverse clinical outcomes such as heart failure, arrhythmias, and sudden cardiac death [22].

CMR is invaluable in monitoring treatment response to chelation therapies demonstrated by improvements in T2* and LVEF [23]. Pennell et al. [24] demonstrated a significantly reduced risk of developing heart failure with improvement in T2* with only minimal improvement in LVEF suggesting LVEF may underestimate the clinical impact of chelation therapies.

CMR is recognized in the AHA Consensus Statement [25] as a critical tool in the diagnosis and clinical management of iron overload cardiomyopathy.

16.5.2 Fabry Disease

Fabry disease is an X-linked recessive disorder of glycosphingolipid metabolism with resultant intracellular accumulation of glycosphingolipids especially in the skin, kidneys, and heart.

There is concentric LV thickening on CMR which can be confused with hypertrophic cardiomyopathy. Mid-myocardial or subepicardial pattern of delayed enhancement may be seen typically involving the basal inferolateral segment. Delayed enhancement has been shown to be associated with development of ventricular arrhythmias as well as sudden cardiac death [26]. Rather than the presence or absence of delayed enhancement, it was the annual increase in fibrosis demonstrated on delayed enhancement images that was an independent predictor of ventricular arrhythmias.

T1 mapping technique has been utilized to characterize Fabry's cardiomyopathy. Reduction in T1 values are associated with reduced longitudinal strain and early diastolic dysfunction prior to the development of LV hypertrophy. This suggests T1 mapping may be valuable in detecting early dysfunction before structural abnormalities [27]. CMR has also been utilized to monitor response to enzyme replacement therapies. One study demonstrated that despite enzyme replacement therapy, there can be progression of delayed enhancement suggesting progressive fibrosis [26].

Key Point

- CMR is a critical tool in the diagnosis and in monitoring treatment of iron overload cardiomyopathy.

16.6 Arrhythmogenic Right Ventricular Cardiomyopathy/Dysplasia (ARVC/D)

Arrhythmogenic right ventricular cardiomyopathy (ARVC) is a heritable heart muscle disease characterized by fibrofatty replacement of predominantly the right ventricular (RV) myocardium. This predisposes patients to potentially life-threatening arrhythmias and ventricular dysfunction. Affected patients typically present between the second and fourth decade of life with arrhythmias coming from the RV2. ARVC is an unusual condition, with an estimated prevalence of 1 in 1000 to 1 in 5000 Caucasian individuals. Approximately 60% of index cases harbor mutations in genes encoding the cardiac desmosome, a structure that provides mechanical connection between cardiomyocytes. The defective mechanical connections in ARVC may structurally be represented by global or regional contraction abnormalities, ventricular enlargement, and/or fibrofatty replacement. As such, accurate evaluation of cardiac morphology and function is essential for ARVC diagnosis and management.

ARVC is generally transmitted as an autosomal dominant trait with incomplete penetrance and variable expressivity. However, it is important to realize that 50–70% of mutation carriers will never develop disease expression and that severity of disease may vary greatly, even among members of the same family or those carrying the same mutation. In contrast, a negative genetic test result in a proband does not exclude the possibility of disease, nor does it exclude the possibility of a genetic process in the individual or family.

The CMR protocol for ARVC is somewhat unique compared to other cardiomyopathies. The primary difference is the addition of axial black blood T1-weighted fast spin echo images. These cover the left and right ventricles from the base to the diaphragm. Cine SSFP axial images are then obtained in the same plane, with the same slice thickness and gap (8 mm × 2 mm is typically used). After this, standard SSFP cine imaging of the ventricles is obtained in the short and long axes. Many sites also obtain a vertical long axis cine view of the right ventricle. After gadolinium administration, short and long axis late gadolinium enhancement images are obtained. In patients with significant ventricular ectopy, a low dose of a beta-blocker (metoprolol 25–50 mg) is recommended for arrhythmia suppression during the CMR scan.

The diagnostic TFC for CMR require the presence of both qualitative findings (RV regional akinesia, dyskinesia, dyssynchronous contraction) and quantitative metrics (decreased ejection fraction or increased indexed RV end-diastolic volume) (Table 16.1).

Besides global reduction in RV function, more subtle regional disease of the RV has been described in the literature using a variety of terms including focal bulges, microaneurysms, segmental dilatation, regional hypokinesis, etc. In

Table 16.1 MRI task force criteria for ARVC

Global or regional dysfunction and structural alterations
Major
Regional RV akinesia or dyskinesia or dyssynchronous RV contraction AND one of the following:
– RV EDV/BSA ≥110 mL/m^2 (male) or ≥100 mL/m^2 (female)
– RV ejection fraction ≤40%
Minor
Regional RV akinesia or dyskinesia or dyssynchronous RV contraction AND one of the following:
– RV EDV/BSA ≥100 to 110 mL/m^2 (male) or ≥90 to 100 mL/m^2 (female)
– RV ejection fraction >40 to ≤45%

EDV end-diastolic volume, *BSA* body surface area, *RV* right ventricle the current TFC, the terms "akinesia" (lack of motion) and "dyskinesia" (abnormal movement, instead of contracting in systole, the myocardium bulges outward in systole) and "dyssynchronous" (regional peak contraction occurring at different times in adjacent myocardium) are used for all imaging modalities (CMR, echocardiography and angiography) to describe regional wall motion abnormalities in ARVC. The RV apex is spared in early ARVC. The so-called accordion sign represents a focal "crinkling" of the myocardium in the subtricuspid region [28] (Fig. 16.4). In terms of TFC, the accordion sign is due to a small region of highly localized myocardium with dyssynchronous contraction.

RV LGE has been observed in up to 88% of ARVC patients, while LV LGE was reported in up to 61% of cases. In ARVC, RV wall thinning is pronounced, which makes the LGE technique less reliable than for the LV. Second, distinguishing fat from fibrosis by LGE sequences is challenging, which makes its interpretation highly subject to the CMR physician's experience.

Some ARVC subjects have early and predominant LV involvement [29]. LV involvement has even been reported in 76% of ARVC subjects, of whom the majority had advanced disease. The disease is, therefore, increasingly being referred to as "arrhythmogenic cardiomyopathy." LV involvement in ARVC typically manifests as LGE, often involving the inferior and lateral walls without concomitant wall motion abnormalities. Figure 16.5 shows an example. Septal LGE is present in more than 50% of cases with left dominant ARVC, in contrast to the right dominant pattern in which septal involvement is unusual. In addition, LV fatty infiltration was shown to be a prevalent finding in ARVC, often involving the subepicardial lateral LV and resulting in myocardial wall thinning [30].

Key Point

- ARVC typically manifests as right heart dysfunction and dilation out of proportion to similar findings in the left heat.

16.7 Concluding Remarks

Nonischemic cardiomyopathy encompasses a heterogeneous group of diseases. Genetic components of these disease are increasingly being recognized. The myocardium responds to injury by accumulation of either fibrotic tissue or fatty replacement or both. MRI is very good at detecting fatty tissue; the detection of myocardial fibrosis is performed using late gadolinium enhancement techniques and/or T1 mapping. While all patients undergo echocardiography screening to assess for myocardial function, tissue characterization remains in the realm of cardiac MRI evaluation.

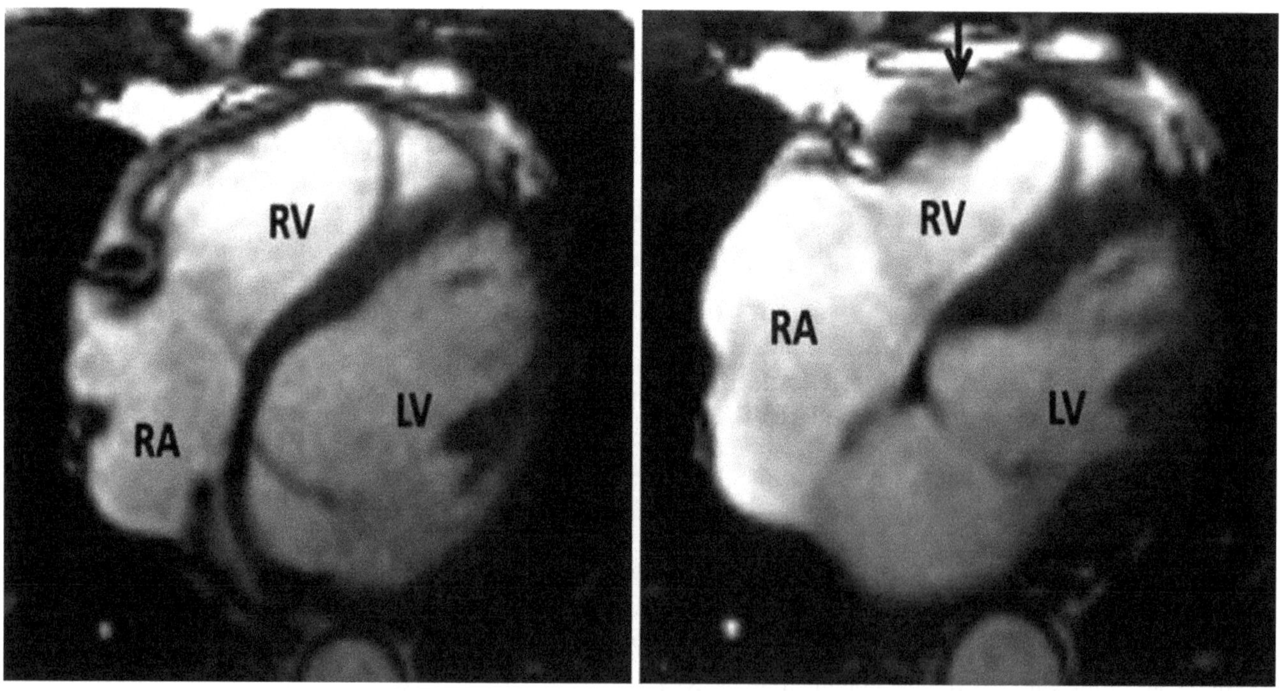

Fig. 16.4 Arrhythmogenic right ventricular cardiomyopathy. End-diastolic (left) and end-systolic (right) images are shown. In systole at the arrows, there is infolding of the right ventricle wall, termed the accordion sign. This is due to dyskinesia of the right ventricle free wall in the subtricuspid region

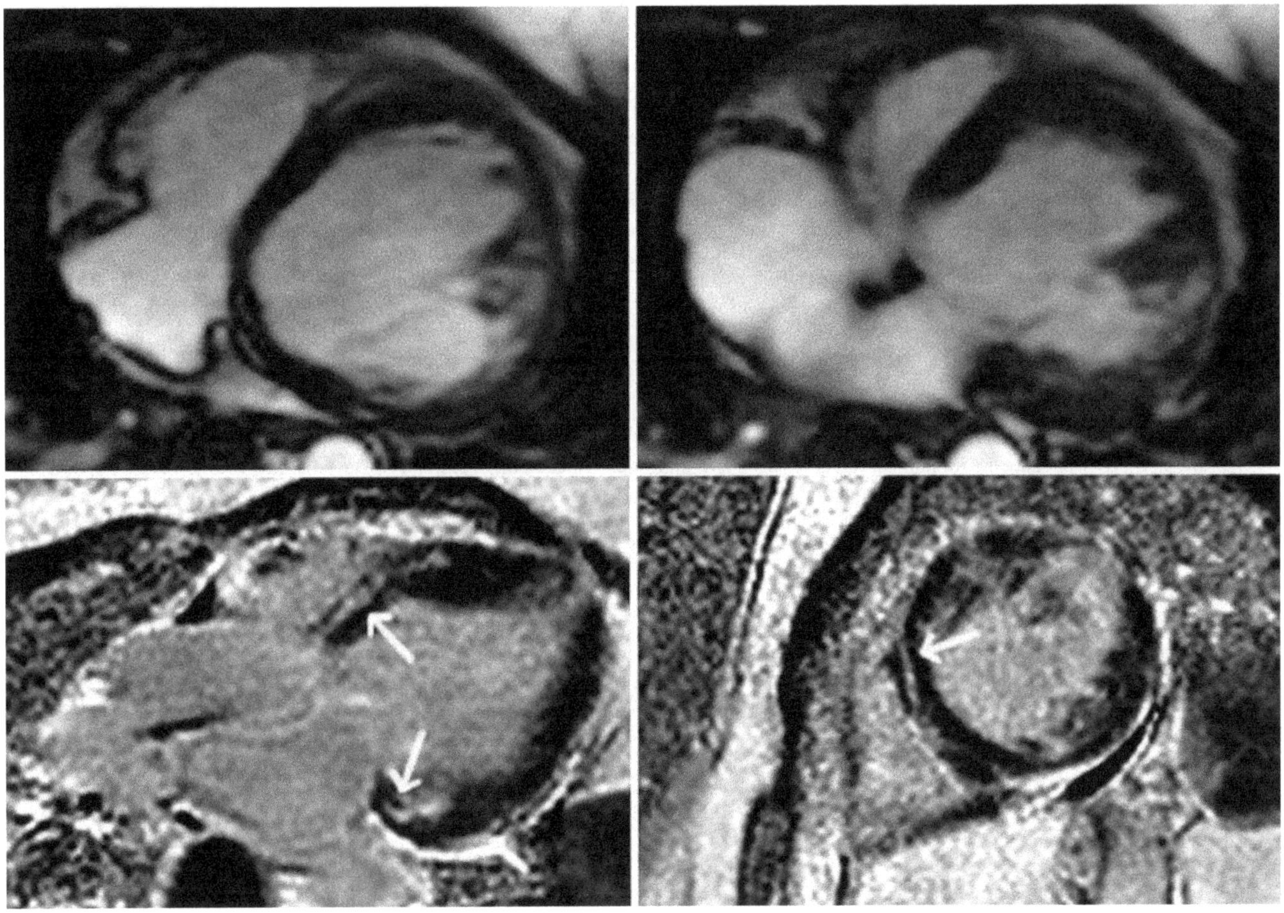

Fig. 16.5 Left ventricular presentation of arrhythmogenic right ventricular cardiomyopathy. Top row shows images at end diastole (left) and end systole (right), with poor left ventricular ejection fraction and left ventricular enlargement. Bottom row shows late gadolinium enhancement images, with focal enhancement on the four-chamber view (left) at the base (arrows) of the left ventricle. The short axis view (right) shows scattered late gadolinium enhancement (arrow)

Take-Home Messages

- Late gadolinium enhancement shows nonischemic pattern of enhancement in cardiomyopathies, characterized by midwall or epicardial enhancement in a noncoronary artery distribution.
- T1 mapping may be used to assess myocardial fibrosis. Typically, native T1 values are elevated due to the presence of fibrosis, while post gadolinium T1 values are lower than expected.
- In addition to late gadolinium enhancement images, myocardial global and regional function is readily assessed to further characterize the myocardial abnormality and extent in nonischemic cardiomyopathy.

Bibliography

1. Karamitsos TD, Francis JM, Myerson S, Selvanayagam JB, Neubauer S. The role of cardiovascular magnetic resonance imaging in heart failure. J Am Coll Cardiol. 2009;54(15):1407–24. https://doi.org/10.1016/j.jacc.2009.04.094.
2. Spirito P, Bellone P, Harris KM, Bernabo P, Bruzzi P, Maron BJ. Magnitude of left ventricular hypertrophy and risk of sudden death in hypertrophic cardiomyopathy. N Engl J Med. 2000;342(24):1778–85. https://doi.org/10.1056/NEJM200006153422403.
3. Green JJ, Berger JS, Kramer CM, Salerno M. Prognostic value of late gadolinium enhancement in clinical outcomes for hypertrophic cardiomyopathy. J Am Coll Cardiol Img. 2012;5(4):370–7. https://doi.org/10.1016/j.jcmg.2011.11.021.
4. Rubinshtein R, Glockner JF, Ommen SR, Araoz PA, Ackerman MJ, Sorajja P, et al. Characteristics and clinical significance of late gadolinium enhancement by contrast-enhanced magnetic resonance imaging in patients with hypertrophic cardiomyopathy. Circ Heart Fail. 2010;3(1):51–8. https://doi.org/10.1161/CIRCHEARTFAILURE.109.854026.
5. Chan RH, Maron BJ, Olivotto I, Pencina MJ, Assenza GE, Haas T, et al. Prognostic value of quantitative contrast-enhanced cardiovascular magnetic resonance for the evaluation of sudden death risk in patients with hypertrophic cardiomyopathy. Circulation. 2014;130(6):484–95. https://doi.org/10.1161/CIRCULATIONAHA.113.007094.
6. Ismail TF, Jabbour A, Gulati A, Mallorie A, Raza S, Cowling TE, et al. Role of late gadolinium enhancement cardiovascular magnetic resonance in the risk stratification of hypertrophic cardiomyopathy. Heart. 2014;100(23):1851–8. https://doi.org/10.1136/heartjnl-2013-305471.
7. Gulati A, Jabbour A, Ismail TF, Guha K, Khwaja J, Raza S, et al. Association of fibrosis with mortality and sudden cardiac death in patients with nonischemic dilated cardiomyopathy. JAMA. 2013;309(9):896–908. https://doi.org/10.1001/jama.2013.1363.

8. Banka P, Robinson JD, Uppu SC, Harris MA, Hasbani K, Lai WW, et al. Cardiovascular magnetic resonance techniques and findings in children with myocarditis: a multicenter retrospective study. J Cardiovasc Magn Reson. 2015;17:96. https://doi.org/10.1186/s12968-015-0201-6.
9. Placido R, Cunha Lopes B, Almeida AG, Rochitte CE. The role of cardiovascular magnetic resonance in takotsubo syndrome. J Cardiovasc Magn Reson. 2016;18(1):68. https://doi.org/10.1186/s12968-016-0279-5.
10. Francone M. Role of cardiac magnetic resonance in the evaluation of dilated cardiomyopathy: diagnostic contribution and prognostic significance. ISRN Radiol. 2014;2014:365404. https://doi.org/10.1155/2014/365404.
11. Maron BJ, Towbin JA, Thiene G, Antzelevitch C, Corrado D, Arnett D, et al. Contemporary definitions and classification of the cardiomyopathies: an American Heart Association Scientific Statement from the Council on Clinical Cardiology, Heart Failure and Transplantation Committee; Quality of Care and Outcomes Research and Functional Genomics and Translational Biology Interdisciplinary Working Groups; and Council on Epidemiology and Prevention. Circulation. 2006;113(14):1807–16. https://doi.org/10.1161/CIRCULATIONAHA.106.174287. CIRCULATIONAHA.106.174287 [pii].
12. Petersen SE, Selvanayagam JB, Wiesmann F, Robson MD, Francis JM, Anderson RH, et al. Left ventricular non-compaction. J Am Coll Cardiol. 2005;46(1):101–5. https://doi.org/10.1016/j.jacc.2005.03.045.
13. Kawel N, Nacif M, Arai AE, Gomes AS, Hundley WG, Johnson WC, et al. Trabeculated (noncompacted) and compact myocardium in adults: the multi-ethnic study of atherosclerosis. Circ Cardiovasc Imaging. 2012;5(3):357–66. https://doi.org/10.1161/CIRCIMAGING.111.971713.
14. Wan J, Zhao S, Cheng H, Lu M, Jiang S, Yin G, et al. Varied distributions of late gadolinium enhancement found among patients meeting cardiovascular magnetic resonance criteria for isolated left ventricular non-compaction. J Cardiovasc Magn Reson. 2013;15:20. https://doi.org/10.1186/1532-429X-15-20.
15. Puntmann VO, D'Cruz D, Smith Z, Pastor A, Choong P, Voigt T, et al. Native myocardial T1 mapping by cardiovascular magnetic resonance imaging in subclinical cardiomyopathy in patients with systemic lupus erythematosus. Circ Cardiovasc Imaging. 2013;6(2):295–301. https://doi.org/10.1161/CIRCIMAGING.112.000151.
16. Mayr A, Kitterer D, Latus J, Steubing H, Henes J, Vecchio F, et al. Evaluation of myocardial involvement in patients with connective tissue disorders: a multi-parametric cardiovascular magnetic resonance study. J Cardiovasc Magn Reson. 2016;18(1):67. https://doi.org/10.1186/s12968-016-0288-4.
17. Banypersad SM, Fontana M, Maestrini V, Sado DM, Captur G, Petrie A, et al. T1 mapping and survival in systemic light-chain amyloidosis. Eur Heart J. 2015;36(4):244–51. https://doi.org/10.1093/eurheartj/ehu444.
18. Vignaux O. Cardiac sarcoidosis: spectrum of MRI features. AJR Am J Roentgenol. 2005;184(1):249–54. https://doi.org/10.2214/ajr.184.1.01840249.
19. Greulich S, Deluigi CC, Gloekler S, Wahl A, Zurn C, Kramer U, et al. CMR imaging predicts death and other adverse events in suspected cardiac sarcoidosis. J Am Coll Cardiol Img. 2013;6(4):501–11. https://doi.org/10.1016/j.jcmg.2012.10.021.
20. Vignaux O, Dhote R, Duboc D, Blanche P, Dusser D, Weber S, et al. Clinical significance of myocardial magnetic resonance abnormalities in patients with sarcoidosis: a 1-year follow-up study. Chest. 2002;122(6):1895–901.
21. Hendel RC, Patel MR, Kramer CM, Poon M, Hendel RC, Carr JC, et al. ACCF/ACR/SCCT/SCMR/ASNC/NASCI/SCAI/SIR 2006 appropriateness criteria for cardiac computed tomography and cardiac magnetic resonance imaging: a report of the American College of Cardiology Foundation Quality Strategic Directions Committee Appropriateness Criteria Working Group, American College of Radiology, Society of Cardiovascular Computed Tomography, Society for Cardiovascular Magnetic Resonance, American Society of Nuclear Cardiology, North American Society for Cardiac Imaging, Society for Cardiovascular Angiography and Interventions, and Society of Interventional Radiology. J Am Coll Cardiol. 2006;48(7):1475–97. https://doi.org/10.1016/j.jacc.2006.07.003.
22. Anderson LJ, Holden S, Davis B, Prescott E, Charrier CC, Bunce NH, et al. Cardiovascular T2-star (T2*) magnetic resonance for the early diagnosis of myocardial iron overload. Eur Heart J. 2001;22(23):2171–9.
23. Ambati SR, Randolph RE, Mennitt K, Kleinert DA, Weinsaft JW, Giardina PJ. Longitudinal monitoring of cardiac siderosis using cardiovascular magnetic resonance T2* in patients with thalassemia major on various chelation regimens: a 6-year study. Am J Hematol. 2013;88(8):652–6. https://doi.org/10.1002/ajh.23469.
24. Pennell DJ, Carpenter JP, Roughton M, Cabantchik Z. On improvement in ejection fraction with iron chelation in thalassemia major and the risk of future heart failure. J Cardiovasc Magn Reson. 2011;13:45. https://doi.org/10.1186/1532-429X-13-45.
25. Pennell DJ, Udelson JE, Arai AE, Bozkurt B, Cohen AR, Galanello R, et al. Cardiovascular function and treatment in beta-thalassemia major: a consensus statement from the American Heart Association. Circulation. 2013;128(3):281–308. https://doi.org/10.1161/CIR.0b013e31829b2be6.
26. Kramer J, Niemann M, Stork S, Frantz S, Beer M, Ertl G, et al. Relation of burden of myocardial fibrosis to malignant ventricular arrhythmias and outcomes in Fabry disease. Am J Cardiol. 2014;114(6):895–900. https://doi.org/10.1016/j.amjcard.2014.06.019.
27. Pica S, Sado DM, Maestrini V, Fontana M, White SK, Treibel T, et al. Reproducibility of native myocardial T1 mapping in the assessment of Fabry disease and its role in early detection of cardiac involvement by cardiovascular magnetic resonance. J Cardiovasc Magn Reson. 2014;16:99. https://doi.org/10.1186/s12968-014-0099-4.
28. Dalal D, Tandri H, Judge DP, Amat N, Macedo R, Jain R, et al. Morphologic variants of familial arrhythmogenic right ventricular dysplasia/cardiomyopathy a genetics-magnetic resonance imaging correlation study. J Am Coll Cardiol. 2009;53(15):1289–99. https://doi.org/10.1016/j.jacc.2008.12.045.
29. Sen-Chowdhry S, Syrris P, Prasad SK, Hughes SE, Merrifield R, Ward D, et al. Left-dominant arrhythmogenic cardiomyopathy: an under-recognized clinical entity. J Am Coll Cardiol. 2008;52(25):2175–87. https://doi.org/10.1016/j.jacc.2008.09.019.
30. Rastegar N, Zimmerman SL, Te Riele AS, James C, Burt JR, Bhonsale A, et al. Spectrum of biventricular involvement on CMR among carriers of ARVD/C-associated mutations. J Am Coll Cardiol Img. 2015;8(7):863–4. https://doi.org/10.1016/j.jcmg.2014.09.009.

17

Modern Diagnosis in the Evaluation of Pulmonary Vascular Disease

Alexander A. Bankier and Carole Dennie

Learning Objectives

- To provide clinical background information about the most relevant vascular disorders of the thorax
- To elucidate the role of imaging in the work-up of these disorders
- To discuss the role of diagnostic imaging in patient management and clinical decision-making

17.1 Introduction

The conventional chest radiograph, computed tomography (CT), and, with restrictions, magnetic resonance imaging (MRI) are the three most commonly used imaging modalities for evaluating patients with suspected pulmonary vascular disease. Additionally, in the very recent past, fluorodeoxyglucose positron emission tomography (FDG-PET) and FDG-PET/CT have been attributed clinical usefulness in the evaluation of large vessel vasculitis. In general clinical routine, however, CT remains the imaging modality of choice for evaluation of patients with suspected pulmonary vascular disease. This is currently emphasized by new technical developments, such as dual-source and dual-energy scanners, that enable to simultaneously generate morphological and functional information from a sole data set. Therefore, CT has become crucial for evaluating the pulmonary vasculature. This is based on the following: Among the various imaging modalities available in recent decades, computed tomography (CT) has remained the core technique for evaluating respiratory disorders. Over the last few years, this central position has been reinforced by the possibility of deriving morphological and functional information from the same data set. This approach is of major interest for evaluating pulmonary vascular diseases for three main reasons: (1) Pulmonary vascular disorders require good morphological evaluation, not only for the vascular tree per se but also the surrounding lung parenchyma; (2) given that we have reached an upper limit in terms of morphologic image resolution, but simultaneously can provide functional information, CT is the ideal combination of high-end morphologic imaging with perfusion and ventilation imaging; and (3) it is becoming increasingly important to evaluate the cardiac consequences or causes of pulmonary vascular diseases, which requires all advantages tha t CT can provide. Because of these reasons, and given the general importance of CT, this course will focus on CT. Other imaging modalities will not be disregarded but rather discussed in the case-based presentations and framed in their distinct clinical context.

A. A. Bankier (✉)
Department of Radiology, Beth Israel Deaconess Medical Center, Harvard Medical School, Boston, MA, USA
e-mail: abankier@bidmc.harvard.edu

C. Dennie
Department of Medical Imaging, The Ottawa Hospital, University of Ottawa, Ottawa, ON, Canada
e-mail: Cdennie@toh.ca

17.2 Optimized Evaluation of Pulmonary Vessels on Chest CT Examinations

17.2.1 Temporal Resolution of Pulmonary CT Angiograms

Given the anatomical complexity of the lungs, the most crucial prerequisite for optimal chest imaging is a high spatial resolution, required not only to detect subtle morphologic abnormalities but also to adequately image thoracic vessels on CT angiography (CTA) and to differentiate between normal and abnormal vascular structures and dimensions. However, high spatial resolution is optimally employed when short overall examination times and high temporal resolution (i.e., short acquisition times of the individual axial image planes) are available simultaneously. This allows for the analysis of high-resolution images with a minimum of motion artifacts. The technical progress in development of multidetector-row CT (MDCT) has enabled radiologists to image the entire thorax with increasing spatial resolution in decreasing time durations. As a consequence, more patients are able to hold their breath throughout the entire period of data acquisition. This results in a substantial decrease in number and frequency of respiratory motion artifacts. Shorter CT rotation times have furthermore enabled shorter acquisition times and significantly artifacts caused by cardiac motion. These have, in the past, not only decreased image quality in the proximity of cardiac structures but could also cause pulsation artifacts at the anatomical level of systemic and pulmonary vessels, thus mimicking endovascular abnormalities, such as thrombi or neoplastic tissue. In order to image patients with the highest temporal resolution and shortest examination time, it is preferable to choose the shortest rotation time possible and the highest pitch, defined as the table feed per rotation, divided by the nominal beam width at the isocenter of the scanner. For example, on a 64-slice MDCT using a single X-ray source, rotation times range from 0.30 to 0.40 s, resulting in a temporal resolution per image not better than half the rotation time, and the pitch values usually do not exceed 1.5 [1]. The introduction of dual-source 64-slice MDCT technology offers the possibility of improving the technical requirements for CT. When both available tubes are operated at the same kilovoltage, the temporal resolution of each image is 1/4 of the rotation time, each of the two detectors contributing 90° of data in parallel-ray geometry to each image plane [2]. Moreover, the second measurement system of dual-source CT allows for a higher pitch mode than those available with a single-source CT, but without image distortion inside the field of view of the second detector. In a recent study, Tacelli et al. showed that this scanning mode provides CT angiographic examinations of excellent quality for thoracic applications in routine clinical practice, including those referred for pulmonary vascular diseases such as acute pulmonary embolism (PE) [3].

17.3 Improved Morphological Evaluation of the Peripheral Pulmonary Vasculature

With the introduction of MDCT, CTA is now recognized as the reference standard for diagnosing acute PE [4]. The advantages of MDCT over single-slice CT result from the opportunity of scanning the entire volume of the thorax with submillimetric collimation in a very short periods of time, most often under the duration of a single breath-hold, which is particularly useful when evaluating dyspneic patients. These technological advances have improved the evaluation of peripheral pulmonary arteries and the accuracy of CT in the work-up of acute PE. Simultaneously, MDCT allows radiologists to scan patients at a low kilovoltage with two subsequent advantages, in particular, the possibility of reducing the doses of contrast material and reducing the overall radiation dose. This is of particular importance in young female patients who may be exposed to substantial levels of radiation to breast tissue. In the context of acute PE, the latter concern is clinically relevant when keeping in mind the lower prevalence of acute PE, which has dropped from 33% on angiographic studies to <20% on CT/MDCT scans. To date, several studies have investigated the clinical benefits of low-kilovoltage techniques [i.e., 80–100 kV(p) vs 120–140 kV(p)], the parameters at which most CT angiograms are performed. However, for obvious ethical reasons, these studies were based on the comparative analysis of different populations scanned with single-source CT [5–8]. The limitations of these comparisons include the lack of systematic adjustment for individual patient morphology, cardiac hemodynamics, and potential underlying respiratory disease. With the introduction of dual-source CT, it is now possible to two tubes being set at different kilovoltages. In addition to the opportunity to evaluate lung perfusion, standard CT angiograms can also benefit from this scanning mode, which has been shown to improve the ability to analyze small pulmonary arteries with 80 kV(p) [9].

17.4 Perfusion Imaging with Dual-Energy CT

Lung perfusion with dual-energy CT does not reflect blood flow analysis per se, as it represents a measurement at only one time point, but it rather reflects an iodine map of the lung microcirculation at this particular time point. There are numerous parameters known to influence the iodine distribution within pulmonary capillaries. Some are technique-related, whereas others are due to the anatomical and/or physiological circumstances under which data acquisition was performed. Dual-energy CT angiographic examinations can be obtained using a scanning protocol similar to that utilized in clinical practice. The acquisitions are acquired from top to bottom of the chest, with an injection protocol similar to that of a standard CT angiogram obtained with single energy on a 64-slice scanner. Two categories of images can be reconstructed. Diagnostic scans correspond to contiguous 1-mm-thick transverse CT scans generated from the raw spiral projection data of tube A and tube B (60% from the acquisition with tube A, 40% from the acquisition with tube B). Lung perfusion scans (i.e., images of the perfused blood volume of the lung parenchyma) are generated after determination of the iodine content of every voxel of the lung parenchyma on the separate 80- and 140-kV(p) images. They can be rendered as gray-scale or color-coded images. All images can be displayed as transverse scans, complemented as needed by coronal and sagittal reformats. Even though a dual-energy acquisition does not correspond to true perfusion imaging, several applications of this pulmonary micro-CTA have been investigated [10].

17.5 Acute Pulmonary Embolism

Dual-energy CT can detect endoluminal clots on averaged images of tubes A and B as reliably as can single-source CTA [11]. In a preliminary study, the authors validated the detectability of perfusion defects beyond obstructive clots. Perfusion defects in the adjacent lung parenchyma have the typical perfusion-territorial triangular shape well known from pulmonary angiographic, scintigraphic, and magnetic resonance imaging (MRI) perfusion studies. Dual-energy CTA can help predict perfusion defects without directly identifying peripheral endoluminal clots that may be located in subsegmental or more distal pulmonary arterial branches. Dual-energy CT can help differentiate lung infarction from less specific peripheral lung consolidation.

17.6 Chronic Thromboembolic Pulmonary Hypertension (CTEPH)

Dual-energy CTA may depict perfusion defects distal to chronic clots (Fig. 17.1). In a study of 40 patients referred with PH of whom 14 were diagnosed with CTEPH, the sensitivity of DECT was 100% with a specificity of 92% compared to planar VQ [12]. DECT still has limitations with regard to imaging artifacts, but these are expected to improve with technical advancements.

Three vascular characteristics of chronic PE may manifest on dual-energy CT imaging. First, chronic PE causes a mosaic pattern of lung attenuation, characterized by areas of ground-glass attenuation, with enlarged vascular segments intermingled with areas of normal lung attenuation and smaller vascular segments (Fig. 17.2). When present, these findings are suggestive of blood flow redistribution, but are not consistently seen on conventional CT in patients with chronic PE. In such patients, dual-energy CT has the potential to detect ground-glass attenuation of vascular origin via high iodine content within the areas of ground-glass attenuation, thus

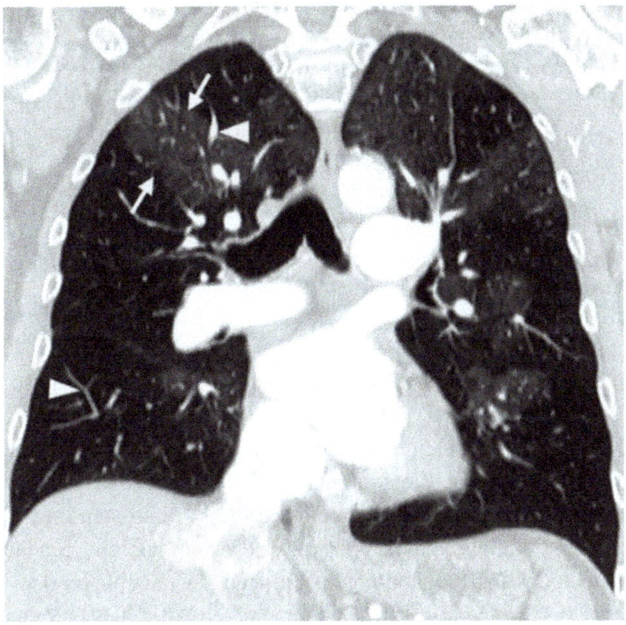

Fig. 17.2 Mosaic attenuation pattern. Coronal reformat (lung window) shows areas of high attenuation (arrows) which contain larger vessels than those within areas of lower attenuation (arrowheads)

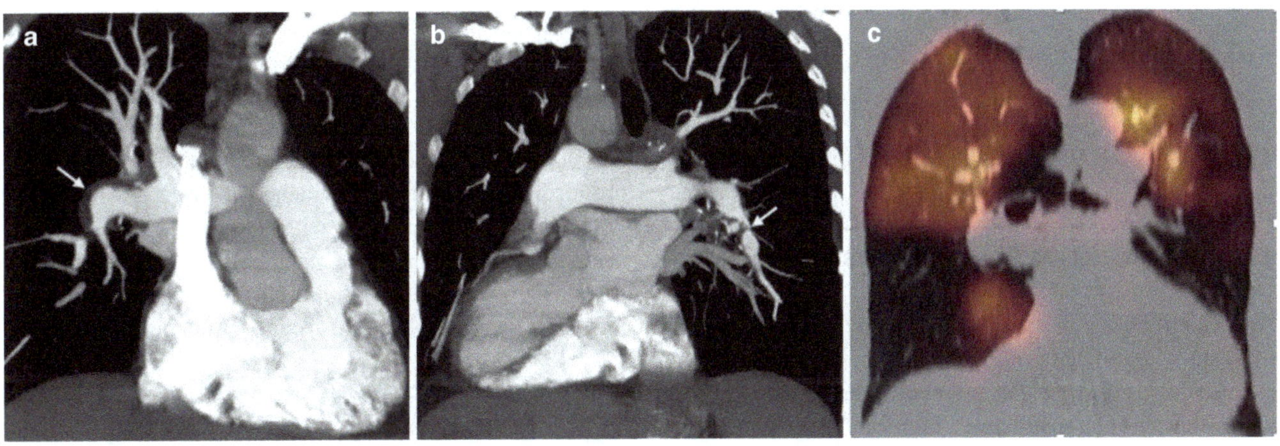

Fig. 17.1 (**a–c**) Chronic thromboembolic disease. Oblique coronal MIP CTPA image (**a**) shows a mural filling defect in the right interlobar artery (arrow). Oblique coronal MIP CTPA image (**b**) in the same patient depicts focal stenosis (arrow) and post-stenotic dilatation involving a segmental artery in the left lower lobe. DECT coronal reformatted image (**c**) in a different patient reveals almost completely absent perfusion in the lower lobes

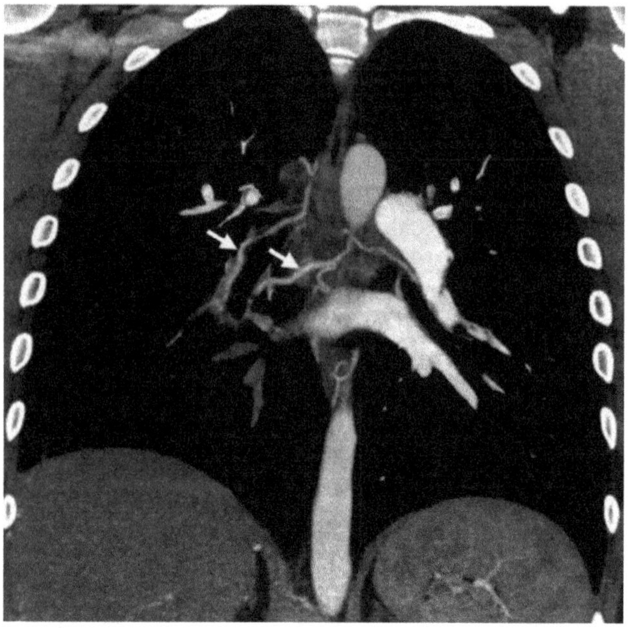

Fig. 17.3 Systemic collateral supply. Coronal reformat CTPA image reveals bronchial artery collaterals (arrows)

enabling their distinction from ground-glass attenuation secondary to bronchial or alveolar diseases [13]. Second, chronic PE can cause calcifications within partially or completely occlusive chronic clots as well as within pulmonary artery walls, when chronic PE is complicated by long-standing or severe pulmonary hypertension. Such calcifications can be detected via virtual non-contrast imaging, accessible by dual-energy CT imaging. Third, the images generated at 80 kV can improve visualization of the systemic collateral supply present in chronic PE that originates from bronchial and non-bronchial systemic arteries (Fig. 17.3).

Key Point

- With technical advancements, DECT may replace VQ in the future in the detection of chronic pulmonary embolism.

17.7 Obstructive Airway Diseases

Abnormalities of pulmonary perfusion are present in numerous smoking-related respiratory diseases. Investigating endothelial dysfunction in pulmonary arteries of patients with mild chronic obstructive pulmonary disease (COPD), Peinado et al. showed that endothelial dysfunction of pulmonary arteries is present even in patients with mild COPD [14]. In these patients, as well as in smokers with normal lung function, some arteries show a thickened intima, suggesting that tobacco consumption may play an important role in the pathogenesis of pulmonary vascular pathologies in COPD. Several structural changes in early stages of COPD have been described in experimental and animal models, including proliferation of smooth muscle fibers within peri-bronchiolar arterioles and collagen and elastin deposition in the thickened intima of vessels [15, 16]. In preliminary studies, Hoffman et al. [17] showed an increased heterogeneity of local mean transit times of the contrast material within pulmonary microvasculature of smokers with normal pulmonary function tests. More recently, Pansini et al. studied pulmonary lobar perfusion with dual-source, dual-energy CTA in COPD patients [18]. These authors found that nonsmokers had no alterations in lung structure and that there is a uniform distribution of iodine content within upper and lower lobes and between right and left lungs. Perfusion scans of emphysematous patients showed significantly lower iodine content within lung microcirculation of the upper lobes, as compared to smokers without emphysema, and a significantly lower perfusion in the upper lung zones as compared with lower lung zones, thus matching lung parenchymal destruction. These structural abnormalities are substantial observations, given the epidemiologic and socioeconomic burden of COPD.

17.8 Restrictive Airway Diseases

The substantial importance of pulmonary hypertension on the clinical course and prognosis of patients with fibrotic lung disease has been extensively recognized. Similar to obstructive lung disorders, MDCT and DSCT have a role to play in the evaluation of these disorders. Recent research suggests that the mere measurement of pulmonary artery diameters might not be a reliable parameter for disease severity assessment, given the potentially confounding role of parenchymal traction on central and peripheral pulmonary vessels. Moreover, given the age of the population in which these diseases usually occur, age-related changes have to be taken into account of any morphometric-based clinical decision-making and classification. Overall, and despite promising initial scientific evidence, the role of MDCT and DSCT in assessing patients with fibrotic lung diseases still needs to be determined. The many ongoing pharmacological trials, notably in patients with usual interstitial pneumonitis, may provide an ample study ground in this field.

17.9 Pulmonary Hypertension

Once left heart causes and intracardiac shunts have been ruled out with echocardiography, CT can play a key role in the classification of patients with pulmonary hypertension

Table 17.1 Abbreviated Nice classification of pulmonary hypertension

1. Pulmonary arterial hypertension (PAH)
   a. Idiopathic
   b. Heritable
   c. Drugs and toxins induced
   d. Associated with connective tissue disease, HIV infection, portal hypertension, congenital heart disease, schistosomiasis
   - Pulmonary veno-occlusive disease and/or pulmonary capillary hemangiomatosis
   - Persistent pulmonary hypertension of the newborn
2. Pulmonary hypertension due to left heart disease
3. Pulmonary hypertension due to lung disease and/or hypoxia
4. Chronic thromboembolic pulmonary hypertension and other pulmonary artery obstructions
5. Pulmonary hypertension with unclear and/or multifactorial mechanisms

(PH) (Table 17.1) [19]. There are vascular, cardiac, and pulmonary parenchymal features of pulmonary hypertension on CT. A main pulmonary artery (MPA) diameter of greater than 29.5 mm has a sensitivity of 70.8% and specificity of 79.4% for the detection of pulmonary hypertension [20]. However, there is no correlation between the degree of PH and MPA diameter. The specificity is lower in patients who have interstitial fibrosis which is postulated to cause MPA dilatation due to traction without PH [21]. A ratio of diameter of MPA to that of ascending aorta in the same axial plane of ≥1.0 is also indicative of PH, especially in younger patients (<50), and may be a more useful predictor of PH in those with advanced interstitial fibrosis [22]. In one study, the segmental artery-to-bronchus diameter ratio of >1:1 in three or four lobes along with a dilated MPA had almost 100% specificity in the diagnosis of PH [23].

Other CT features of PH include right ventricular dilatation and hypertrophy (>4 mm), straightening or bowing of the interventricular septum, and reflux of contrast into a dilated inferior vena cava ± hepatic veins. Pulmonary parenchymal features include the mosaic attenuation pattern most commonly seen in patients with chronic thromboembolic pulmonary hypertension (CTEPH). Other less common findings include centrilobular ground-glass nodules due to the presence of cholesterol granulomas, plexogenic arteriopathy or capillary proliferation, and serpiginous centrilobular arterioles as a sign of neovascularity [24].

Electrocardiograph (ECG)-gated MDCT acquisitions of the entire thorax enable the evaluation of novel functional parameters in addition to the standard morphology. In patients with PH, right pulmonary artery distensibility has been reported as an accurate predictor for PH on ECG-gated 64-slice MDCT scans of the chest [25]. In this study, its diagnostic value was superior to that of the single measurement of PA diameter.

17.10 Right Ventricular Function

Fast rotation speed and dedicated cardiac reconstruction algorithms designed to extend the conventional multislice acquisition data scheme have opened new opportunities for cardiac and thoracic imaging applications. However, cardiac MRI (CMR) has become the gold standard for the assessment of right function due to superior reproducibility in comparison to echo and its superior temporal resolution compared to CT. CMR also provides prognostic information and can be performed at baseline and in follow-up without the use of ionizing radiation.

Multiple MR parameters have been assessed in patients with PH. Increased right ventricular volumes and reduced stoke volumes at baseline have been shown to be predictors of treatment failure and increased mortality [26]. On velocity-encoded phase contrast imaging, an average velocity in the MPA of <11.7 cm/s has a 92.9% sensitivity and 82.4% specificity for the detection of PH, and interventricular septal bowing has been correlated with a systolic pulmonary artery pressure (PAP) of >67 mm Hg [76]. Swift retrospectively analyzed CMR and right heart catheterization in 233 patients with suspected PH. Ventricular mass index (VMI) was the CMR measurement with the strongest correlation with mean PAP ($r = 0.78$) and the highest diagnostic accuracy (area under ROC = 0.91) for the detection of PH. Late gadolinium enhancement (Fig. 17.4), VMI ≥ 0.4, and pulmonary artery relative area change ≤15% predicted the presence of PH with ≥ 94% positive predictive value [27]. Recently, 4D flow MRI has revealed turbulent vortices

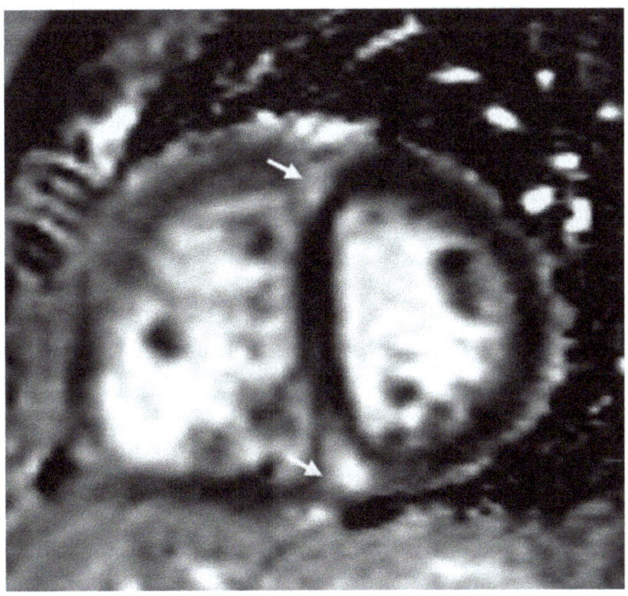

Fig. 17.4 Late gadolinium enhancement short axis image shows the typical enhancement pattern seen in PH with enhancement at the superior and inferior insertion points of the right ventricle into the interventricular septum (arrows)

in the central pulmonary arteries and has enabled measurement of wall shear stress [28, 29]. Other novel CMR techniques include right ventricular T1 mapping and strain imaging [30].

Key Point

- Although CT can be very useful in determining the cause of PH, CMR is the gold standard for the assessment of right ventricular function and can provide information on pulmonary artery dynamics. Importantly, it can also impart prognostic information.

17.11 Imaging of Pulmonary Vasculitis

Systemic primary vasculitides are idiopathic diseases causing an inflammatory injury to the vessel walls. Pulmonary involvement is frequent, and chest CT often in combination with PET/CT is the reference imaging technique in its assessment. Pulmonary vasculitis occurs in a wide variety of systemic and pulmonary vascular disorders. Most vasculitic entities affecting the lung induce overlapping disease patterns such as pneumonitis with or without capillaritis, diffuse alveolar damage and acute pulmonary hemorrhage, or inflammatory obstruction of central pulmonary arteries down to small vessels with chronic secondary pulmonary hypertension with or without interstitial lung disease, and therefore the clinical symptoms per se or the CT morphology alone is often nonspecific.

Owing to their complementary value in imaging of central and peripheral vascular territories and their secondary parenchymal or interstitial abnormalities, CT angiography (CTA), high-resolution CT (HRCT), and fusion imaging play key roles in the noninvasive work-up of patients with suspected pulmonary vasculitis. They enable indicative for further clinical tests, imaging, or invasive diagnostics and direct medical treatment during follow-up. This course will familiarize radiologists with CT diagnostic key features that reflect pulmonary vasculitic pathology inherent to the underlying disease.

17.12 The Role of CT in the Differential Diagnosis of Pulmonary Vasculitis

A wide variety of CT pathology of the lung parenchyma, vessels, and airways has been described, and diagnosis is a challenging interdisciplinary field. Clinical and laboratory data have to be included in close cooperation with the referring physician. This course will describe the most common typical and atypical CT features of pulmonary vasculitis and their possible changes over time and therapy, focusing on the differential diagnosis with other inflammatory/infectious hereditary and neoplastic disorders.

In large vessel vasculitis, CT is the method of choice often in combination with PET to discriminate macroscopic vascular abnormality presenting key pathological features such as pulmonary arterial wall thickening with late enhancement, steno-occlusive or thrombo-obliterating disease with resulting oligemia, infarction in the dependent lung, or arterial aneurysms as a facultative cause of massive pulmonary hemorrhage. CT is the modality of choice to demonstrate effects of peripheral small vessel pulmonary vasculitis on the central pulmonary arteries such as secondary chronic pulmonary hypertension due to reduction of the total cross-sectional area with arteriolar remodeling or narrowing of the capillary bed in capillaritis. The variety of peripheral vascular bronchial and parenchymal CT patterns of small vessel vasculitis is great, often complex requiring interpretation in combination with clinical symptoms and laboratory test results. However, many vasculitic disorders present CT features, which are suggestive of a vasculitic disorder. CT-pathologic correlates of the peribronchovascular axial interstitium, pulmonary hemorrhage, types of inflammatory parenchymal infiltration, and secondary pathologies such as organizing pneumonia are discussed with reference to the revised 2012 International Chapel Hill Consensus Conference on pulmonary vasculitis and the American College of Rheumatology (ACR) [31].

17.13 Concluding Remarks

Pulmonary vascular diseases are a complex group of conditions with various potential causes. Radiological techniques play a key role in diagnosing and managing these diseases. A thorough knowledge is required from the radiologist about the manifestations of these diseases, and about the reasonable use of the various imaging techniques available, to facilitate the diagnostic process and to streamline patient management.

Take-Home Messages

- Thorough knowledge of pulmonary vascular diseases is required from radiologists to contribute to diagnosis and work-up.
- The imaging armamentarium plays a key role in the diagnosis and management of these disorders.

References

1. Rogalla P, Kloeters C, Hein PA. CT technology overview: 64-slice and beyond. Radiol Clin N Am. 2009;47:1–11.
2. Petersilka M, Bruder H, Krauss B, et al. Technical principles of dual source CT. Eur J Radiol. 2008;68:362–8.
3. Tacelli N, Remy-Jardin M, Flohr T, et al. Dual-source chest CT angiography with high temporal resolution and high pitch modes: evaluation of image quality in 140 patients. Eur Radiol. 2010;20:1188–96.
4. Remy-Jardin M, Pistolesi M, Goodman LR, et al. Management of suspected acute pulmonary embolism in the era of CT angiography: a statement from the Fleischner Society. Radiology. 2007;245:315–29.
5. Holmquist F, Nyman U. Eighty-peak kilovoltage 16-channel multidetector computed tomography and reduced contrast medium doses tailored to body weight to diagnose pulmonary embolism in azotaemic patients. Eur Radiol. 2006;16:1165–76.
6. Sigal-Cinqualbre AB, Hennequin R, Abada H, et al. Low-kilovoltage multi-detector row chest CT in adults: feasibility and effect on image quality and iodine dose. Radiology. 2004;231:169–74.
7. Schueller-Weidekamm C, Schaefer-Prokop CM, Weber M, et al. CT angiography of pulmonary arteries to detect pulmonary embolism: improvement of vascular enhancement with low kilovoltage settings. Radiology. 2006;241:899–907.
8. Heyer CM, Mohr PS, Lemburg SP, et al. Image quality and radiation exposure at pulmonary CT angiography with 100- or 120-kVp protocol: prospective randomized study. Radiology. 2007;245:577–83.
9. Gorgos AB, Remy-Jardin M, Duhamel A, et al. Evaluation of peripheral pulmonary arteries at 80 kV and at 140 kV: dual-energy computed tomography assessment in 51 patients. J Comput Assist Tomogr. 2009;33:981–6.
10. Remy-Jardin M, Faivre JB, Pontana F, et al. Thoracic applications of dual energy. Radiol Clin N Am. 2010;48:193–205.
11. Pontana F, Faivre JB, Remy-Jardin M, et al. Lung perfusion with dual-energy multidetector-row CT (MDCT): Feasibilityfor the evaluation of acute pulmonary embolism in 117 consecutive patients. Acad Radiol. 2008;15:1494–504.
12. Dournes G, Verdier D, Montaudon M, et al. Dual-energy CT perfusion and angiography in chronic thromboembolic pulmonary hypertension: diagnostic accuracy and concordance with radionuclide scintigraphy. Eur Radiol. 2014;24(1):42–51.
13. Pontana F, Remy-Jardin M, Duhamel A, et al. Lung perfusion with dual energy multidetector-row CT: can it help recognize ground glass opacities of vascular origin? Acad Radiol. 2010;17:587–94.
14. Peinado VI, Barberà JA, Ramirez J, et al. Endothelial dysfunction in pulmonary arteries of patients with mild COPD. Am J Phys. 1988;274:L908–13.
15. Yamato Y, Sun JP, Churg A, et al. Guinea pig pulmonary hypertension caused by cigarette smoke cannot be explained by capillary bed destruction. J Appl Physiol. 1997;82:1644–53.
16. Santos S, Peinado VI, Ramirez J, et al. Characterization of pulmonary vascular remodelling in smokers and patients with mild COPD. Eur Respir J. 2002;19:632–8.
17. Hoffman EA, Simon BA, McLennan G. A structural and functional assessment of the lung via multidetector-row computed tomography. Proc Am Thorac Soc. 2006;3:519–34.
18. Pansini V, Remy-Jardin M, Faivre JB, et al. Assessment of lobar pulmonary perfusion in COPD patients: preliminary experience with dual-energy CT angiography. Eur Radiol. 2009;19:2834–43.
19. Simonneau G, Gatzoulis MA, Adatia I, et al. Updated clinical classification of pulmonary hypertension. J Am Coll Cardiol. 2013;62:D34–41.
20. McLaughlin VV, Archer SL, Badesch DB, et al. ACCF/AHA 2009 expert consensus document on pulmonary hypertension: a report of the American College of Cardiology Foundation Task Force on Expert Consensus Documents and the American Heart Association developed in collaboration with the American College of Chest Physicians; American Thoracic Society, Inc.; and the Pulmonary Hypertension Association. J Am Coll Cardiol. 2009;53:1573–619.
21. Devaraj A, Wells AJ, Meister MG, et al. The effect of diffuse pulmonary fibrosis on the reliability of CT signs of pulmonary hypertension. Radiology. 2008;249:1042–9.
22. Mahammedi A, Oshmyansky A, Hassoun PM, et al. Pulmonary artery measurements in pulmonary hypertension: the role of computed tomography. J Thorac Imaging. 2013;28(2):96–103.
23. Tan RT, Kuzo R, Goodman LR, et al. Utility of CT scan evaluation for predicting pulmonary hypertension in patients with parenchymal lung disease. Medical College of Wisconsin Lung Transplant Group. Chest. 1998;113(5):1250–6.
24. Peña E, Dennie C, Veinot J, Hernandez Muñiz S. Pulmonary hypertension: how the radiologist can help. Radiographics. 2012;32:9–32.
25. Revel MP, Faivre JB, Remy-Jardin M, et al. Pulmonary hypertension: ECG-gated 64-section CT angiographic evaluation of new functional parameters as diagnostic criteria. Radiology. 2009;250:558–66.
26. Benza R, Biederman R, Murali S, et al. Role of cardiac magnetic resonance imaging in the management of patients with pulmonary arterial hypertension. J Am Coll Cardiol. 2008;52(21):1683–92.
27. Swift AJ, Rajaram S, Condliffe R, Capener D, et al. Diagnostic accuracy of cardiovascular magnetic resonance imaging of right ventricular morphology and function in the assessment of suspected pulmonary hypertension results from the ASPIRE registry. J Cardiovasc Magn Reson. 2012;4:40.
28. Reiter G, Reiter U, Kovacs G, et al. Blood flow vortices along the main pulmonary artery measured with MR imaging for diagnosis of pulmonary hypertension. Radiology. 2015;275(1):71–9.
29. Barker AJ, Roldán-Alzate A, Entezari P, et al. 4D flow assessment of pulmonary artery flow and wall shear stress in adult pulmonary arterial hypertension: results from two institutions. Magn Reson Med. 2015;73(5):1904–13.
30. Freed BH, Collins JD, François CJ, et al. Magnetic resonance and computed tomography imaging for the evaluation of pulmonary hypertension. JACC Cardiovasc Imaging. 2016;9(6):715–32.
31. Jennette JC, Falk RJ, Bacon PA, et al. Revised international chapel hill consensus conference nomenclature of vasculitides. Arthritis Rheum. 2012;65(1):1–11.

18

Imaging of Acute Aortic Syndromes

Thomas M. Grist and Geoffrey D. Rubin

Learning Objectives

- Understand the pathological classification of acute aortic disease causing acute aortic syndromes.
- Describe eight key imaging findings in the evaluation of acute aortic syndrome.
- Prescribe and implement the correct protocols for accurate diagnosis using CT and MR imaging of the acute aorta.

The accurate detection and evaluation of acute aortic syndrome is one of the radiologist's most important and immediately impactful opportunities to avoid unnecessary death and disability. Acute aortic syndrome is often a clinical emergency and a situation that demands accurate radiologic diagnosis and intervention to provide lifesaving care. The diagnosis of acute aortic syndrome has evolved significantly over the last two decades, evolving from an arteriographic diagnosis to a diagnosis based upon multi-detector CT angiography [1] and, to a limited extent, MRI. With the advent of these new techniques for diagnosis, investigators have revisited the questions and pathologies surrounding acute aortic syndromes.

T. M. Grist (✉)
Department of Radiology, University of Wisconsin School of Medicine and Public Health, Madison, WI, USA
e-mail: tgrist@uwhealth.org

G. D. Rubin
Department of Radiology, Duke University School of Medicine, Durham, NC, USA
e-mail: grubin@duke.edu

18.1 Anatomic and Pathological Considerations

Acute aortic syndromes are principally diseases of the aortic wall. As a result, it is useful to review the fundamental features of the aortic wall in order to categorize the acute aortic syndromes.

The aorta is composed of three layers. From inner to outer, they are the intima, media, and adventitia. The intima is made up of a single layer of flattened epithelial cells with a supporting layer of elastin-rich collagen, fibroblasts, and myointimal cells. The latter myointimal cells tend to accumulate lipid with aging resulting in intimal thickening which is the earliest sign of atherosclerosis. The majority of the aortic wall thickness is composed of the media which itself is broad and elastic with concentric fenestrated sheets of elastin, collagen, and sparsely distributed smooth muscle fibers. The predominance of elastin arrayed as elastic lamina reflects the fact that the aorta and the pulmonary arteries are considered to be the only elastic arteries of the body. Because the aorta and the pulmonary arteries receive the entirety of the cardiac output, they undergo substantial deformation in order to accommodate large volume changes with each cardiac contraction. The remaining arteries of the body are considered muscular arteries with minimal elastin and a predominance of smooth muscle allowing for the body to regulate regional blood flow. The boundary between the intima and media is not readily defined. The division between the intima and media is defined histologically at the internal elastic lamina, which represents the innermost of the many elastic lamellae within the aortic media. The adventitia lacks elastic lamellae and is predominantly composed of loose connective tissue and blood vessels or vasa vasorum.

Anatomically, the aorta can be divided longitudinally into five zones—the aortic root, ascending thoracic aorta, aortic arch, descending thoracic aorta, and abdominal aorta. Acute aortic syndromes can involve any of these five anatomic zones; however they only rarely originate within the abdominal aorta. An important principle in the management of acute aortic syndromes is the classification of lesions into Stanford type A or type B. Type A lesions, defined as those involving the ascending aorta or aortic root, are considered lesions that demand urgent surgical intervention with replacement of the diseased ascending aortic segment. The rationale for this urgent intervention is a high risk of aortic rupture, which can lead to pericardial tamponade or frank exsanguination. Type B lesions do not involve the ascending aorta and as a result can occur within the aortic arch or the descending thoracic aorta. If there is evidence for active aortic rupture, then these patients too should be referred for urgent surgical intervention with endografting becoming an increasingly important option, for treating descending thoracic aortic leaks and pseudoaneurysms [2, 3]. In the absence of active bleeding, they are typically managed with blood pressure reduction and regular monitoring to assess the evolution of aortic dimension and disease extension.

18.2 Definitions and Classifications

Collectively, acute aortic syndromes represent life-threatening conditions that are associated with a high risk of aortic rupture and sudden death. The typical presentation is the sudden onset of chest pain, which may be accompanied by signs or symptoms of hypoperfusion or ischemia to distal organs, extremities, or the brain.

Traditionally, acute aortic syndromes are categorized as aortic dissection, intramural hematoma, and penetrating atherosclerotic ulcer.

Aortic dissection (AD) is characterized by a separation of the aortic media creating an intimal medial complex, which separates from the remaining aortic wall. Blood flowing between the intimal medial complex or flap and the remaining wall is considered to be within a false lumen, whereas blood flow bounded by the intima is considered to be within a true lumen. Multiple communication points can be observed between the true and false lumen. The proximal most communication is considered to be the "entry tear" with the remaining points of communication are considered to be "exit tears" implying flow directionality from true to false lumen and from false to true lumen, respectively. The actual incidence of AD is difficult to define, since AD involving the ascending aorta is often a fatal disease and patients frequently die prior to hospitalization. Likewise, AD is sometimes misdiagnosed on initial presentation, and these patients are also at risk for death outside of the hospital. Nevertheless, various population-based studies suggest that the incidence of AD ranges from 2 to 4 case per 100,000 patients [4].

The temporal definition of acute AD is a dissection that is identified less than 2 weeks after the onset of symptoms, while subacute ranges from 2 to 6 weeks following initial painful episode, and a chronic AD more than 6 weeks after the onset of pain.

Intramural hematoma (IMH) is an entity that was first described approximately 30 years ago as a stagnant collection of blood within the aortic wall. The common association of IMH with pathologically detected intimal defects led to the hypothesis that most are sequelae of penetrating atherosclerotic ulcer. An alternative cause of IMH, typically invoked in the absence of an intimal defect, is rupture of the vasa vasorum. This hypothetical cause of IMH has never been definitively proven. IMH is treated similar to dissections in terms of initial diagnosis as well as clinical management. Most IMH occur in the descending thoracic aorta and can be associated with severe pain. The imaging features vary depending on the amount of blood accumulated in the wall of the aorta, but typically the normal wall measures less than 7 mm in thickness. The natural history of IMH can be quite variable. Roughly one third of them will progress to aortic dissection, whereas one third will be stable and one third will resolve [5]. The mortality for patients with IMH involving the ascending aorta is similar to that of classic dissection, and therefore these patients are treated as though they have a classic AD with emergent surgery [6]. On the other hand, IMH involving the descending thoracic aorta can be followed, given appropriate therapy for hypertension.

Penetrating atherosclerotic ulcer (PAU) is a condition that originates with atherosclerotic plaque involvement of the aorta, primarily the descending thoracic aorta (Fig. 18.1). As the plaque evolves, the ulceration "penetrates" through the internal elastic lamina into the media of the aortic wall. Overtime the PAU may extend through all three layers of the aortic wall to form a false or pseudoaneurysm. A finding of PAU does not necessarily imply the existence of an acute aortic syndrome. Signs of IMH or extravasation indicate acuity.

There are two limitations to this traditional classification. One concerns the omission of a rupturing true aortic aneurysm, as the nature of the presentation and the severity of the event are similar to that of the other acute aortic syndromes. The other limitation is that IMH, defined as a stagnant intramural collection of blood, can be observed in the setting of AD, PAU, and rupturing aortic aneurysm. As such, it is a feature or characteristic associated with any of the acute aortic syndromes reflecting degradation of the aortic wall as a harbinger of impending aortic rupture.

In consideration of these two points, a new classification scheme has been proposed based upon the primary location of the lesion within the aortic wall. In this new classification scheme, there are three pathological entities: AD, PAU, and rupturing aortic aneurism [7]. These three entities are differentiated by the fact that AD principally involves the aortic media, PAU originates within the aortic intima, and aortic aneurysm is a disease of all three layers. The presence of IMH is an observation or epiphenomenon to be applied to

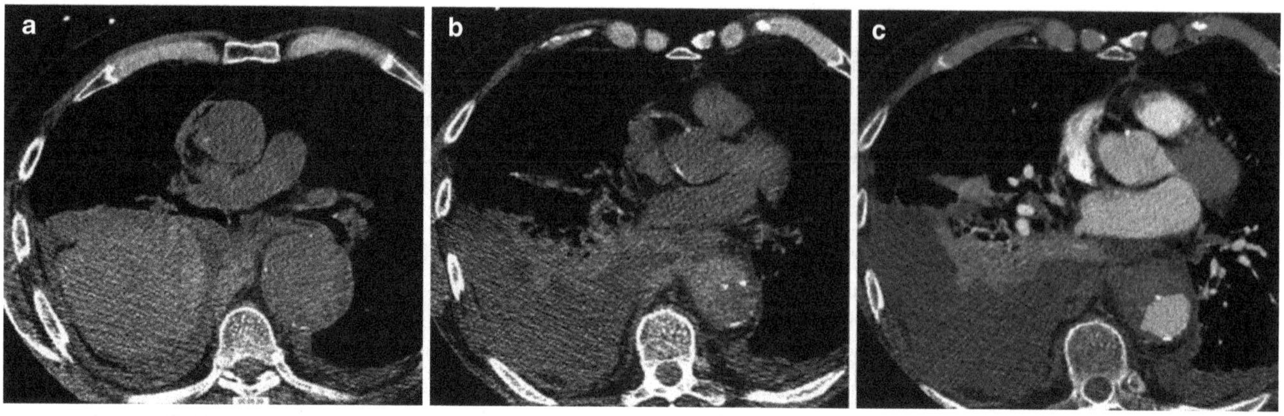

Fig. 18.1 Rupturing thoracic aortic aneurysm: (**a**) Unenhanced CT demonstrates high-attenuation hematoma in the right pleural space and the middle mediastinum. There is an aneurysm of the descending aorta. (**b**) Unenhanced CT section 5 cm inferior to (**a**) reveals an IMH at the inferior margin of the aneurysm with extravasation of blood into the middle mediastinum. Note displacement of intimal calcium along the inner wall of the IMH. (**c**) Following administration of IV contrast material, the IMH is harder to visualize owing to the wider window used to display the CT angiogram

any of these three fundamental pathologies. In the setting of an isolated IMH without PAU, "non-communicating dissection" has been proposed as a descriptor, although most people will associate the term "IMH" with this lesion. Recently, a subtype of aortic dissection has been described as "limited intimal tears" [8], which has similar natural history as AD and IMH, but can be particularly subtle to detect given their limited extent along the length of the thoracic aorta.

18.3 Essential Elements of Aortic Imaging Reports

In 2010, a group of medical organizations representing the disciplines of cardiology, radiology, thoracic surgery, and anesthesia published guidelines for the diagnosis and management of patients with thoracic aortic diseases. In this report, the authors identified eight essential elements that should be addressed in aortic imaging reports [4]. While these guidelines are not comprehensive, nor do they imply the necessity of reporting every element in every case, they are a useful construct from which to build any formalized description of the imaging findings of an acute aortic syndrome. They are:

1. The location at which the aorta is abnormal
2. The maximum diameter of any dilation, measured from the external wall of the aorta, perpendicular to the axis of flow and the length of the aorta that is abnormal
3. For patients with genetic syndromes at risk for aortic root disease, measurements of aortic valve, sinuses of Valsalva, sinotubular junction, and ascending aorta
4. The presence of internal filling defects consistent with thrombus or atheroma
5. The presence of IMH, PAU, or calcification
6. Extension of aortic abnormality inter-branch vessels, including dissection and aneurism, and secondary evidence of end-organ injury (e.g., renal or bowel hypoperfusion)
7. Evidence of aortic rupture, including periaortic and mediastinal hematoma, pericardial, and pleural fluid, and contrast extravasation from the aortic lumen (Fig. 18.2)
8. When a prior examination is available, direct image-to-image comparison to determine if there has been any increase in diameter

Recently, predication models have been developed to identify predictors of late adverse events following Type B AD. In particular, false luminal circumferential coverage and maximum aortic diameter at the time of index presentation and a diameter increase of 5 mm or more in the first 6 months following presentation have been associated with a significant increase in adverse events [9, 10].

18.4 Imaging Approaches to Acute Aortic Syndromes Using CT

High-quality and comprehensive aortic and end-organ assessment should be performed using multi-detector row CT with at least 16 detector rows. This scanner configuration allows for imaging from the neck through the pelvis, acquiring $\leq$1.5 mm thick transverse sections during the arterial phase of enhancement from an intravenous contrast administration. It also allows for the use of electrocardiographic gating of the scan when appropriate, as described below.

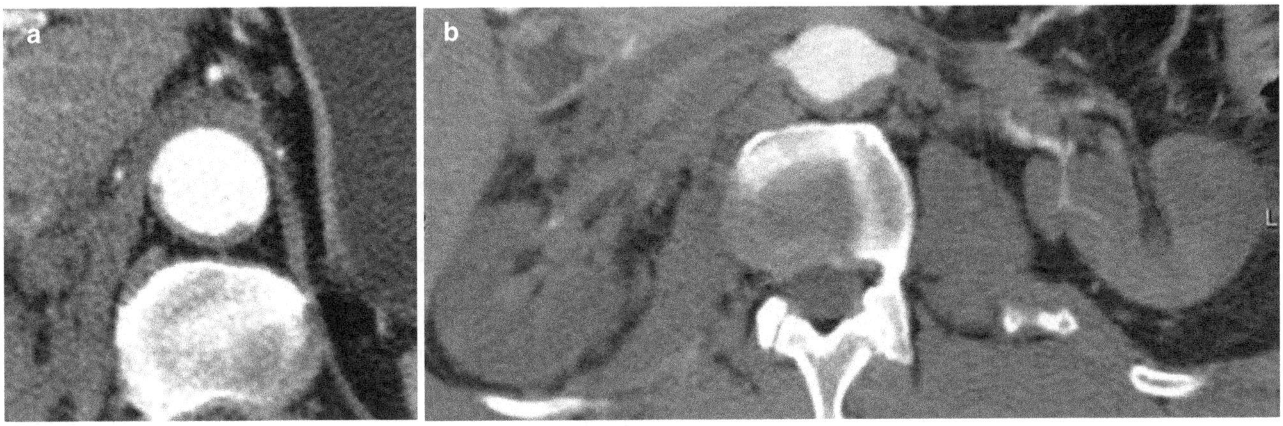

Fig. 18.2 Type B aortic dissection. (**a**) The true lumen is completely collapsed posteriorly, and only the true lumen fills with contrast material. The entry tear was (not shown) in the proximal descending aorta. (**b**) Because of their supply from the aortic true lumen, the renal arteries do not opacity, and the kidneys are not perfused

18.5 Unenhanced CT

An unenhanced scan can be valuable prior to the administration of intravenous contrast for the detection of what can be subtle intramural and periaortic blood. It can also be useful for mapping the specific regions of the aorta that are abnormal and thus guide the mode of subsequent CT angiographic acquisition. While an associated increase in radiation exposure results from this approach, the potential value of the information almost always outweighs the risk. It has been hypothesized that using dual energy scanning, a virtual unenhanced scan might obviate the need for a separate unenhanced acquisition. However, this approach has not been comprehensively validated in acute aortic syndromes.

18.6 CT Angiography

While unenhanced imaging can reveal aortic dilation, intramural and extra-aortic hemorrhage, and in uncommon circumstances directly visualize an intimal flap, the use of intravenously administered contrast medium is required for a complete assessment in suspected acute aortic syndrome (Fig. 18.3). The volume and flow rate of the contrast material should be adjusted based on patient size. A concentrated iodine solution of ≥350 mg of iodine/ml should be used in order to assure adequate intravenous delivery of iodine with a safe and reliable flow rate of the contrast material into the peripheral vein. Typical volumes and injector flow rates for iodinated contrast range between 60 and 115 mL at flow rates between 3.5 and 6 mL/sec.

To assure diagnostic aortic enhancement throughout the CT acquisition, the duration of the contrast injection should exceed the scan duration by 5–10 s, and the initiation of the CT angiographic acquisition should be based upon the active

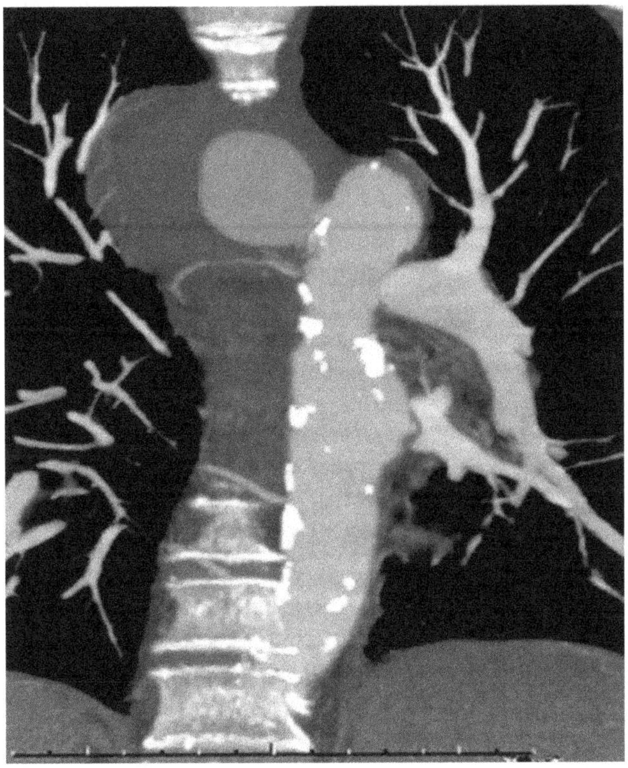

Fig. 18.3 PAU with pseudoaneurysm formation in the proximal descending aorta

monitoring on the arrival of iodine within the descending thoracic aorta.

18.7 Imaging the Abdominal Aorta and Iliac Arteries

Because of the likelihood of direct extension of thoracic aortic disease into the abdominal aorta and iliac arteries, unrelated but important abdominal aortoiliac pathology, the value of assessing the caliber of a transfemoral delivery route to intra-aortic repair devices, and the possibility for abdominal visceral ischemia, scan ranges that extend through the abdomen and pelvis are highly recommended as a routine approach to imaging acute aortic syndromes. By beginning the scan in the neck and extending inferiorly below the lesser trochanters of the femurs, the scan range will comfortably include several centimeters of the cervical carotid arteries through the bifurcation of the femoral artery. Scan ranges that include less anatomy risk the possibility that important observations will be missed, and additional CT scans with further injections of iodinated contrast material may be required.

18.8 ECG Gating

When the ascending aorta is involved with an acute aortic syndrome, electrocardiographic (ECG) gating can be valuable. ECG gating allows for clear delineation of the position of the intimal flap across the cardiac period, distinction of the involvement of the structures of the aortic root including the coronary artery ostia and the aortic annulus, elimination of pulsation-related artifacts that can blur the aortic wall, and subtle regions of extravasation. Unlike the use of ECG gating in the setting of coronary artery disease assessment, the strategy for using ECG gating in acute aortic syndromes does not rely upon the manipulation of heart rate or coronary artery dimension using beta-blockers or nitrates. Regardless of the basal heart rate, the placement of ECG leads and acquisition of a retrospectively gated CT scan (with judicious use of ECG directed X-ray tube current pulsing to minimize radiation exposure) allows for a four-dimensional assessment of the aortic root, aortic valve, coronary arteries, and ascending aorta. It is sufficient to reconstruct ten phases every 10% of the R-R interval. Gating is only beneficial through the thoracic aorta. For patients with heart rates less than 80 beats per minute, prospective triggering of multiple axial slabs, a single wide area acquisition, or a single high-pitch dual source may suffice to delineate the structures of the aortic root, depending upon the type of CT scanner available. The abdomen and pelvis are acquired after the chest using a non-gated acquisition with minimization of delay between the two scans so that only one contrast injection is required.

ECG gating is not required for all patients; however, it can be critical in patients with aortic root involvement. Review of preliminary unenhanced CT sections by a radiologist can help to identify patients for whom gating may be of value. Otherwise a second CT scan may be required and could delay treatment.

18.9 Clinical Indications for MRI in Acute Aortic Syndrome

While CT remains the mainstay for the initial diagnosis of patients with acute aortic syndrome, MRI may play a limited role in patients who cannot have a contrast-enhanced CTA, as well as in the follow-up of patients for complications following prior aortic dissection. However, due to the immediate availability of non-contrast CT in most emergency rooms, a non-contrast CT in patients who have a severe allergy to iodinated contrast may still be the method of choice for evaluating the potential complications of acute aortic syndrome, including IMH, ruptured aorta, pericardial or pleural effusions, and a displaced, calcified intimomedial flap.

Nevertheless, in patients who cannot have iodinated contrast associated with CT, MR may plan a useful role in the diagnosis of patients with acute aortic dissection. Investigators have demonstrated the value of rapid MRI using steady-state free precession (SSFP) for detecting the intimal media flap associated with dissection [11, 12]. Using SSFP, it is possible to perform the diagnostic exam with minimal MRI table time in the acutely ill patient. In addition, contrast-enhanced MRA may be performed quickly and will provide information regarding branch vessel involvement, the presence of intraluminal abnormalities, PAU, and for demonstrating the intimomedial flap location and the entry and exit tears in dissection. We have successfully performed a rapid MR evaluation of the thoracic aorta and great vessels in the acutely ill patient presenting with chest pain in less than 15-minute room time using a rapid MR evaluation protocol in patients presenting to the emergency room [13]. Nevertheless, it should be emphasized the CTA remains the mainstay for evaluating patients with suspected acute aortic syndrome also in part related to the ease of evaluation of the entire thoracic and abdominal aorta.

18.10 MRI Technique and Imaging Findings

Evaluation of thoracic pathology with MRI begins with rapid SSFP imaging of the aorta and its major branches (Table 18.1). This technique, when high-performance gradients are used to acquire images using a short repetition time (TR) and short echo time (TE), is especially helpful for imaging aortic vascular pathology in the absence of gadolinium contrast media. These images are typically acquired initially in axial and oblique sagittal projections and gated to the diastolic phase of the cardiac waveform. In addition, for more complete characterization of intimal flap motion in the setting of aortic dissection, cine SSFP MRI can be used to further delineate the entry and exit zones of the intimal media

Table 18.1 MRI techniques for diagnosis and monitoring AAS

Sequence	Plane	TR/TE (MS)	Matrix	Accel factor	Gating	+Gd
MRI in the acute setting						
SSFP	2D axial/SAG	3/1.5	256 × 192	1–2	Yes	No
High-res CE MRA	3D SAG	3/1	320 × 256 × 128	4	No	0.1 mmol/ kg
Spin echo for characterization of IMH						
T_1 fast spin echo	2D axial	~600/10	256 × 192	n/a	No	No
T_2 fast spin echo	2D axial	~2500/60	256 × 192	n/a	No	No
For characterization of flow abnormalities in complicated subacute or chronic dissection						
4D flow phase contrast	3D SAG	10/4	256 × 128 × 64	6–10	Yes	Yes

flap, as well as potential dynamic compression of branch vessels. Likewise, cine MRI can be used to further characterize the relationship of a type A dissection flap to the aortic valve and any resultant aortic valve insufficiency.

Gadolinium contrast-enhanced MRA is used to characterize the luminal pathology associated with acute aortic syndrome [14]. Contrast-enhanced MRA is usually acquired during the arterial phase of contrast as well as during the delayed "steady-state" phase of contrast enhancement. Some authors describe the use of time-resolved 3D MRA during a small bolus of GBCA first, thus allowing the radiologist to delineate filling pathways of the true and false lumen and branch vessels dynamically [15]. However, time-resolved images are typically followed by high-resolution 3D images for more precise characterization of the anatomy.

Extracellular Gd contrast agents are the primary diagnostic enhancement agents, and higher relaxivity contrast agents are preferred due to their greater signal at a lower dose as well as their protein binding, which facilitates delayed imaging in the steady state. For delayed imaging, we typically use a fat-suppressed post-contrast T1-weighted gradient echo image with spoiling of the transverse magnetization. The delayed images are particularly helpful for evaluation of extra luminal pathology affecting the aorta, including aortic leaks, arteritis, and infection, and characterizing the size and extent of hematoma outside of the wall.

The arterial phase contrast-enhanced MRA findings in classic aortic dissection are similar to those identified on CT, including displaced intimal flap, thrombosed lumen, and demonstration of entry and exit tears [12]. One key finding on CT that is not reliable on MR is the displaced intimal calcifications associated with a displaced intimal flap. Contrast-enhanced MRA demonstrates filling patterns in aortic dissection and is helpful in delineating branch vessel involvement and assessing end-organ perfusion.

The exquisite soft tissue contrast in delayed contrast-enhanced MR images may be helpful for delineating penetrating aortic ulceration. The immediate arterial phase images on contrast-enhanced MR may show the size and extent of ulceration; however the delayed images add enhanced visualization of the aortic adventitia and surrounding soft tissues, thus allowing more definitive characterization of the aortic enlargement and associated structures in penetrating aortic ulceration (Fig. 18.4).

In the setting of suspected intramural hematoma, SSFP MRI or contrast-enhanced MRA alone is inadequate for detecting hemorrhage in the wall of the aorta. In this clinical scenario, T1- and T2-weighted spin-echo technique is typically necessary for diagnosis. MRI using fast spin-echo technique is useful for detecting IMH and characterizing its age or confirming and dating suspected IMH identified on an unenhanced CT scan. IMH exhibits the expected signal characteristics associated with the transition of hemorrhage from deoxyhemoglobin (low T1 and T2) in the hyperacute stage to intracellular methemoglobin (high T1, intermediate T2) in the subacute stage and extracellular methemoglobin (high T1 and T2) in the late stage of IMH (Fig. 18.5).

Finally, phase contrast MR may be helpful for delineating entry and exit zone sites in classic aortic dissection, as well as for documenting flow patterns in the true and false lumen. In addition, in the setting of suspected branch vessel ischemia, phase contrast MR may demonstrate and quantify the abnormal aortic and branch vessel flow associated with dissection. Future work may allow the use of computational fluid dynamics to predict the likelihood of vascular rupture in patients with aortic aneurysm or dissection; however additional validation of the predictive power of these techniques is necessary.

18.11 Summary

High-resolution CT and MR imaging have fundamentally changed the diagnosis and treatment of acute aortic syndrome in the modern era. Multi-detector CTA has streamlined the early diagnosis and management of these patients and has allowed us to rethink the classification of the syndrome as a manifestation of specific pathologies involving the aortic wall. Recent improvements in understanding of this entity contribute to the improved survival with broader

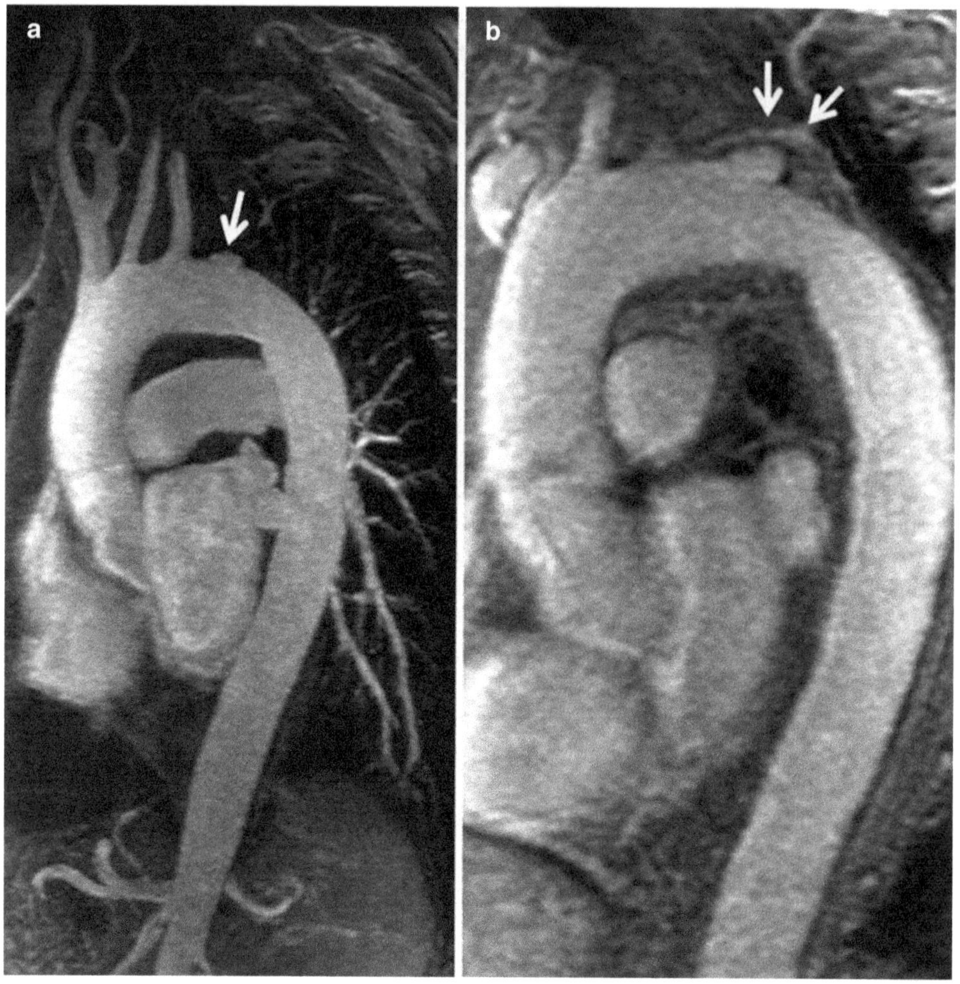

Fig. 18.4 Penetrating aortic ulcer. (**a**) Early arterial-phase and (**b**) delayed "steady-state" phase MRA demonstrating penetrating aortic ulceration involving the superior surface of the aortic arch. Note the excellent delineation of the aortic adventitia on the delayed images due to the contrast enhancement that occurs in the steady-state imaging phase

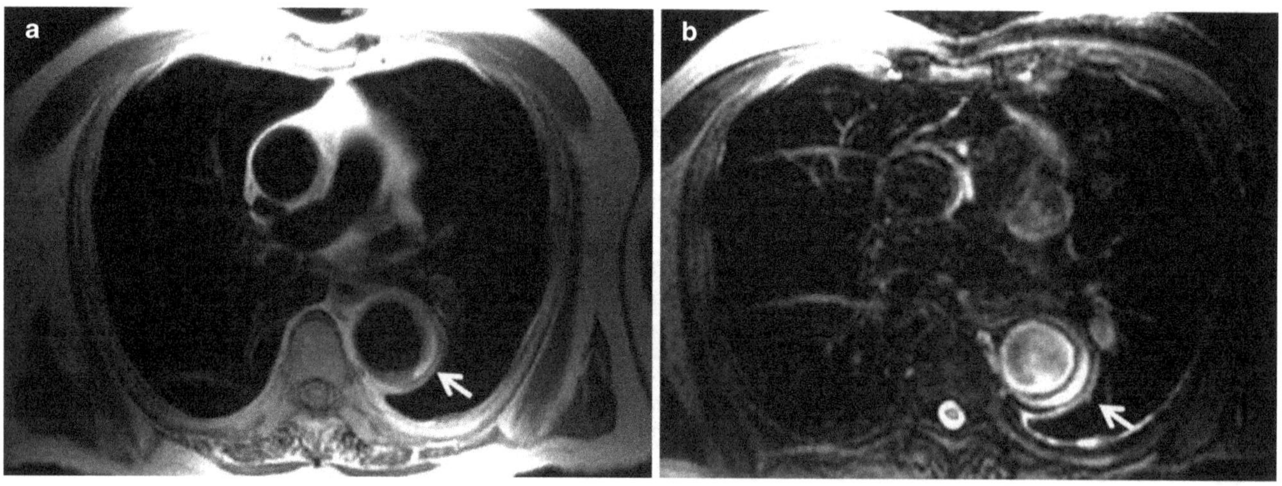

Fig. 18.5 (**a**) T1-weighted MRI demonstrating IMH with mixed signal intensity components including low signal intensity corresponding to deoxyhemoglobin and high signal intensity extracellular methemoglobin suggesting an IMH of subacute or chronic duration. (**b**) T2-weighted image demonstrating high signal intensity associated with extracellular methemoglobin due to chronic IMH

treatment options for patients who are correctly diagnosed, including significant advances in endovascular therapy for complicated type B dissections over the last decade. The role of MRI in patients with aortic disease is more limited to the diagnosis and management of complications, follow-up studies, and in the initial diagnosis in patients who cannot undergo CTA. The accurate detection and evaluation of acute aortic syndrome is one of the radiologist's most immediately impactful opportunities to reduce morbidity and mortality associated with this spectrum of diseases.

Key Points

- A new classification scheme has been proposed based upon the primary location of the lesion within the aortic wall: aortic dissection principally involves the aortic media, penetrating aortic ulcer originates within the aortic intima, and aortic aneurysm is a disease of all three layers.
- The presence of intramural hematoma is an observation or epiphenomenon to be applied to any of these three fundamental pathologies.
- An unenhanced CT scan is important to perform prior to the administration of intravenous contrast for the detection of what can be subtle intramural and periaortic blood and for characterizing the post-operative aorta.
- MRI is useful for specific problem-solving, post-dissection surveillance, and hemodynamic assessment in patients with mal-perfusion syndromes.

Take-Home Messages

- Radiologists can save lives by accurate and immediate diagnosis of acute aortic syndromes.
- Unenhanced and contrast-enhanced CTA is the quickest, most available, and accurate method to determine the pathological cause of acute aortic syndrome.
- An understanding of the pathological origin of aortic disease is important to accurate description of the key imaging findings identified in the setting of acute aortic syndrome.

References

1. Rubin GD, Leipsic J, Joseph Schoepf U, Fleischmann D, Napel S. CT angiography after 20 years: a transformation in cardiovascular disease characterization continues to advance. Radiology. 2014;271(3):633–52.
2. Arafat A, Roselli EE, Idrees JJ, et al. Stent grafting acute aortic dissection: comparison of DeBakey extent IIIA versus IIIB. Ann Thorac Surg. 2016;102(5):1473–81.
3. Geisbusch P, Kotelis D, Weber TF, Hyhlik-Durr A, Kauczor HU, Bockler D. Early and midterm results after endovascular stent graft repair of penetrating aortic ulcers. J Vasc Surg. 2008;48(6):1361–8.
4. Hiratzka LF, Bakris GL, Beckman JA, et al. 2010 ACCF/AHA/AATS/ACR/ASA/SCA/SCAI/SIR/STS/SVM guidelines for the diagnosis and management of patients with thoracic aortic disease: a report of the American College of Cardiology Foundation/American Heart Association task force on practice guidelines, American Association for Thoracic Surgery, American College of Radiology, American Stroke Association, Society of Cardiovascular Anesthesiologists, Society for Cardiovascular Angiography and Interventions, Society of Interventional Radiology, Society of Thoracic Surgeons, and Society for Vascular Medicine. Circulation. 2010;121(13):e266–369.
5. Ganaha F, Miller DC, Sugimoto K, et al. Prognosis of aortic intramural hematoma with and without penetrating atherosclerotic ulcer: a clinical and radiological analysis. Circulation. 2002;106(3):342–8.
6. Evangelista A, Mukherjee D, Mehta RH, et al. Acute intramural hematoma of the aorta: a mystery in evolution. Circulation. 2005;111(8):1063–70.
7. Fleischmann D, Mitchell RS, Miller DC. Acute aortic syndromes: new insights from electrocardiographically gated computed tomography. Semin Thorac Cardiovasc Surg. 2008;20(4):340–7.
8. Chin AS, Willemink MJ, Kino A, et al. Acute limited intimal tears of the thoracic aorta. J Am Coll Cardiol. 2018;71(24):2773–85.
9. Sailer AM, van Kuijk SMJ, Nelemans PJ, et al. CT imaging features in acute uncomplicated stanford type-B aortic dissection predict late adverse events. Circ Cardiovasc Imaging. 2017;10(4):e005709.
10. Sailer AM, Nelemans PJ, Hastie TJ, et al. Prognostic significance of early aortic remodeling in acute uncomplicated type B aortic dissection and intramural hematoma. J Thorac Cardiovasc Surg. 2017;154(4):1192–200.
11. Pereles FS, McCarthy RM, Baskaran V, et al. Thoracic aortic dissection and aneurysm: evaluation with nonenhanced true FISP MR angiography in less than 4 minutes. Radiology. 2002;223(1):270–4.
12. Gebker R, Gomaa O, Schnackenburg B, Rebakowski J, Fleck E, Nagel E. Comparison of different MRI techniques for the assessment of thoracic aortic pathology: 3D contrast enhanced MR angiography, turbo spin echo and balanced steady state free precession. Int J Cardiovasc Imaging. 2007;23(6):747–56.
13. Schiebler ML, Nagle SK, Francois CJ, et al. Effectiveness of MR angiography for the primary diagnosis of acute pulmonary embolism: clinical outcomes at 3 months and 1 year. J Magn Res Imaging. 2013;38(4):914–25.
14. Prince MR, Narasimham DL, Jacoby WT, et al. Three-dimensional gadolinium-enhanced MR angiography of the thoracic aorta. AJR Am J Roentgenol. 1996;166(6):1387–97.
15. Finn JP, Baskaran V, Carr JC, et al. Thorax: low-dose contrast-enhanced three-dimensional MR angiography with subsecond temporal resolution - initial results. Radiology. 2002;224(3):896–904.

19

Pre- and Post-aortic Endovascular Interventions: What a Radiologist Needs to Know?

Thorsten Bley and Justus Roos

Learning Objectives
- To discuss elements of vascular anatomy pertinent to endovascular aneurysm repair of the thoracic and abdominal aorta
- To understand common complications of post-endovascular stent-graft placement

19.1 Introduction

Aortic aneurysmal disease of the thoracic and abdominal aorta is a potentially life-threatening disease and requires besides preventive measures early detection of the disease and if present for the patient-tailored interventional treatment. Per definition, an abdominal aortic aneurysm is present if the abdominal aorta exceeds 1.5 times the normal diameter of 2.5–3 cm [1]. Many AAA remain asymptomatic and are found incidentally on routine imaging. Among a variable number of risk factors, such as arterial hypertension, inherited diseases, connective tissue diseases, and age, smoking appears to be the most important risk factor. Since rupture of an AAA is related with a very high mortality, repair is recommended with a size exceeding more than 5.0–5.5 cm, if a patient turns symptomatic or an interval annual growth rate of >1 cm is detected [2]. Endovascular aneurysmal repair (EVAR) surpassed the method of open surgical repair since approximately a decade and became the method of choice to treat AAA [3]. Newest generations of EVAR devices allow to exclude the vast majority of AAA, despite their sometimes challenging anatomical morphology. Pre-procedural imaging is pivotal and important for EVAR to adequately assess the aneurysm size and anatomical configuration and with this to choose an adequate device and access site [4]. Post-procedural complications are relatively frequent (e.g., endoleaks) and demand regular post-EVAR surveillance [5]. Different imaging modalities, such as conventional radiography (CR), ultrasound (US), magnetic resonance angiography (MRA), and computed tomography angiography (CTA), play a role in pre- and post-procedural EVAR assessment with their relative strengths and weaknesses. In this article we focus on CTA as being the workhorse imaging modality used in the vast majority of institutions due to its high accuracy for pre- and post-procedural imaging [6].

Key Point
- An abdominal aortic aneurysm is present if the abdominal aorta exceeds 1.5 times the normal diameter of 2.5–3 cm. CT angiography is considered the workhorse imaging modality used in the vast majority of institutions due to its high accuracy for pre- and post-procedural imaging.

EVAR devices are basically bifurcated metallic stents with a mounted layer of nonporous graft material. Their modular design normally includes one aortoiliac limb with an ipsilateral long component and a contralateral short limb that is secondly joined with a uniiliac component [4]. Different design variants are available to help to circumvent anatomical challenges. In general, EVAR endografts are placed with attention to the proximal and distal landing zones, where proper sealing of the device to the native aorta is crucial to exclude blood flow into the aneurysmal sac, thereby resulting in lowered sac pressures and decreased risk of further expansion. In case of incomplete exclusion of

T. Bley (✉)
Institut für Diagnostische und Interventionelle Radiologie, Universitätsklinikum Würzburg, Würzburg, Deutschland
e-mail: bley_t@ukw.de

J. Roos
Radiologie und Nuklearmedizin, Institut für Radiologie und Nuklearmedizin, Luzerner Kantonsspital, Luzern, Switzerland
e-mail: justus.roos@luks.ch

the blood flow influx into the aneurysmal sac, the AAA remains pressurized. Different sources, so-called endoleaks, are causative for a persistent blood flow into the aneurysmal sac [7, 8].

Similar to the EVAR procedure, several pathologies of the thoracic aorta and the aortic arch such as thoracic aortic aneurysm (TAA), penetrating aortic ulcer (PAU), intramural hemorrhage (IMH), traumatic aortic rupture, and aortic dissection (AD) can be treated with the so-called thoracic endovascular aortic repair (TEVAR) [9]. Technical success of TEVAR reaches <90% in studies with substantially lower rates of neurologic complications and mortality as compared to open surgery [10–13]. No sternotomy or thoracotomy is necessary for the TEVAR procedure. TEVAR devices may consist of a short section of bare metal stent for better conformity and alignment in the aortic arch in order to reduce the risk of endoleak [14].

Key Point

- Indications for endovascular aneurysmal repair of the abdominal aorta (EVAR) or the thoracic aorta (TEVAR) include besides aneurysmal disease, penetrating aortic ulcer (PAU), intramural hemorrhage (IMH), and (non-)traumatic aortic rupture or aortic dissection (AD).

19.2 Pre-procedural Imaging

Figure 19.1 summarizes a number of anatomic and morphologic parameters every pre-procedural CTA report needs to address, in order to reliably select the right EVAR device, to anticipate procedural challenges, and to plan for ancillary

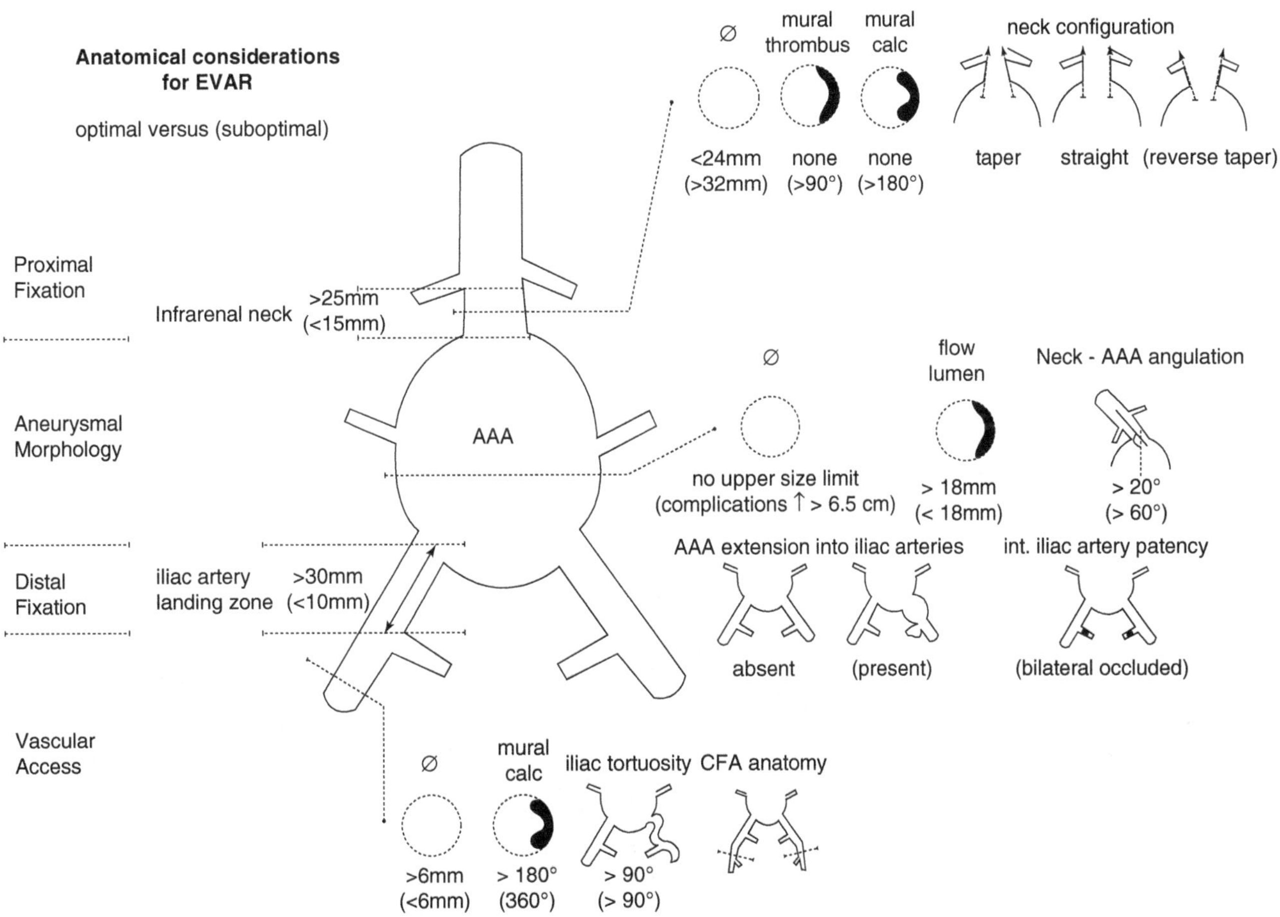

Fig. 19.1 Anatomical considerations to be addressed at pre-procedural imaging: Description of the **proximal fixation site** with infrarenal neck length, diameter, and configuration (mural thrombus, mural calcifications, shape). Description of the **aneurysm morphology** (saccular, fusiform), aneurysm size (largest diameter), aneurysm length, aneurysm flow lumen, aorta diameter at the level of the lowest renal artery and aortic bifurcation, and angle between supra-renal aorta and AAA. Description of the **distal fixation site** with the length of the iliac landing zone, iliac artery minimal diameter, iliac tortuosity and mural calcifications, extension of AAA into common iliac artery (CIA) aneurysms, and patency of internal iliac arteries. Description of the **vascular access site** with minimal luminal diameter, tortuosity, mural calcifications, location, and status of common femoral artery CFA (e.g., anterior luminal calcifications). **Note:** Optimal anatomical configurations for EVAR are indicated with letters, whereas suboptimal or unfavorable anatomical parameters are indicated within parentheses

procedures during or after EVAR [15, 16]. In general, four anatomical areas thereby have to be addressed: (a) proximal fixation site, (b) aneurysm morphology, (c) distal fixation site, and (d) access vessel evaluation.

In general, optimal anatomical AAA configuration for EVAR includes an infrarenal aortic neck length of >25 mm; no mural neck thrombus/calcifications; no reverse taper infrarenal neck; lack of AAA tortuosity or angulation; patent non-tortuous, non-stenotic iliac arteries with a distal landing zone of >30 mm; patient internal iliac arteries; and normal common femoral artery non-calcified anatomy.

As with EVAR a suitable landing zone is of utmost importance for the success of the TEVAR procedure. A proximal landing zone of 15–25 mm is desirable [17]. Depending on the anatomic conditions, a sufficient proximal landing zone may need to be generated by supra-aortic debranching surgery, in which, for example, the left subclavian artery is transposed to the brachiocephalic trunk (Fig. 19.2). By doing so the left subclavian ostium can be overstented, and the proximal landing zone will be enlarged. Overstenting the left subclavian artery without prior debranching increases the risk of a type II endoleak, a subclavian steal phenomenon or ischemia of the vertebral artery territory, of the left upper extremity or spinal ischemia. Variants of the supra-aortic arteries must be taken into account when evaluating the proximal landing zone [9].

Thrombotic plaques in the aortic arch increase the risk of embolic stroke since catheter and stent-graft maneuvers in the arch may loosen the plaque [18]. Assessing the plaque burden of the thoracic aorta with focus on mobile atheromas is important to estimate the risk of embolic stroke which is as high in TEVAR as in open surgery with 4–10% [6, 19].

The risk of spinal ischemia with paraplegia due to overstenting the artery of Adamkiewicz feeding intercostal artery, which is of variable location, is lower in TEVAR procedures than open surgery [20]. Extensive coverage of the thoracic aorta by the stent-graft and coverage of the left subclavian artery are recognized risks of spinal ischemia following TEVAR. Occurrence of stroke following TEVAR with left subclavian coverage is almost twice as high as following TEVAR without left subclavian coverage (6.3% vs 3.2%) [21, 22].

Proper alignment of the stent graft to the aortic wall depends on the curvature of the aortic arch and on the conformability of the stent-graft material. In a sharp angulating aortic arch, the forces on the stent graft will hamper proper alignment, and the risk of a type I endoleak increases. Proper and in some cases adaptive radial forces of the stent-graft enable seamless adaption of the stent-graft to the inner and outer curvature of the aortic arch without leaving space for an endoleak and without damaging the aortic wall.

For better adaption to the aortic wall, tapered stent grafts are also available that have a conic architecture and adapt to the aortic wall despite different luminal diameters of the proximal and distal landing zones. Low-profile stent-graft systems enable better handling of the graft and access through smaller or via kinging iliac vessels.

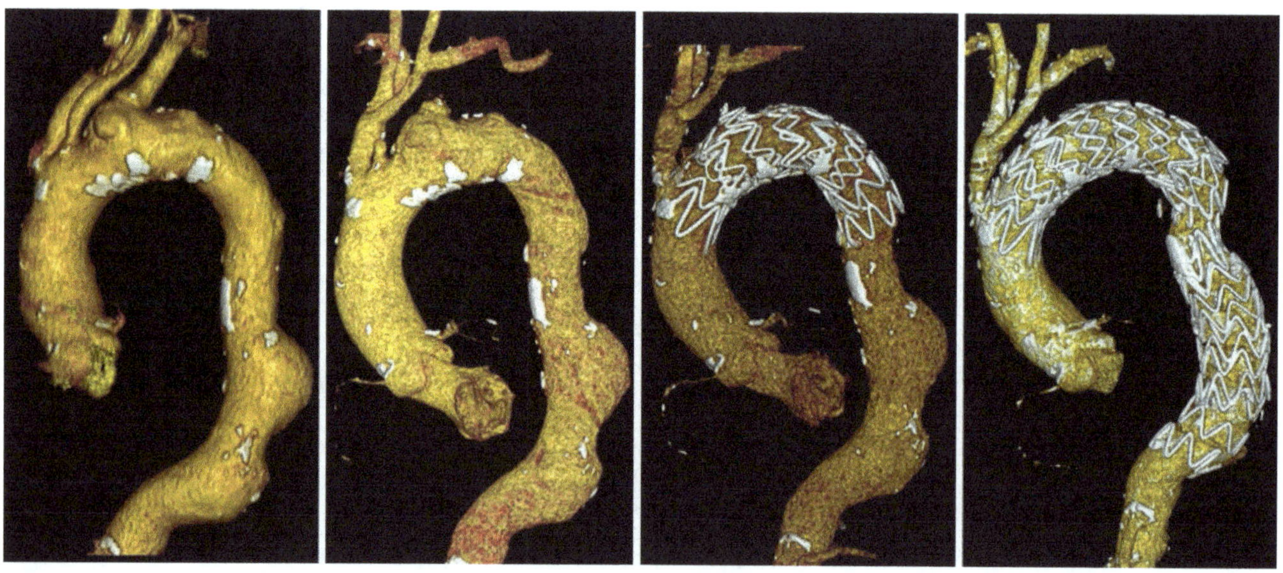

Fig. 19.2 Volume-rendered CT images of a 72-year-old lady with aneurysmal aortic disease readily reveal penetrating aortic ulcer of the aortic arch at the level of the ostium of the left subclavian artery and two sequential aneurysms of the descending thoracic aorta (**a**). Debranching surgery with transposition of the left subclavian and left common carotid artery to the brachiocephalic trunk created a suitable proximal landing zone (**b**) for TEVAR placement (**c**). In the second step, the descending aortic aneurysms were treated with TEVAR extension (**d**)

Key Point

- Every radiology pre-procedural imaging report has to address specific anatomical and morphological parameters allowing to accurately select the right EVAR device, to anticipate procedural challenges, and to plan for ancillary procedures during or after EVAR.

19.3 Post-procedural Imaging

Post-procedural surveillance imaging primarily focuses on early detection of EVAR stent-graft complications and failures. The complications may manifest immediately flowing EVAR, may resolve or persist over time, or appear at a time remote from the procedure itself.

The most common complication is the development of an endoleak following EVAR. With an endoleak, part of the blood flow remains outside the endograft and goes into the native aneurysmal sac. Endoleaks are classified by their source of blood flow and subclassified based on their location (Fig. 19.3). Approximately 25% of patients within 30 days post EVAR develop an endoleak; however, endoleaks can first occur years after EVAR continued surveillance imaging is required. Five types of endoleaks have been classified [7, 8].

Type I endoleak (Fig. 19.4) occurs due to an incomplete endograft seal at the proximal (type Ia) or distal (type Ib) fixation site or due to a leak around an iliac occludes plug in a patient with a aorto-uniiliac device and fem-fem crossover device [23]. With an endoleak type I, CTA detects contrast flow passing outside the fixation seal directly into the aneurysmal sac. Predisposing factors for type I endoleak are suboptimal infrarenal neck configurations (e.g., mural thrombus, reverse taper neck), neck dilatation from EVAR remodeling, complex chimney graft installations, or endograft migration to due insufficient endograft fixation (e.g., endograft fracture). Type I endoleaks are normally treated with reinforcement of the proximal/distal seal with placement of extender cuffs/stents.

Type II endoleak (Fig. 19.4) is the most common type of endoleaks occurring in patients post EVAR [24–26]. The incidence to develop an endoleak type II is approx. 25% per year [27]. They are fed by one (type IIa) or multiple (type IIb) collateral arterial pathways, such as lumbar arteries or inferior mesenteric artery (IMA). With an endoleak type II, CTA detects contrast flow within the aneurysmal sac, which can be traced back to an offending feeding/draining native vessel. Since approx. 40% of type II endoleaks spontaneously occlude and are often not associated with aneurysm sac enlargement in the first year, they do not require prompt treatment and are rather observed. In contrast, type II endoleaks occurring later than 1 year require often treatment since they are associated with aneurysm enlargement. Interventional vascular radiology offers various methods to halt blood flow of the type II feeder vessels.

Type III endoleak (Fig. 19.5) is rare and related to structural failure of the device. Endograft factures have been described in earlier generations of devices. Disconnection between the aortic body component and the uniiliac contralateral limb is the most common cause of a type III endoleak [28]. CTA may detect the endograft fracture site resulting into a direct contrast influx in the aneurysm sac [5, 29]. Treatment occurs normally promptly by placing an extender

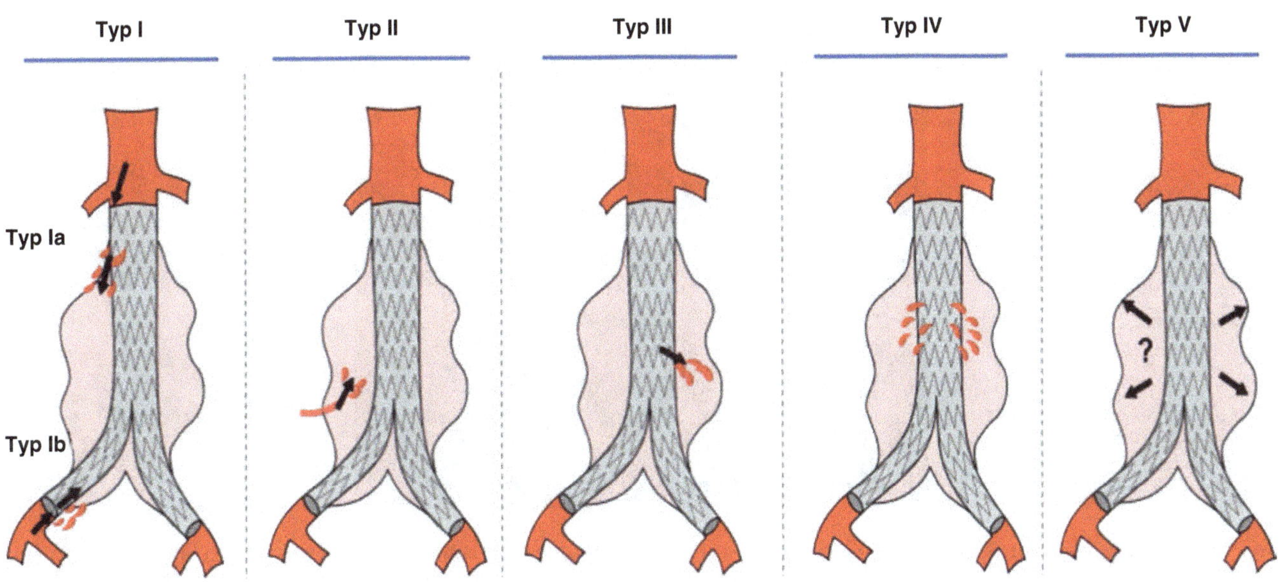

Fig. 19.3 Schematic drawing of the five types of endoleaks after aortic stent-graft placement

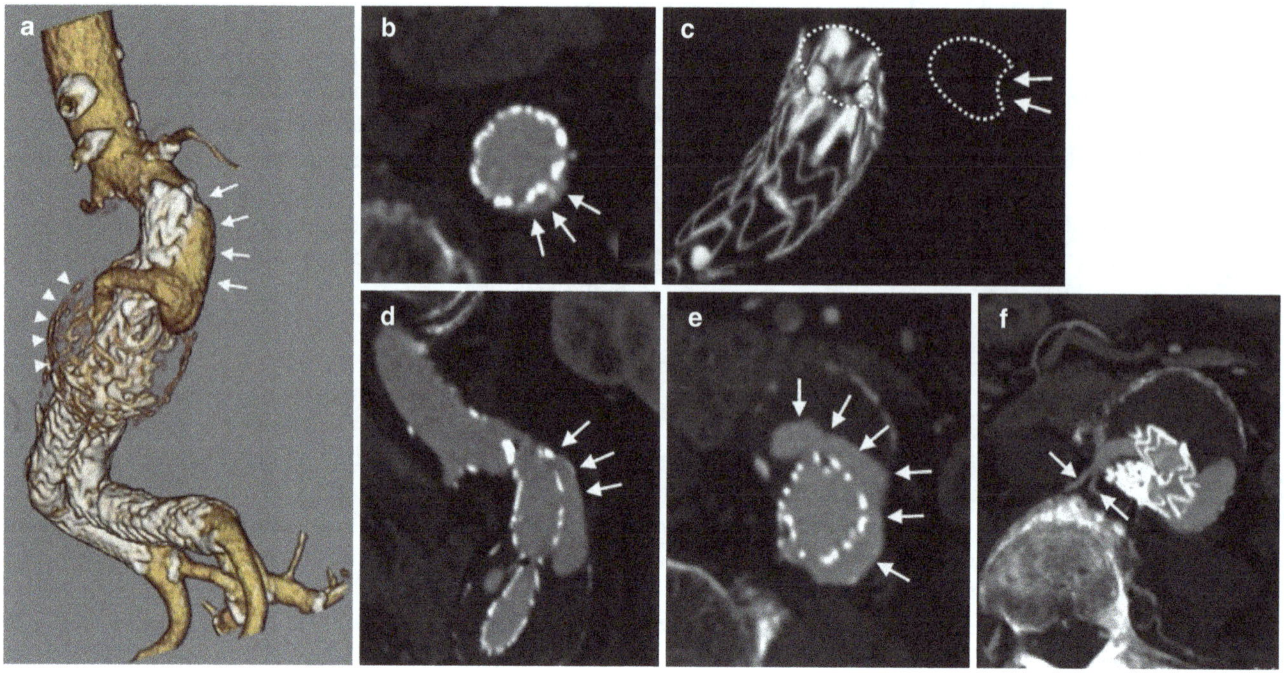

Fig. 19.4 Demonstration of type Ia and IIa endoleak in a patient 30 days post EVAR. (**a**) Volume-rendered image demonstrates contrast leaking along the proximal endograft fixation site (arrows) tracking into the aneurysm sac (aneurysm wall calcifications indicated by arrowheads). (**b**) Axial image at the uppermost proximal end of the endograft depicts contrast flowing outside the endograft lumen due to incomplete seal of the endograft device within the infrarenal neck. (**c**) Volume-rendered image visualizes deformed stent-struts forming a channel for contrast and blood causing a type Ia endoleak (arrows). (**d**) Coronal reformatted image reveals the contrast column flowing outside and (**e**) around the endograft device within the aneurysm sac. (**f**) Axial thin slab MIP image demonstrates the communication of the type I endoleak with a type II endoleak fed by lumbar arteries

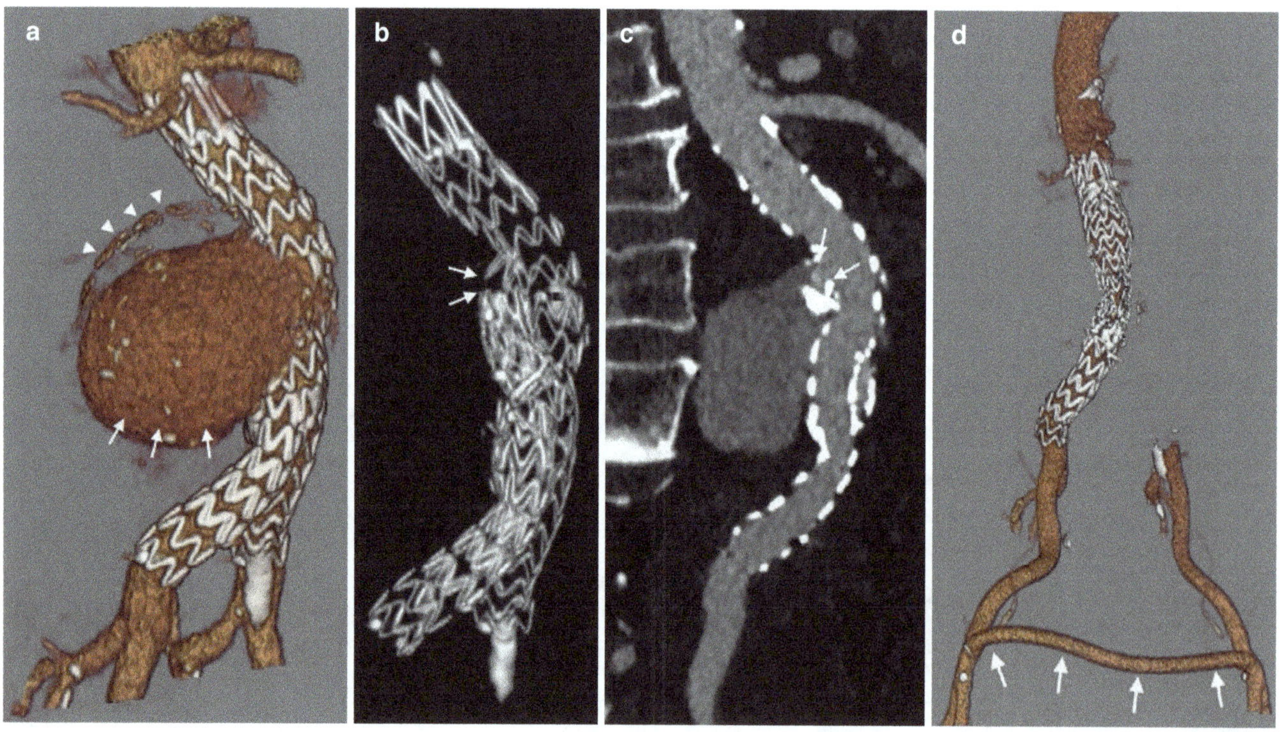

Fig. 19.5 Demonstration of type III endoleak in the first post-EVAR control. (**a**) Volume-rendered image demonstrates contrast leaking into the aneurysm sac (aneurysm wall calcifications indicated by arrowheads) at approx. Mid level of the endograft device. (**b**) Corresponding volume-rendered image reveals a stent-graft fracture at the proximal limb of the left uniiliac endograft limb (arrows). (**c**) Curved planar reformatted image shows active contrast extravasation at the level of the structural failure (arrows) flowing into the aneurysmal sac. (**d**) Volume-rendered image demonstrates result of immediate repair with placement of aorto-uniiliac endograft to seal the leak. Contralateral endograft limb is occluded; femoro-femoral bypass (arrows) provides blood flow to the pelvis and leg

cuffs/stents. Since type III endoleaks may easily occur several years post EVAR, continuous surveillance is of paramount importance.

Type IV endoleak has never been seen with newer-generation devices. It is related to a transient graft fabric porosity, where contrast penetrating the fabric component can be seen as a blush with intra-arterial contrast injection. Type IV endoleak is typically of no clinical significance and rarely to never seen with CTA [30].

Type V endoleak, also called endotension, represents the group of growing aneurysms without any identifiable endoleak [31]. Endotension theories include systemic pressure transmittance across the graft to the aneurysm sac, present but not detectable type I–IV endoleaks, slow-grade infection, and difference in osmotic pressures among compartments [32]. Type V endoleaks normally occur later after EVAR, and surgical repair becomes necessary if aneurysm size becomes critical.

Other complications post EVAR include early complications at the vascular access site (thrombosis, dissection, pseudoaneurysm or AV fistula formation, infection), embolic mesenteric or renal disease related to migrated thrombotic material from the aneurysm sac, renal insufficiency, and endograft infection [33]. Endograft migration may occur several years after stent-graft placement (Fig. 19.6) [34].

Lifelong surveillance and meticulous attention to any possible endograft dysfunction are the goals to prevent the catastrophic event of a delayed rupture of EVAR. Mehta et al.

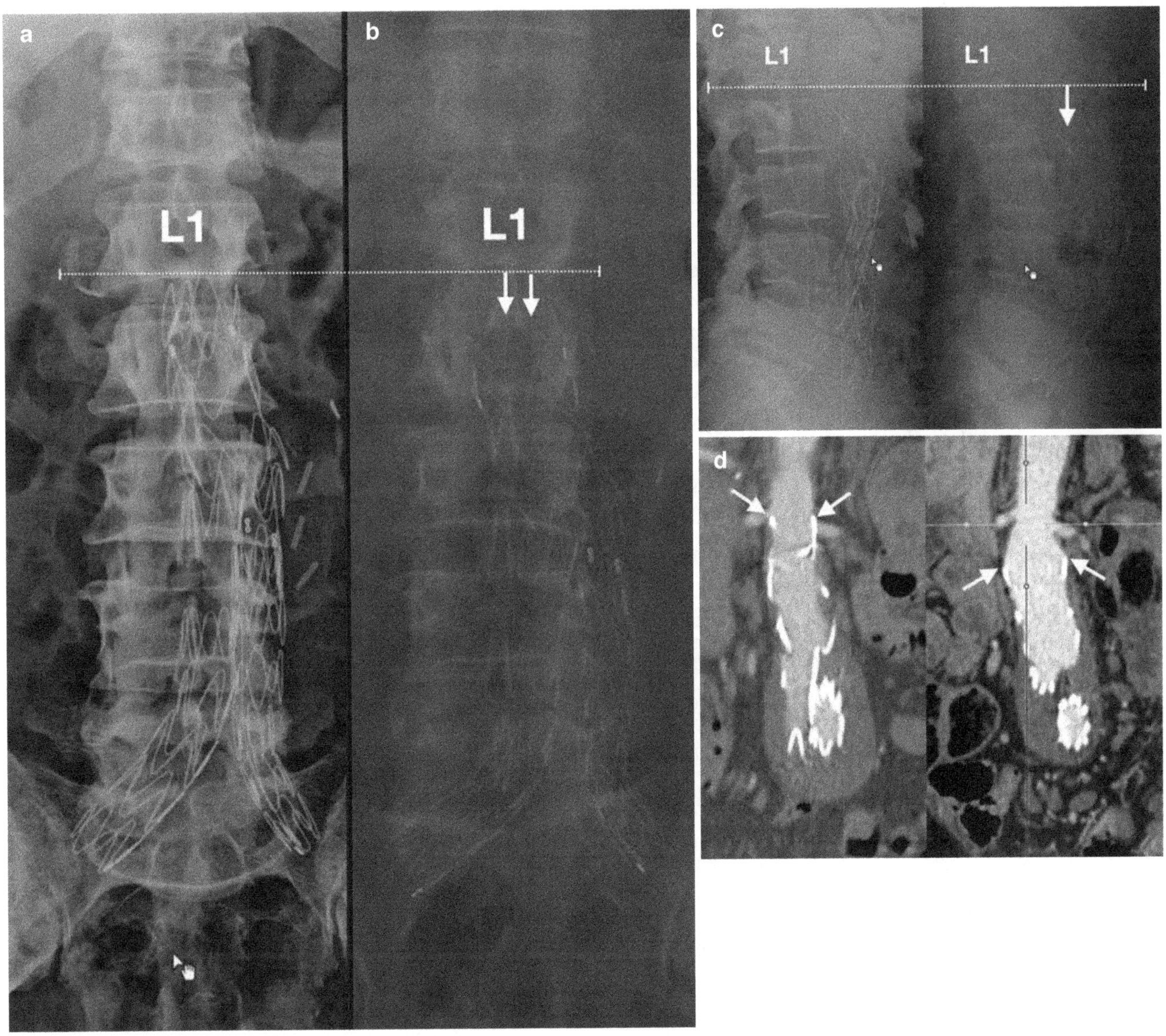

Fig. 19.6 Demonstration of slow endograft migration over a period of 6 years. (**a**) Abdominal ap plain film immediately post EVAR demonstrates endograft device in appropriate location with the proximal device end at the level of L1 lumbar inferior endplate. (**b**) Abdominal ap plain film demonstrates gradually inferior migration (arrows) of the endograft device. (**c**) Corresponding lateral views demonstrate significant inferior migration (arrow) of the endograft device. (**d**) Coronal multiplanar reformatted images confirm inferior migration of the proximal endograft device initially located at the orifice of the renal arteries (arrows)

reported an incidence of delayed rupture after EVAR at 1.5% occurring at mean 29 months. The majority of patients had a type I endoleak (74%), and endograft migration was present in 90% of patients [35]. Important to note is that patients with delayed ruptures may not show increasing aneurysm size on surveillance imaging. In case of rupture, unlike in native AAA rupture, the patients mostly remained hemodynamically stable and were able to undergo imaging. Emergent CTA imaging has to determine the underlying cause of rupture and to guide subsequent open surgical or endovascular repair.

Key Point

- Reliable detection of potential endoleaks, aneurysm sack volume increase, stent-graft migration, infection, and false aneurysm in the access vessel has to be assured for post-interventional surveillance of EVAR.

19.4 Concluding Remarks

CT angiography is the most valuable modality for pre- and post-imaging of aortic endovascular interventions. Assessment of the proximal and distal landing zones with meticulous attention to details of the branching vessels, aortic geometry, atheromatous plaques, and suitable access vessels are of utmost importance in the planning scan. Detection of potential endoleaks, aneurysm sack volume increase, stent-graft migration, infection, and false aneurysm in the access vessel are the main focus of post-intervention surveillance.

Take-Home Messages

- Aortic aneurysmal disease of the thoracic and abdominal aorta is a potentially life-threatening disease and requires besides preventive measures early detection of the disease and patient-tailored interventional treatment.
- Endovascular aneurysmal repair (EVAR) surpassed the method of open surgical repair since approximately a decade and became the method of choice to treat thoracic and abdominal aortic aneurysmal disease.
- Pre-procedural imaging reports have to address specific anatomical and morphological parameters in order to accurately select the right EVAR device, to anticipate procedural challenges, and to plan for ancillary procedures during or after intervention.
- In general, four anatomical areas have to be assessed: (a) proximal fixation site, (b) aneurysm morphology, (c) distal fixation site, and (d) access vessel evaluation.
- Post-interventional surveillance is of paramount importance in order to detect potential life-threatening early and late complications, such as stent-graft migration, endoleaks, aneurysm sack volume increase, delayed aortic rupture, or endograft infection.

References

1. Aggarwal S, Qamar A, Sharma V, et al. Abdominal aortic aneurysm: a comprehensive review. Exp Clin Cardiol. 2011;16:11–5.
2. Lederle FA, Johnson GR, Wilson SE, et al. Rupture rate of large abdominal aortic aneurysms in patients refusing or unfit for elective repair. JAMA. 2002;287:2968–72.
3. Ng TT, Mirocha J, Magner D, et al. Variations in the utilization of endovascular aneurysm repair reflect population risk factors and disease prevalence. J Vasc Surg. 2010;51:801–9, 809.e1.
4. Bryce Y, Rogoff P, Romanelli D, et al. Endovascular repair of abdominal aortic aneurysms: vascular anatomy, device selection, procedure, and procedure-specific complications. Radiographics. 2015;35:593–615.
5. Hallett RL, Ullery BW, Fleischmann D. Abdominal aortic aneurysms: pre- and post-procedural imaging. Abdom Radiol (NY). 2018;43:1044–66.
6. Riambau V, Böckler D, Brunkwall J, et al. Editor's choice—Management of Descending Thoracic Aorta Diseases: clinical practice guidelines of the European Society for Vascular Surgery (ESVS). Eur J Vasc Endovasc Surg. 2017;53:4–52.
7. White GH, Yu W, May J. Endoleak–a proposed new terminology to describe incomplete aneurysm exclusion by an endoluminal graft. J Endovasc Surg. 1996;3:124–5.
8. Shah A, Stavropoulos SW. Imaging surveillance following endovascular aneurysm repair. Semin Interv Radiol. 2009;26:10–6.
9. Bean MJ, Johnson PT, Roseborough GS, et al. Thoracic aortic stent-grafts: utility of multidetector CT for pre- and postprocedure evaluation. Radiographics. 2008;28:1835–51.
10. Bavaria JE, Appoo JJ, Makaroun MS, et al. Endovascular stent grafting versus open surgical repair of descending thoracic aortic aneurysms in low-risk patients: a multicenter comparative trial. J Thorac Cardiovasc Surg. 2007;133:369–77.
11. Chan YC, Cheng SW, Ting AC, et al. Supra-aortic hybrid endovascular procedures for complex thoracic aortic disease: single center early to midterm results. J Vasc Surg. 2008;48:571–9.
12. Makaroun MS, Dillavou ED, Wheatley GH, et al. Five-year results of endovascular treatment with the Gore TAG device compared with open repair of thoracic aortic aneurysms. J Vasc Surg. 2008;47:912–8.
13. Matsumura JS, Melissano G, Cambria RP, et al. Five-year results of thoracic endovascular aortic repair with the zenith TX2. J Vasc Surg. 2014;60:1–10.
14. Maeda K, Ohki T, Kanaoka Y. Endovascular treatment of various aortic pathologies: review of the latest data and technologies. Int J Angiol. 2018;27:81–91.

15. Chaikof EL, Fillinger MF, Matsumura JS, et al. Identifying and grading factors that modify the outcome of endovascular aortic aneurysm repair. J Vasc Surg. 2002;35:1061–6.
16. Picel AC, Kansal N. Essentials of endovascular abdominal aortic aneurysm repair imaging: preprocedural assessment. AJR Am J Roentgenol. 2014;203:W347–57.
17. Coady MA, Ikonomidis JS, Cheung AT, et al. Surgical management of descending thoracic aortic disease: open and endovascular approaches: a scientific statement from the American Heart Association. Circulation. 2010;121:2780–804.
18. Feezor RJ, Martin TD, Hess PJ, et al. Risk factors for perioperative stroke during thoracic endovascular aortic repairs (TEVAR). J Endovasc Ther. 2007;14:568–73.
19. Buth J, Harris PL, Hobo R, et al. Neurologic complications associated with endovascular repair of thoracic aortic pathology: incidence and risk factors. A study from the European collaborators on stent/graft techniques for aortic aneurysm repair (EUROSTAR) registry. J Vasc Surg. 2007;46:1103–10.. discussion 1110.
20. Cheng D, Martin J, Shennib H, et al. Endovascular aortic repair versus open surgical repair for descending thoracic aortic disease a systematic review and meta-analysis of comparative studies. J Am Coll Cardiol. 2010;55:986–1001.
21. Hajibandeh S, Antoniou SA, Torella F, et al. Meta-analysis of left subclavian artery coverage with and without revascularization in thoracic endovascular aortic repair. J Endovasc Ther. 2016;23:634–41.
22. Cooper DG, Walsh SR, Sadat U, et al. Neurological complications after left subclavian artery coverage during thoracic endovascular aortic repair: a systematic review and meta-analysis. J Vasc Surg. 2009;49:1594–601.
23. Stavropoulos SW, Clark TW, Carpenter JP, et al. Use of CT angiography to classify endoleaks after endovascular repair of abdominal aortic aneurysms. J Vasc Interv Radiol. 2005;16:663–7.
24. Arko FR, Rubin GD, Johnson BL, et al. Type-II endoleaks following endovascular AAA repair: preoperative predictors and long-term effects. J Endovasc Ther. 2001;8:503–10.
25. van Marrewijk CJ, Fransen G, Laheij RJ, et al. Is a type II endoleak after EVAR a harbinger of risk? Causes and outcome of open conversion and aneurysm rupture during follow-up. Eur J Vasc Endovasc Surg. 2004;27:128–37.
26. Jones JE, Atkins MD, Brewster DC, et al. Persistent type 2 endoleak after endovascular repair of abdominal aortic aneurysm is associated with adverse late outcomes. J Vasc Surg. 2007;46:1–8.
27. Veith FJ, Baum RA, Ohki T, et al. Nature and significance of endoleaks and endotension: summary of opinions expressed at an international conference. J Vasc Surg. 2002;35:1029–35.
28. Maleux G, Poorteman L, Laenen A, et al. Incidence, etiology, and management of type III endoleak after endovascular aortic repair. J Vasc Surg. 2017;66:1056–64.
29. Roos JE, Hellinger JC, Hallet R, et al. Detection of endograft fractures with multidetector row computed tomography. J Vasc Surg. 2005;42:1002–6.
30. Pandey N, Litt HI. Surveillance imaging following endovascular aneurysm repair. Semin Interv Radiol. 2015;32:239–48.
31. Ricotta JJ. Endoleak management and postoperative surveillance following endovascular repair of thoracic aortic aneurysms. J Vasc Surg. 2010;52:91S–9S.
32. Trocciola SM, Dayal R, Chaer RA, et al. The development of endotension is associated with increased transmission of pressure and serous components in porous expanded polytetrafluoroethylene stent-grafts: characterization using a canine model. J Vasc Surg. 2006;43:109–16.
33. Wilt TJ, Lederle FA, Macdonald R, et al. Comparison of endovascular and open surgical repairs for abdominal aortic aneurysm. Evid Rep Technol Assess (Full Rep). 2006:1–113.
34. Sampaio SM, Panneton JM, Mozes G, et al. AneuRx device migration: incidence, risk factors, and consequences. Ann Vasc Surg. 2005;19:178–85.
35. Mehta M, Paty PS, Roddy SP, et al. Treatment options for delayed AAA rupture following endovascular repair. J Vasc Surg. 2011;53:14–20.

20

Noninvasive Angiography of Peripheral Arteries

Tim Leiner and James C. Carr

Learning Objectives

- To describe the most commonly used clinical classification systems for peripheral arterial disease
- To describe the technical principles of both MRA and CTA of peripheral arteries
- To learn about the diagnostic accuracy of both MRA and CTA for detection of peripheral arterial disease
- To name several causes of non-atherosclerotic peripheral arterial disease

Technical advances over the past decade have facilitated fast and robust noninvasive imaging of the peripheral vascular tree in routine clinical practice for the entire spectrum of peripheral arterial disease (PAD). Both magnetic resonance angiography (MRA) and computed tomography angiography (CTA) are highly accurate methods that enable high-fidelity depiction of arterial anatomy, atherosclerotic plaque, and narrowing of the peripheral vasculature from the aorta down to the feet. In addition, due to their ability to depict extra-arterial anatomy of the entire lower extremity, both methods are well suited for the detection of non-atherosclerotic peripheral arterial disease.

Below, we first detail the clinical context and technical background of both MRA and CTA since high-quality peripheral vascular imaging demands careful attention to proper patient positioning and acquisition. We include suggestions for imaging protocols for both modalities. Subsequently, we discuss the most common clinical applications of both MRA and CTA. We conclude with a short discussion of the clinical efficacy of both methods.

20.1 Epidemiology and Different Manifestations of Peripheral Arterial Disease

Peripheral arterial disease refers to conditions affecting blood flow to the lower extremities due to obstruction of some part of the arterial system from the infrarenal aorta or further distally. Total disease prevalence based on objective testing has been evaluated in several epidemiologic studies and is in the range of 3–10%, increasing to 15–20% in persons over 70 years [1].

Although atherosclerosis is the underlying cause in the vast majority of cases, there are many diseases that can cause PAD (see below). It is important to keep in mind that causes of arterial obstruction vary primarily as a function of age. Identification of the underlying cause necessitates careful review of the patients' history, symptoms, risk factors, and other medical conditions. In patients below 45 years of age, one should always consider non-atherosclerotic causes of PAD such as vasculitis, fibromuscular dysplasia, popliteal entrapment, cystic adventitial disease, and other uncommon entities, especially if there are little or no risk factors for atherosclerosis.

Key Point

- Peripheral arterial disease is highly prevalent in older patients. In patients <45 years old, alternative causes should be considered.

T. Leiner (✉)
Department of Radiology, Utrecht University Medical Center, Utrecht, The Netherlands
e-mail: t.leiner@umcutrecht.nl

J. C. Carr
Department of Radiology, Northwestern Memorial Hospital, Chicago, IL, USA
e-mail: jcarr@northwestern.edu

20.2 Clinical Background and Classification Systems

There are various classification systems for PAD. Clinically the primary distinction is between patients with *intermittent claudication* (IC) and patients with the more severe form of PAD, *chronic critical ischemia* (CCI). The former is usually limited to "single-level" disease, i.e., a stenosis or short occlusion in the iliac or femoral arteries. IC is a lifestyle limiting disease, and first-line treatment consists of treatment of risk factors and supervised exercise therapy [1]. There is a relative indication for invasive therapy, and the risk for major complications such as amputations is very low. This is opposed to patients with CCI, who have high-grade stenoses and/or occlusions at multiple levels of the vascular tree. In CCI resting perfusion is inadequate to meet basic metabolic demand, and patients suffer from rest pain and sometimes even tissue loss. Patients with CCI have an absolute indication for invasive treatment to restore adequate perfusion to the tissues subtended by the stenosed or occluded arteries. If perfusion is not restored, major complications such as permanent loss of function and amputation can result.

The simplest and most commonly used system to classify chronic hypoperfusion of the lower extremity is that described by *Fontaine* in 1954, who distinguishes four categories of PAD (Table 20.1). A more elaborate system with six categories is the one described by *Rutherford* (Table 20.2). The distinction between the two systems is primarily based on the addition of objective findings such as Doppler signals, arterial brachial index (ABI), and pulse volume recordings, in addition to anamnestic pain-free walking distance. Rutherford also described a system for classification of acute limb ischemia (Table 20.3). There are various other clinical classification systems, all refinements of the systems by Fontaine and Rutherford. Hardman et al. review these additional PAD classification systems in [2].

Key Point

- The Fontaine and Rutherford classifications are important clinical tools to communicate the severity of peripheral arterial disease.

Table 20.1 The Fontaine classification system for peripheral arterial disease as first described in [28]

Grade	Symptoms
Stage I	Asymptomatic, incomplete blood vessel obstruction
Stage II	Mild claudication pain in the limb
Stage IIA	Claudication at a distance >200 m
Stage IIB	Claudication at a distance <200 m
Stage III	Rest pain, mostly in the feet
Stage IV	Necrosis and/or gangrene of the limb

20.3 Technical Background of Peripheral MRA and Imaging Protocol

Magnetic resonance angiography of the peripheral vascular tree (pMRA) is a highly reliable method to identify arterial stenoses and obstructions, and several meta-analyses reported high sensitivities and specificities for the detection of angiographically proven arterial narrowing [3, 4]. Currently, two methods are used: contrast-enhanced pMRA and non-contrast-enhanced pMRA. Contrast-enhanced techniques are most commonly used although the latter method is potentially more attractive because no injection of contrast agent is needed.

20.3.1 Contrast-Enhanced Techniques

The typical pMRA imaging protocol consists of imaging of three consecutive fields of view (FOV) in rapid succession during infusion of a gadolinium-based contrast agent. Imaging parameters and spatial resolution are optimized for each FOV to balance the required time to complete the acquisition versus

Table 20.2 Rutherford classification for chronic limb ischemia [29, 30]

Grade	Category	Clinical description	Objective criteria
0	0	Asymptomatic—no hemodynamically significant occlusive disease	Normal treadmill or reactive hyperemia test
	1	Mild claudication	Completes treadmill exercise; AP after exercise >50 mmHg but at least 20 mmHg lower than resting value
I	2	Moderate claudication	Between categories 1 and 3
	3	Severe claudication	Cannot complete standard treadmill exercise and AP after exercise <50 mm Hg
II	4	Ischemic rest pain	Resting AP <40 mm Hg, flat or barely pulsatile ankle or metatarsal PVR; TP < 30 mm Hg
III	5	Minor tissue loss—nonhealing ulcer, focal gangrene with diffuse pedal ischemia	Resting AP < 60 mm Hg, ankle or metatarsal PVR flat or barely pulsatile; TP < 40 mm Hg
	6	Major tissue loss—extending above TM level, functional foot no longer salvageable	Same as category 5

Table 20.3 Rutherford classification for acute limb ischemia

Category	Description/prognosis	Findings		Doppler signal	
		Sensory loss	Muscle weakness	Arterial	Venous
I. Viable	Not immediately threatened	None	None	Audible	Audible
II. Threatened					
(a) Marginally	Salvageable if promptly treated	None or minimal (toes)	None	Inaudible	Audible
(b) Immediately	Salvageable with immediate revascularization	More than toes, associated rest pain	Mild or moderate	Inaudible	Audible
III. Irreversible	Major tissue loss or permanent nerve damage inevitable	Profound, anesthetic	Profound, paralysis	Inaudible	Inaudible

the level of detail required to optimize detection of arterial narrowing with high sensitivity and specificity.

The arterial system is imaged with a heavily T_1-weighted sequence during the first arterial passage of the contrast agent. Because the length of the peripheral vascular tree exceeds the FOV of the MRI scanner, it takes three to four acquisitions to depict the abdominal aorta and the lower extremities. In patients with IC a "top-to-bottom" approach whereby the acquisition commences in the abdomen followed by acquisitions of the upper and lower leg stations usually suffices to obtain the necessary information for clinical decision-making. Occasionally, venous enhancement is encountered in the lower leg station that may hamper detection of stenosis in the lower leg arteries. Although this may degrade image quality, it almost never leads to a study that yields insufficient information for clinical management since treatment is primarily focused on the aortoiliac and superficial femoral arteries. In patients with CCI, this is usually supplemented with a dedicated dynamic acquisition with a separate contrast agent injection to depict lower leg arterial anatomy. High-fidelity depiction of the outflow vasculature is essential in patients with CCI because treatment options may involve percutaneous transluminal angioplasty (PTA) or bypass surgery involving lower leg or pedal arteries.

Injection of contrast agent renders the vascular system bright, while signal from the background is suppressed due to the short repetition time (TR). The vascular tree is typically displayed using maximum intensity projections (MIP) to provide a complete overview of the vascular system at a glance. In order to obtain sufficient background suppression to identify small peripheral arteries, it is essential to suppress signal from fat, since this has the lowest T_1 of any tissue in the body. The most commonly used strategy to suppress fat is to use *subtraction*. This approach requires acquisition imaging the peripheral vascular tree without the injection of contrast agent with identical imaging parameters [5]. The acquired images are subtracted from the images with contrast agent with the aim to suppress signal from fat and background tissue (Fig. 20.1a). Advantages of this approach are the high vessel-to-background contrast and the simplicity (i.e., it can be applied on virtually any MRI scanner). Disadvantages are the $\sqrt{2}$ drop in signal to noise and the additional time it takes to acquire the images without contrast agent. Also, the resulting subtracted images may suffer from misregistration artifacts in case of patient motion between the acquisition with and without contrast agent of the same anatomical location. To avoid false-positive diagnosis of stenosis, contrast-enhanced source images always need to be evaluated. A second approach to suppress signal from fat is to combine the acquisition with *Dixon-based water-fat decomposition techniques* [6]. In contrast to subtraction, there is no need to acquire to same anatomy twice. Instead, images are acquired with two instead of one echoes for every TR, which allows to decompose the signal of protons in water and fat in each voxel. Subsequently, images can be reconstructed in which only the water component is shown and the signal from fat is disregarded (Fig. 20.1b).

Key Point
- In MRA the signal of fat is suppressed using either subtraction or Dixon techniques.

20.3.2 Non-contrast-Enhanced Techniques

There has been considerable interest in non-contrast or native MR angiography in recent years. The excellent review by Lim and Koktzoglou [7] will provide the interested reader with a technical overview. An in-depth discussion of the different techniques is beyond the scope of this chapter because of the wide variety of methods offered by different vendors. To date most experience in the peripheral vasculature has been obtained with quiescent interval single-shot magnetic resonance angiography (QISS). QISS angiography is particularly useful for imaging the lower extremities because the technique allows for large anatomical coverage in short imaging times (Fig. 20.2). Also, good results have been obtained versus standard of reference techniques [8].

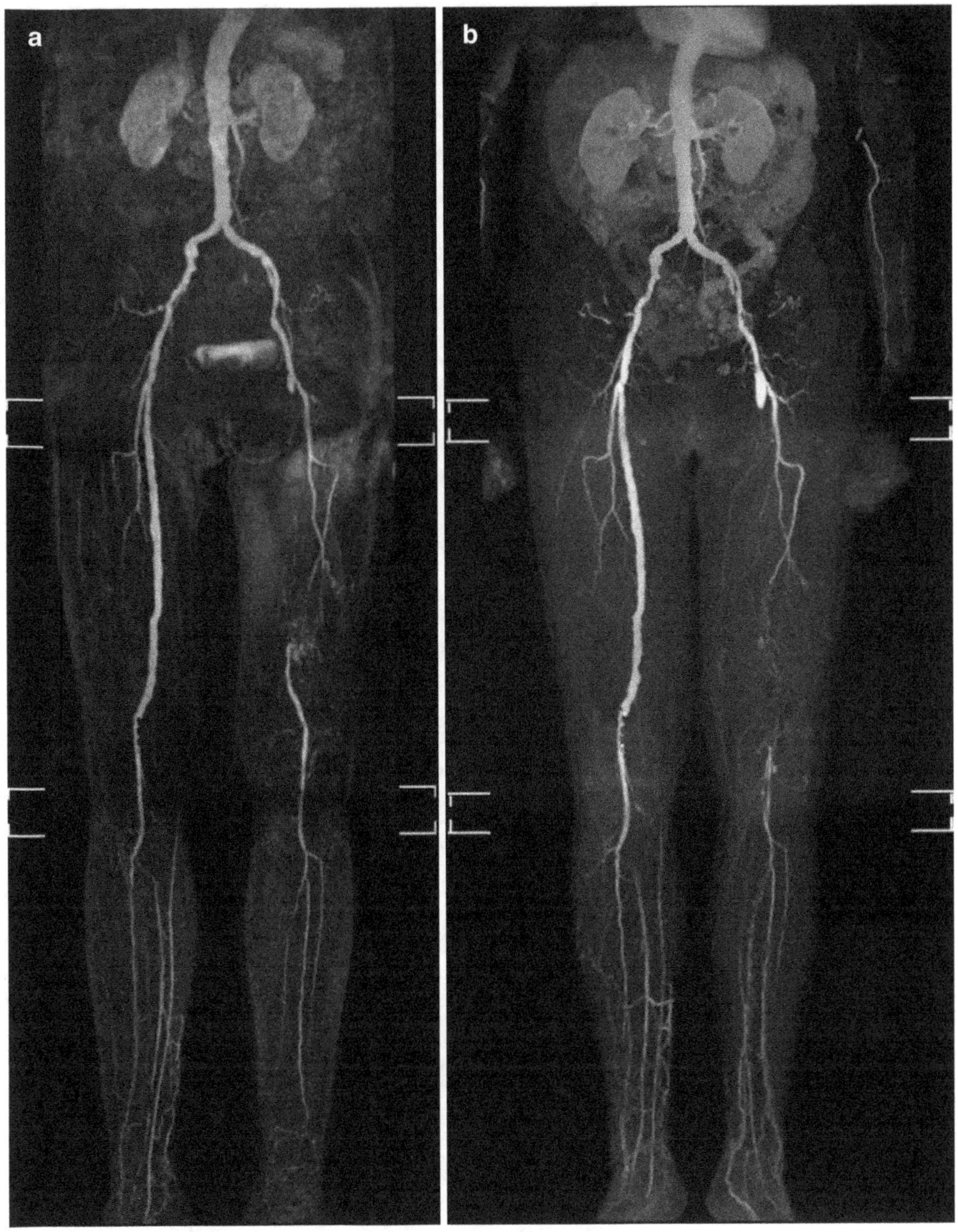

Fig. 20.1 Maximum intensity projection (MIP) of three-station MRA of the peripheral arteries in a 67-year-old female. Image on the left (**a**) is obtained using subtraction. Image on the right (**b**) is obtained using a non-subtracted Dixon technique

> **Key Point**
> - Non-contrast MRA refers to a variety of different MRA techniques.

20.4 Technical Background of Peripheral CTA and Imaging Protocol

Multi-detector CTA (MDCTA) has revolutionized vascular imaging due to its larger volumetric extent of coverage, rapid acquisition speeds, and high spatial resolution. Modern multi-detector CT scanners have tube rotation speeds as low as 0.28 s and slice thickness of 0.33 mm allowing submillimeter isotropic imaging, which is comparable to the gold standard digital subtraction angiography (DSA). Multi-detector CTA produces a larger volume of coverage per gantry rotation permitting rapid acquisitions from the abdomen to the toe in a matter of seconds. One advantage of this, in addition to patient comfort, is the potential for lowering contrast doses; however, contrast timing also becomes more critical with these devices due to higher acquisition speeds.

20.4.1 Technical Aspects

Image quality in CT angiography is dependent on both spatial resolution and temporal resolution. Axial in-plane spatial resolution within the scan plane is increased by smaller field

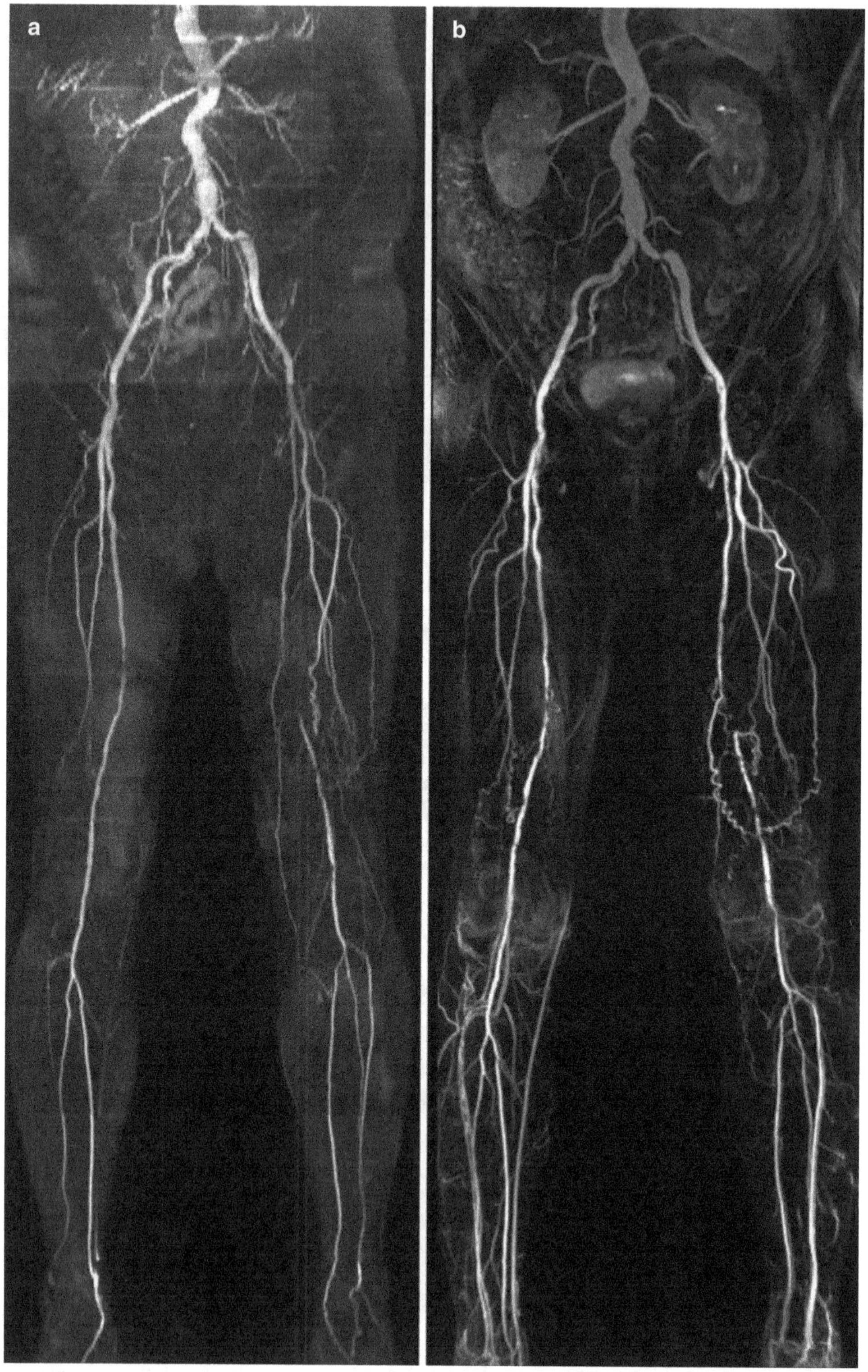

Fig. 20.2 Maximum intensity projection (MIP) images of non-contrast MRA (**a**) and corresponding contrast-enhanced MRA (**b**) in a 66-year-old male with intermittent claudication. The number and severity of arterial stenoses correspond well between the two methods. *Image courtesy of Robert R. Edelman, MD, Department of Radiology, North Shore Hospital, Evanston, IL*

of view, larger matrix size, and smaller focal spot. Through plane z-axis resolution is improved by having a greater number of smaller detectors. High isotropic spatial resolution with modern MDCTA has regular square-shaped voxels of 0.3–0.4 mm or less, allowing full reconstruction of the entire 3D dataset in any arbitrary orientation, making this technique arguably more powerful than DSA [9]. Noise, caused by random fluctuations in radiation exposure, is another important factor affecting image quality in MDCTA, reducing overall image contrast, and can be remedied by increasing tube current/voltage or increasing voxel size. Finally, image contrast which is the difference in intensity between one tissue and another can be improved by lower kVp but is also amplified in MDCTA by use of an iodinated contrast agent.

20.4.2 Scanner Design

Modern CT scanners have a wide array of detectors, with as many as 500–600 in a single row, which absorb the X-ray exposure from the X-ray tube during a single rotation. This allows greater anatomic coverage at high spatial resolution. This is combined with spiral CT mode, where the table and patient are moved steadily through the scanner gantry, as the tube is rotated around the patient. The relationship between patient and gantry motion is referred to as pitch, which is defined as table movement (mm) per tube rotation divided by collimator width (mm). A higher pitch, which is frequently used with CTA of the peripheral arteries, results in lower z-axis resolution but faster coverage and lower radiation exposure. Dual source CT technology consists of two X-ray tubes orientated at right angles to each other and two corresponding sets of detectors. This design improves temporal resolution and overall image quality. Dual-energy CT is when each of the two X-ray tubes on the dual source CT scanner emits X-rays at different energy levels and is detected by the corresponding detector array. The unique absorptive spectra allow discrimination of different tissues. In peripheral CTA, this may have a role in improved characterization of pathology in the vessel wall. Other manufacturers offer alternative scanner designs with rapid kV switching or dual-layer detector technology. Apart from the increased temporal resolution, the improved capability to discriminate tissues is similar.

20.4.3 Radiation Dose

CT is responsible for a significant share of overall radiation dosage to the patient population in medical imaging and MDCTA of the peripheral vasculature, with its extensive anatomic coverage, may result in higher than normal radiation exposure [10]. Radiation dose is dependent on tube current (mAs) and tube voltage (kV). Increasing mAs may improve image quality by increasing contrast to noise and lowering overall noise; however, radiation dose doubles with a doubling of mAs. Lower kV results in lower radiation exposure, but higher kV may be required to attain adequate penetration of the X-ray beam in larger patients. Adaptive scanning, whereby tube current is either reduced or switched off during rotations over sensitive body parts, such as the breast, can result in significant decreases in radiation dose. It has also been shown that peripheral CTA at tube currents as low as low as 50 mAs results in decreased radiation dose without a compromise in diagnostic efficacy [11].

20.4.4 Contrast Administration

With the more rapid acquisition speeds of MDCTA, contrast administration becomes challenging, and timing takes on added importance [12, 13]. High-quality CTA typically necessitates contrast densities of greater than 200 HU in vessels of interest. There are several factors affecting contrast enhancement and time to peak following contrast administration including iodine content [14], injection rate, and patient's cardiac status. In general, higher injection rates will produce a higher peak of enhancement with a tighter bolus; injection rates of 4–5 mL/s are typical with CTA. Similarly, higher iodine content contrast medium will produce a greater enhancement peak, although when adjusted for iodine delivery rate differences are minimized. One disadvantage of modern scanners is that the scanner may "overshoot" the contrast bolus so that for peripheral CTA it may be necessary to slow down the acquisition by slowing the table speed [15].

Accurate contrast timing is typically achieved with either bolus tracking or test bolus techniques. With bolus tracking, scan acquisition is triggered when contrast density reaches a predefined threshold (e.g., 150 HU in abdominal aorta for peripheral CTA), as defined by operator (Fig. 20.3). The test bolus technique involves injecting a small dose of contrast (e.g., 20–30 mL) first to accurately measure the contrast transit time beforehand.

20.4.5 Lower Extremity CTA Technique

A scout view is typically carried out initially. A pre-contrast scan from the upper abdomen to the feet is optional and may be desirable in patients who may have extensive calcifications (e.g., diabetics, dialysis-dependent chronic renal failure) or those with metal in soft tissues (e.g., prior surgery, trauma with metallic foreign body) [16]. Bolus tracking is usually used for contrast timing in CTA of lower extremities. A region of interest (ROI) is placed in the abdominal aorta at the level of the celiac origin, and the scan acquisition is triggered when the density within the vascular lumen reaches more than 150 HU. Contrast agent is injected at 5 mL/s via a large bore (i.e., 18G) intravenous cannula. Images are acquired in a cranial to caudal direction with slice thickness of 1 mm or less and collimator thickness of 0.4–0.6 mm.

Typically, a slower scan time is preferable for lower extremity CTA so as not to overshoot the contrast bolus. Table pitch of 1.1, gantry rotation of 0.37 s, table increment of 21.1 mm/360° rotation, and table speed of 63 mm/s will have a scan time of 23 s; a fast contrast injection is preferred. If there is suspected severe disease with slow flow, then a slower contrast injection bolus and longer scan time may be preferred. This can be achieved by reducing the table speed

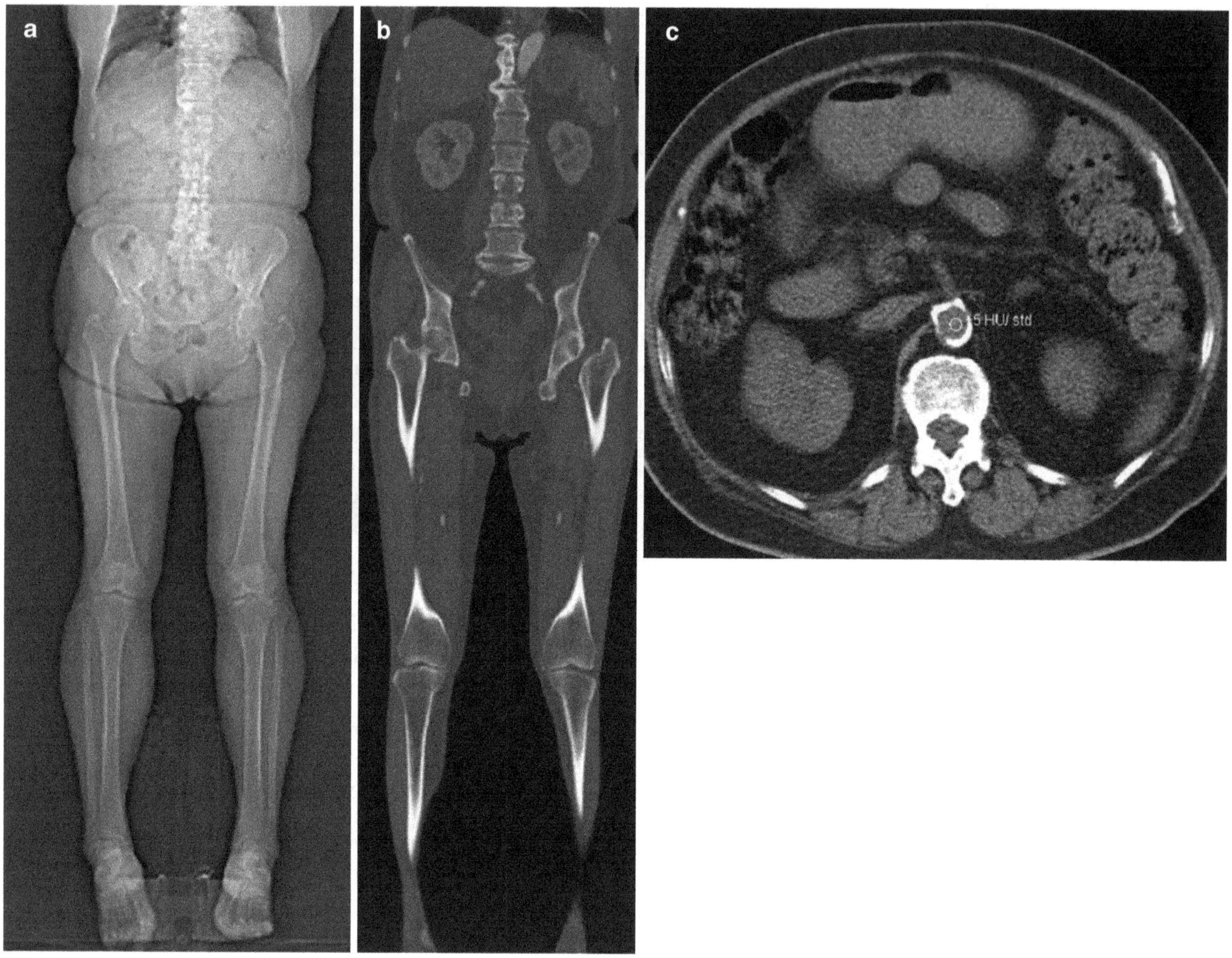

Fig. 20.3 Scout image of the abdomen and lower extremities is used for planning the CT scan (**a**). Source CT images from CTA study of the abdomen, pelvis, and lower extremities following intravenous injection of iodinated contrast (**b**). Bolus tracking technique where region of interest placed in abdominal aorta detects contrast arrival; scan is automatically triggered when density rises above a predefined threshold (**c**)

through the scanner, i.e., the pitch, and by slowing the gantry rotation time.

Dual-energy MDCTA may have advantages at separating calcium from contrast in the vessel lumen. Subtraction of both datasets will produce a contrast only luminal image. Additionally, the calculation of a "virtual" non-contrast dataset will avoid the need for a separate acquisition and may reduce overall radiation exposure. Dual-energy MDCTA has shown high sensitivity for detecting stenosis compared to the gold standard DSA [17].

Dynamic CT, whereby multiphase CT acquisitions are acquired to follow contrast filling and drainage in a time-resolved manner, may have benefits for evaluating the infrapopliteal vessels, particularly in patients with slow or asymmetric flow. Dynamic CTA has been shown to have higher contrast and diagnostic confidence compared to conventional CTA [18]. Limitations of this technique include higher radiation dose and increased volumes of contrast.

Key Point

- In CTA of the peripheral arteries, images are acquired during continuous infusion of contrast agent. Acquisition is initiated by bolus tracking software. The exact CTA protocol for imaging the peripheral arteries depends on the hardware used.

20.4.6 Image Processing

With fully isotropic submillimeter spatial resolution, it is possible to reconstruct the acquired CTA 3D dataset in any anatomic orientation. The 3D data is reconstructed with multiplanar reformatted (MPR), maximum intensity projection (MIP) and volume rendered (VR) algorithms (Fig. 20.4). Basic axial, coronal, and sagittal MPR images are recon-

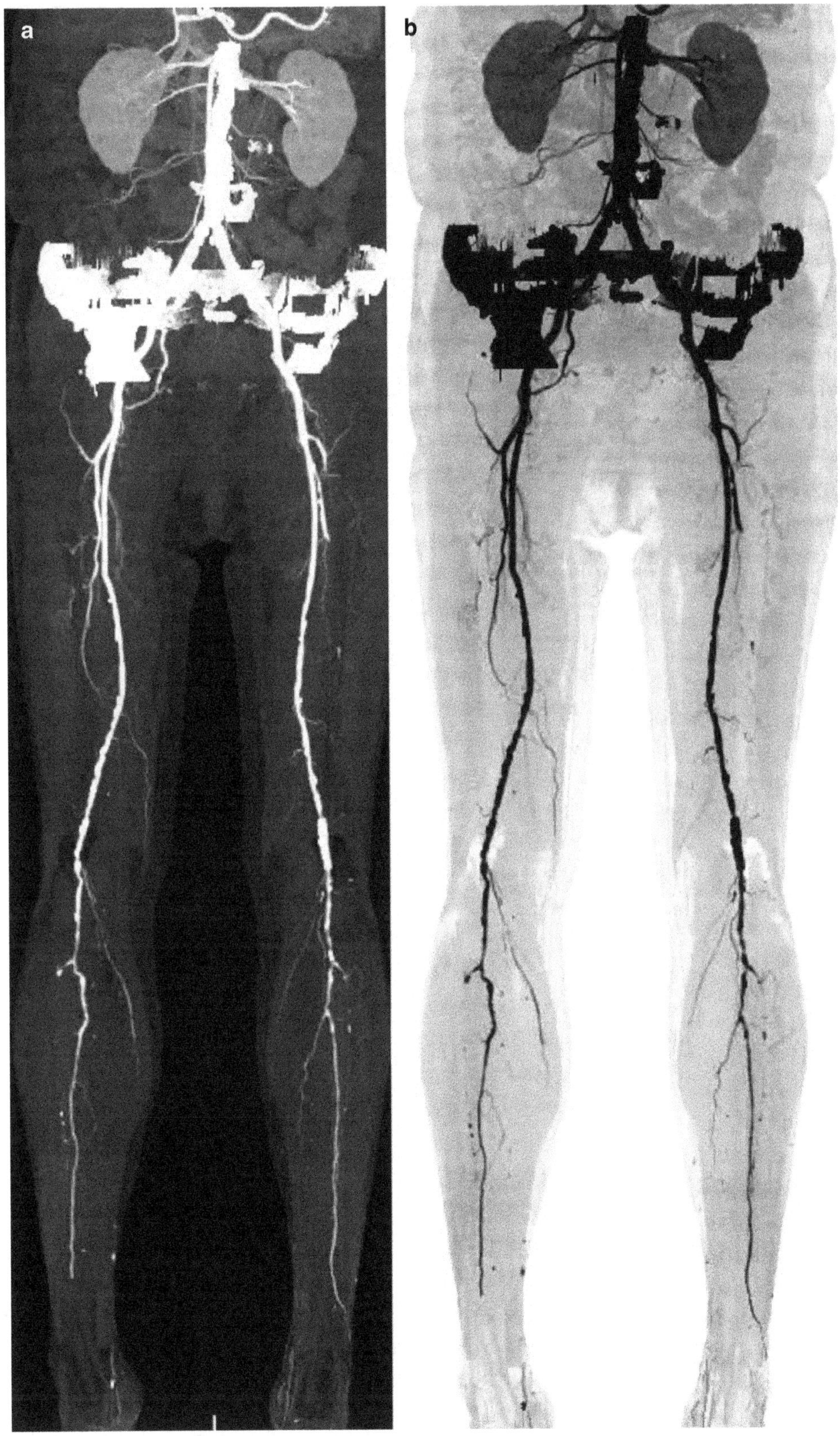

Fig. 20.4 Coronal MIP images with positive (**a**) and negative (**b**) contrast from a patient with significant infra-popliteal peripheral vascular disease. Note incomplete bone removal in the pelvis, which is a limitation of automatic image post processing. In this case bone needed to be manually edited away

structed automatically at the scanner immediately following the CT acquisition. Image data is then transferred to dedicated post-processing software where specific MIP and VR images are created. Curved MPR images of the vessel may be useful to accurately quantify the degree of stenosis and interrogate the vessel wall (Fig. 20.5).

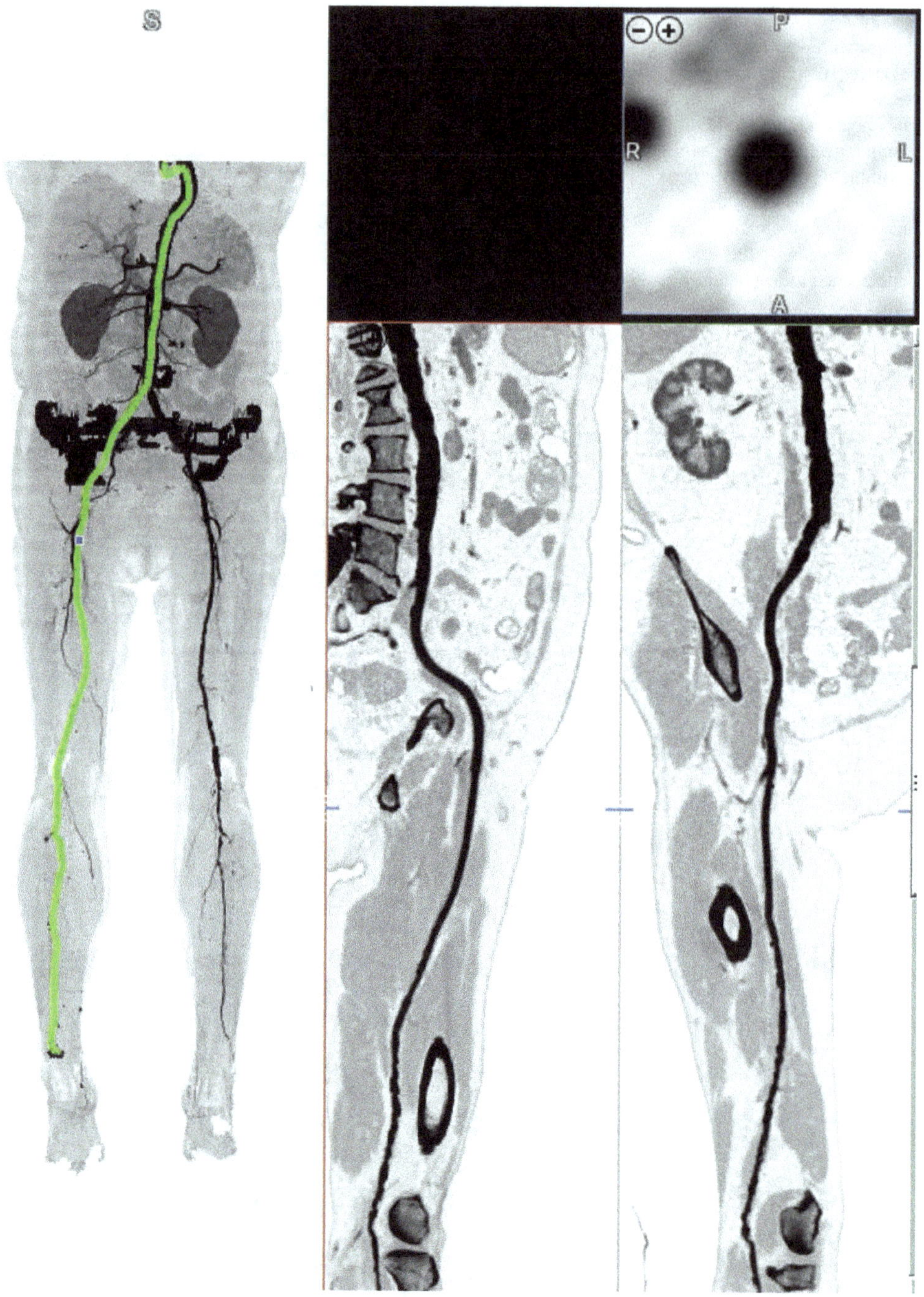

Fig. 20.5 Curved MPR displays the vessel along its entire length and allows accurate measure of stenosis and depiction of vessel wall, if needed

20.4.7 Diagnostic Accuracy

The diagnostic accuracy of CTA for detection and grading of peripheral arterial disease is high and similar to that of MRA. Several meta-analyses have been performed, and all of these report uniformly high values for sensitivity, specificity, and accuracy in patients with intermittent claudication [19–21]. There is a relative lack of data on the diagnostic accuracy of CTA in patients with CCI.

20.5 Clinical Applications

20.5.1 Atherosclerotic Peripheral Arterial Disease

In patients with suspected or known PAD, it is essential to determine and describe the exact location of arterial and extent of arterial lesions. Almost invariably, PAD affects the aorta and iliac and lower extremity arteries. In patients with diabetes mellitus, PAD typically presents with lower leg arterial involvement, while the proximal arteries are relatively spared. Apart from the aortic arch branch vessel origins, the upper extremity is almost never affected. The degree of stenosis is usually described as more or less than 50% luminal narrowing, and occlusions need to be mentioned separately. There is no consensus on how stenosis should be measured (i.e., percentage reduction of luminal diameter or percentage reduction in cross-sectional area); therefore, most observers use visual analysis to estimate the former. Both methods are highly accurate if images of good quality are available. Regardless of which method is used, sensitivity, specificity, and accuracy for detection of angiographically proven stenosis are generally in the range of 90–100% [3, 4, 19–21] with MRA and CTA.

In patients with known stents or metal implants, image quality may be degraded with both MRA and CTA. For pMRA examinations are especially important that the requesting physicians note this on the study request in order to avoid false impression of stenosis. An example of stent artifacts is shown in Fig. 20.6.

Key Point

- Both MRA and CTA have high diagnostic accuracy for detection of location and extent of atherosclerotic narrowing.

20.5.2 Aneurysmal Disease

Aneurysm is defined as a focal enlargement of an artery to more than 1.5 times its normal diameter. For the aorta the general cutoff value that warrants follow-up is 3.0 cm and for the iliac arteries 1.8 cm. Measurements of aneurysms should always be performed perpendicular to the center lumen line and should include any mural thrombus as well as the arterial wall (Fig. 20.7). *True aneurysms* involve the intima, media, and adventitial layers of the vessel. Aneurysm is categorized as *false* when fewer than three layers are involved.

20.5.3 Non-atherosclerotic Peripheral Arterial Occlusive Disease

Although atherosclerosis is by far the most common cause of PAD, there are other causes as well. Any disease process that leads to narrowing or occlusion of peripheral arteries may lead to the typical history and complaints of IC or CCI. Non-atherosclerotic causes of PAD should be considered in young patients or patients without typical risk factors. Depending on the underlying disease process, involvement of specific anatomic sites or characteristic angiographic findings may be seen.

Key Point

- Both MRA and CTA can help identify non-atherosclerotic causes of peripheral arterial disease. These modalities are the technique of choice in patients with incongruencies between symptoms and risk factors for atherosclerotic peripheral arterial disease.

20.5.3.1 Vasculitis

Vasculitis refers to the process of acute or chronic inflammatory changes of small, medium, or large arteries as well as veins. In addition to signs of vascular narrowing or occlusion, patients typically present with systemic signs such as fever,

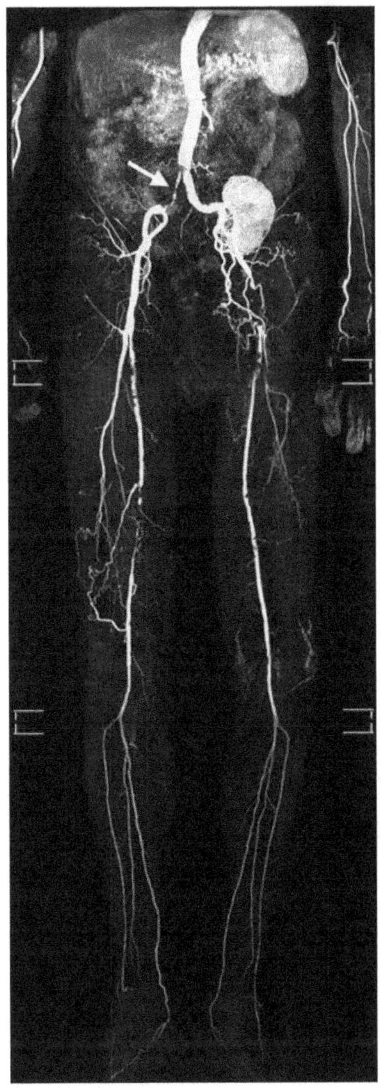

Fig. 20.6 There is signal loss in the right common iliac artery due to the presence of a stainless steel stent (arrow). Artifacts can be recognized by abrupt caliber change of arterial lumen. In this patient it is not possible to assess the degree of stenosis with certainty due to the signal loss

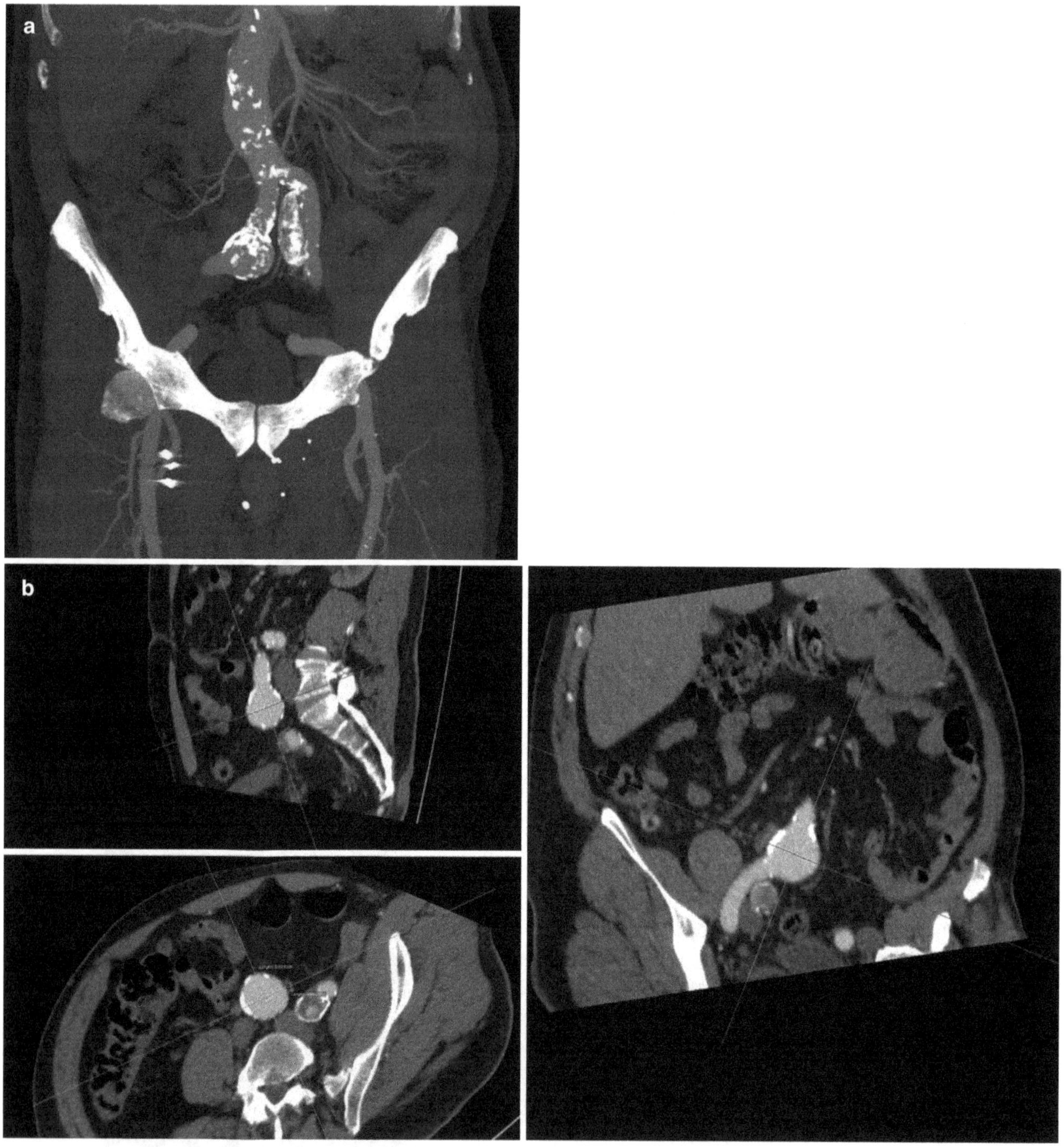

Fig. 20.7 Partial volume maximum intensity projection of bilateral common iliac artery aneurysms in a 68-year-old male (**a**). Diameter measurements of aneurysms should always be performed perpendicular to the center lumen line to avoid over- or underestimation of aneurysm diameters (**b**)

malaise, weight loss, and abnormal laboratory tests such high erythrocyte sedimentation rate (ESR), C-reactive protein (CRP), as well as leukocytosis with granulocytosis, thrombocytosis, and normochromic/normocytic anemia. The latter reflect the acute phase response. It is important to understand that there are no universally accepted diagnostic criteria for large-vessel vasculitides, including giant cell arteritis and Takayasu arteritis. More information about the diagnostic aspects can be found in the excellent review by Keser and Aksu [22]. Both CTA and MRA can suggest the diagnosis of vasculitis, but nowadays whole-body PET imaging is often used in the diagnostic workup. There is a large list of inflammatory arteriopathies that may lead to symptoms of PAD. Below, we discuss the commonly encountered diseases.

20.5.3.2 Takayasu Arteritis

Takayasu arteritis (TA) is a large vessel vasculitis that may affect the aorta, its main branches, as well as the upper extremities. Occasionally, the iliac arteries are involved. The disease mainly affects younger women and can go unrecognized for a prolonged period due to its relatively low prevalence. Besides the typical history of vague, non-specific complaints, TA is characterized by a specific morphological pattern of arterial narrowing; stenoses typically have an elongated "hourglass" aspect (Fig. 20.8). This is in contrast to the more serrated and

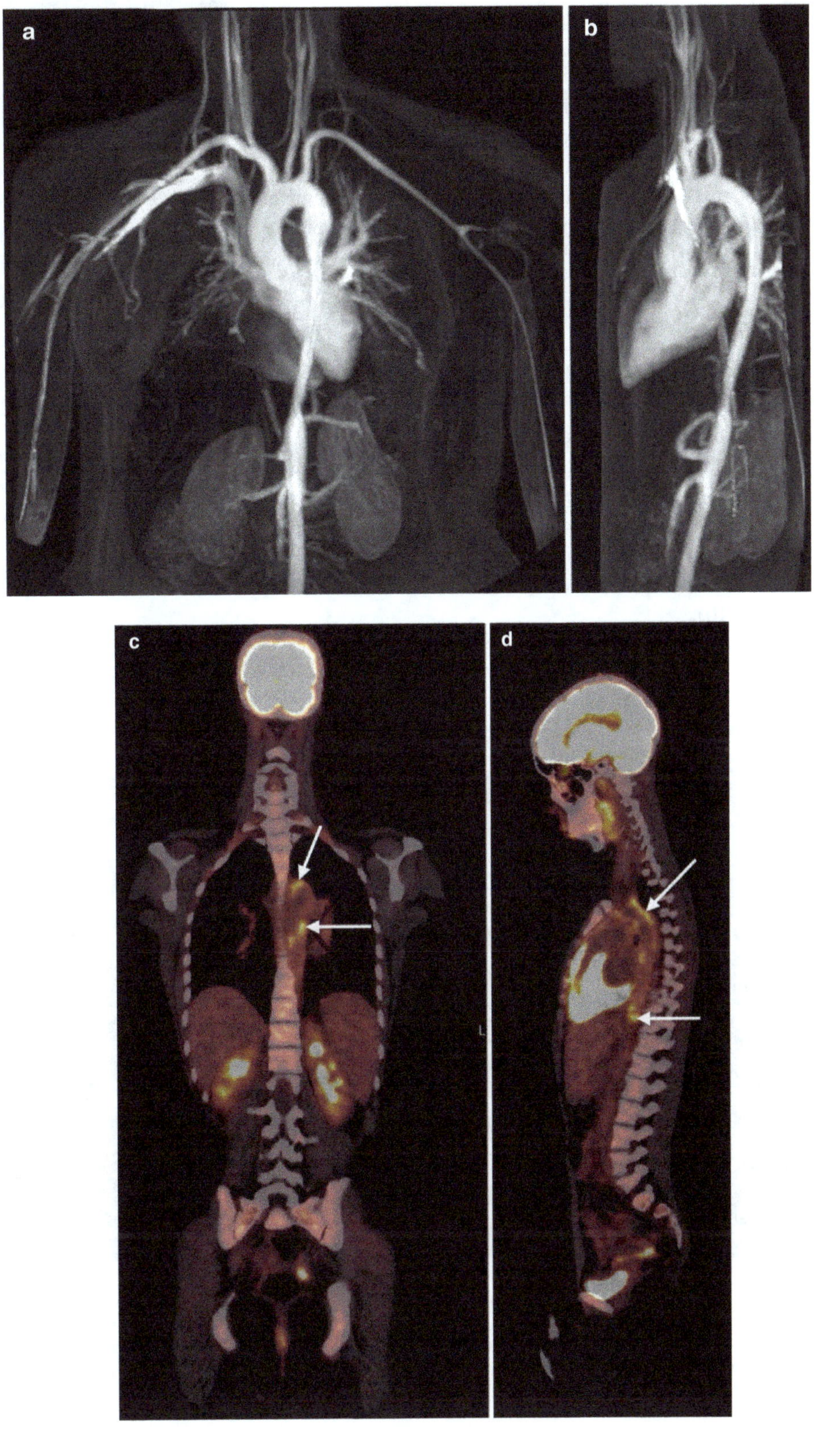

Fig. 20.8 Coronal (**a**) and sagittal (**b**) maximum intensity projections of thoracic MR angiogram show typical smooth elongated "hour-glass" narrowing of the descending thoracic aorta in a 22-year-old female patient with Takayasu disease. PET scanning confirmed active disease in the narrowed segment (**c** and **d**)

abrupt appearance of atherosclerotic stenoses. Both MRA and CTA are excellent diagnostic tools for diagnosis of TA [23].

20.5.3.3 Thromboangiitis Obliterans

Thromboangiitis obliterans (TAO) is an uncommon segmental inflammatory arteriopathy that affects medium- and small-sized arteries, veins, and nerves of the arms and legs. The typical clinical scenario is that of a young male heavy smoker [24]. The main differential diagnosis in case of distal lower extremity involvement is atherosclerotic PAD in diabetes mellitus. However, the presence of diabetes rules out the diagnosis of TAO. Angiographically, TAO is characterized by short segmental occlusions of arteries or veins by inflammatory thrombi. Often, these occlusions are bridged by corkscrew collaterals. This is known as *Martorell's* sign (Fig. 20.9).

20.5.3.4 Fibromuscular Dysplasia

Fibromuscular dysplasia (FMD) is a noninflammatory arteriopathy that usually affects the medium-sized arteries such as the renal, carotid, and iliac arteries in young Caucasian women. Several subtypes are distinguished [25]. The characteristic angiographic appearance is the so-called string of beads which refers to the presence of multiple stenoses interspersed with aneurysmal dilatations (Fig. 20.10).

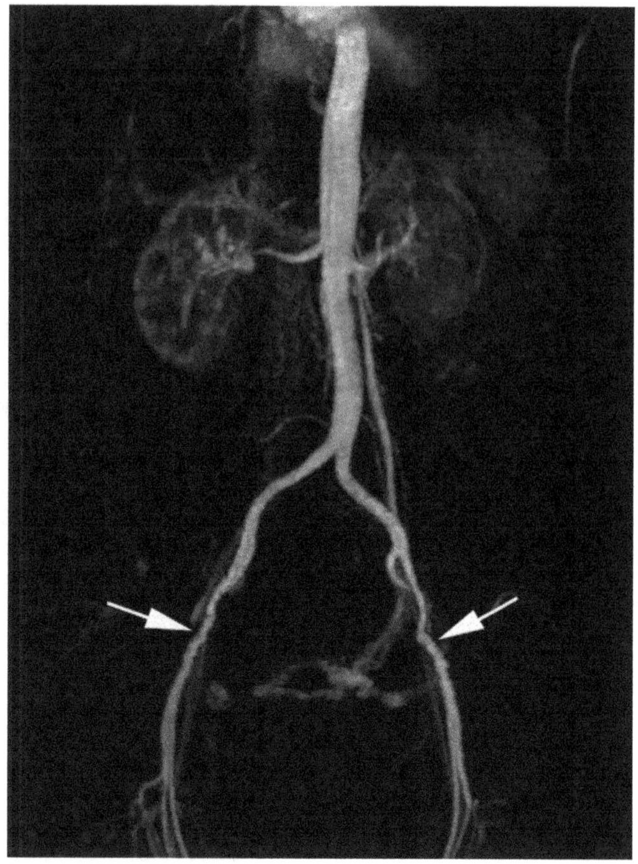

Fig. 20.10 A 37-year-old female patient with bilateral intermittent claudication. In both external iliac arteries, typical "string-of-beads" arterial narrowing can be seen (arrows). This finding is highly suggestive of fibromuscular dysplasia

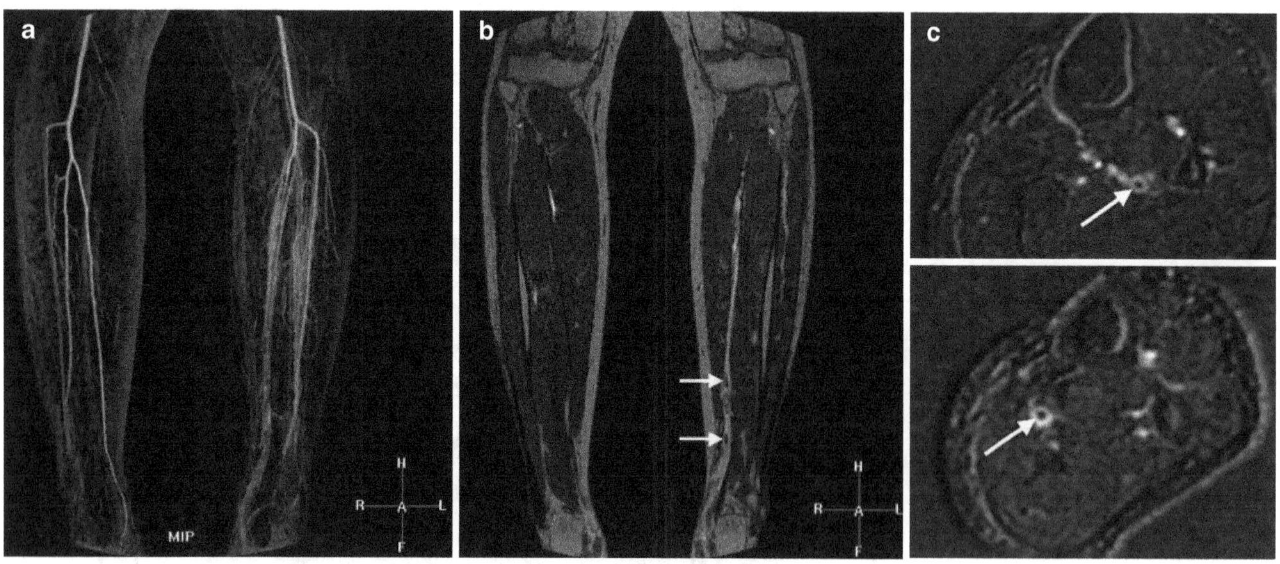

Fig. 20.9 MR angiogram of a 29-year-old male patient with symptoms of critical ischemia in the left lower leg. The patient was a heavy smoker. Left panel (**a**) shows maximum intensity projection with impression of distal lower leg arterial occlusion and moderate to severe venous enhancement. Source images (**b**) show multiple thrombi in posterior tibial artery (arrows). Transverse multiplanar reconstructions at two different levels (**c**) show arterial thombi in posterior tibial and fibular arteries (arrows). *Image courtesy of Roland Bezooijen, MD PhD, Medisch Spectrum Twente, Enschede, The Netherlands*

20.5.3.5 Popliteal Entrapment

Popliteal artery entrapment refers to abnormalities of the popliteal fossa anatomy, whereby the popliteal artery is displaced medially by the medial head of the gastrocnemius muscle or when it courses anterior to the popliteus muscle [26]. The popliteal artery can be dynamically compressed when the gastrocnemius muscle is actively used. There are four types of popliteal entrapment that may be encountered. Types I–III refer to various degrees of medial displacement by the medial head of the gastrocnemius muscle, and in type IV, both the popliteal artery and vein course anterior to the popliteus muscle. Because the diagnosis of popliteal entrapment relies on precise anatomical knowledge of the popliteal fossa, it is necessary to supplement the MR angiography acquisition with high spatial resolution T2-TSE anatomical images of the popliteal fossa to visualize the relationship between the muscles and the vascular structures (Fig. 20.11).

20.5.3.6 Cystic Adventitial Disease

Another non-atherosclerotic cause of PAD is cystic adventitial disease (CAD). In CAD, a mucoid cyst develops in the arterial wall which can lead to compression of the lumen and symptoms of PAD. The disease leads to smooth arterial narrowing of the affected artery. The cyst can easily be diagnosed by ultrasonography, CT, or MRI (Fig. 20.12), although MRI is the technique of choice in case of suspected CAD due to its ability to definitively identify the mucoid cystic source of the arterial narrowing. Although infrequently encountered, treatment consists of simple percutaneous aspiration of the mucoid material which results in immediate relief of symptoms [27].

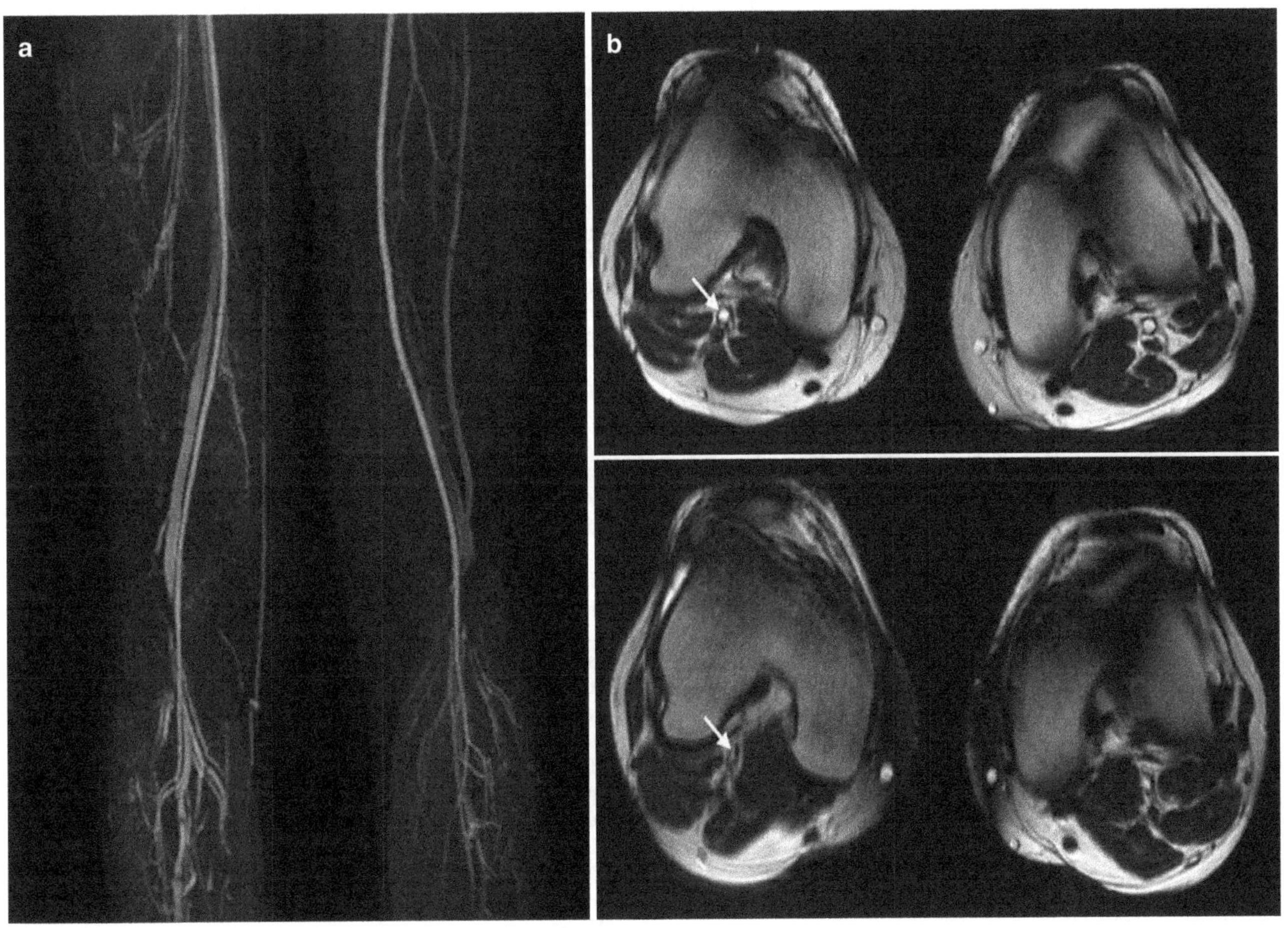

Fig. 20.11 A 39-year-old male patient with complaints of intermittent claudication of the right leg. MR angiogram in neutral position shows normal caliber of popliteal artery on both sides. Supplemental T2-TSE images in neutral position (left) and during plantar flexion (right) show dynamic compression of right popliteal artery (arrows) due to crowding of the right popliteal fossa. Note patent left popliteal artery at rest and during plantar flexion

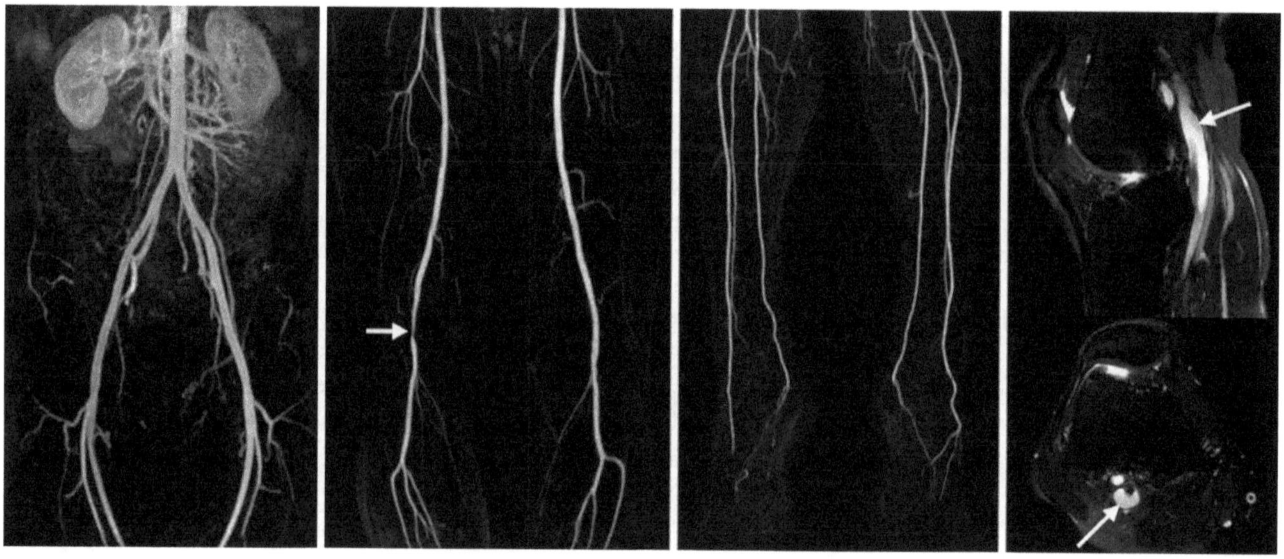

Fig. 20.12 A 41-year-old male patient with intermittent claudication of the right leg. MR angiogram shows smooth luminal narrowing of the right popliteal artery. The age of the patient in combination with the aspect of the stenosis is highly suggestive for non-atherosclerotic peripheral arterial disease. Presence of arterial wall cyst is confirmed on fat-suppressed T2-weighted images (arrows)

Take-Home Messages

- MRA and CTA are highly reliable modalities to noninvasively depict the entire peripheral vascular tree.
- Knowledge about the technical background of both MRA and CTA is helpful to obtain the best possible results with each modality.
- MRA and CTA accurately depict the location and severity of atherosclerotic arterial obstruction.
- Noninvasive imaging of the peripheral arteries can help elucidate the cause of symptoms in symptomatic patients with low likelihood of atherosclerotic peripheral arterial disease.

References

1. Norgren L, Hiatt WR, Dormandy JA, Nehler MR, Harris KA, Fowkes FG, TASC II Working Group. Inter-society consensus for the management of peripheral arterial disease (TASC II). J Vasc Surg. 2007;45(Suppl 1):S5–67.
2. Hardman RL, Jazaeri O, Yi J, Smith M, Gupta R. Overview of classification systems in peripheral artery disease. Semin Interv Radiol. 2014;31:378–88.
3. Nelemans PJ, Leiner T, de Vet HC, van Engelshoven JM. Peripheral arterial disease: meta-analysis of the diagnostic performance of MR angiography. Radiology. 2000;217:105–14.
4. Menke J, Larsen J. Meta-analysis: accuracy of contrast-enhanced magnetic resonance angiography for assessing steno-occlusions in peripheral arterial disease. Ann Intern Med. 2010;153:325–34.
5. Leiner T, Ho KY, Nelemans PJ, de Haan MW, van Engelshoven JM. Three-dimensional contrast-enhanced moving-bed infusion-tracking (MoBI-track) peripheral MR angiography with flexible choice of imaging parameters for each field of view. J Magn Reson Imaging. 2000;11:368–77.
6. Leiner T, Habets J, Versluis B, Geerts L, Alberts E, Blanken N, Hendrikse J, Vonken EJ, Eggers H. Subtractionless first-pass single contrast medium dose peripheral MR angiography using two-point Dixon fat suppression. Eur Radiol. 2013;23:2228–35.
7. Lim RP, Koktzoglou I. Noncontrast magnetic resonance angiography: concepts and clinical applications. Radiol Clin N Am. 2015;53:457–76.
8. Amin P, Collins JD, Koktzoglou I, Molvar C, Markl M, Edelman RR, Carr JC. Evaluating peripheral arterial disease with unenhanced quiescent-interval single-shot MR angiography at 3 T. AJR Am J Roentgenol. 2014;202:886–93.
9. Mahesh M, Cody DD. Physics of cardiac imaging with multiple-row detector CT. Radiographics. 2007;27:1495–509.
10. Mettler FA, Wiest PW, Locken JA, Kelsey CA. CT scanning: patterns of use and dose. J Radiol Prot. 2000;20:353–9.
11. Fraioli F, Catalano C, Napoli A, et al. Low-dose multidetector-row CT angiography of the infra-renal aorta and lower extremity vessels: image quality and diagnostic accuracy in comparison with standard DSA. Eur Radiol. 2006;16:137–46.
12. Bae KT. Peak contrast enhancement in CT and MR angiography: when does it occur and why? Pharmacokinetic study in a porcine model. Radiology. 2003;227:809–16.
13. Bae KT, Tran HQ, Heiken JP. Uniform vascular contrast enhancement and reduced contrast medium volume achieved by using exponentially decelerated contrast material injection method. Radiology. 2004;231:732–6.
14. Fleischmann D. Use of high concentration contrast media: principles and rationale-vascular district. Eur J Radiol. 2003;45(Suppl 1):S88–93.
15. Fleischmann D, Rubin GD. Quantification of intravenously administered contrast medium transit through the peripheral arteries: implications for CT angiography. Radiology. 2005;236:1076–82.
16. Fleischmann D, Hallett RL, Rubin GD. CT angiography of peripheral arterial disease. J Vasc Interv Radiol. 2006;17:3–26.
17. Kau T, et al. Dual-energy CT angiography in peripheral arterial occlusive disease—accuracy of maximum intensity projections in clinical routine and subgroup analysis. Eur Radiol. 2011;21:1677–86.

18. Sommer WH, et al. Diagnostic accuracy of dynamic computed tomographic angiographic of the lower leg in patients with critical limb ischemia. Investig Radiol. 2012;47:325–31.
19. Heijenbrok-Kal MH, Kock MC, Hunink MG. Lower extremity arterial disease: multidetector CT angiography meta-analysis. Radiology. 2007;245:433–9.
20. Met R, Bipat S, Legemate DA, Reekers JA, Koelemay MJ. Diagnostic performance of computed tomography angiography in peripheral arterial disease: a systematic review and meta-analysis. JAMA. 2009;301:415–24.
21. Jens S, Koelemay MJ, Reekers JA, Bipat S. Diagnostic performance of computed tomography angiography and contrast-enhanced magnetic resonance angiography in patients with critical limb ischaemia and intermittent claudication: systematic review and meta-analysis. Eur Radiol. 2013;23:3104–14.
22. Keser G, Aksu K. Diagnosis and differential diagnosis of large-vessel vasculitides. Rheumatol Int. 2018. doi: https://doi.org/10.1007/s00296-018-4157-3.
23. Barra L, Kanji T, Malette J, Pagnoux C. CanVasc. Imaging modalities for the diagnosis and disease activity assessment of takayasu's arteritis: a systematic review and meta-analysis. Autoimmun Rev. 2018;17:175–87.
24. Rivera-Chavarría IJ, Brenes-Gutiérrez JD. Thromboangiitis obliterans (Buerger's disease). Ann Med Surg (Lond). 2016;7:79–82.
25. Narula N, Kadian-Dodov D, Olin JW. Fibromuscular dysplasia: contemporary concepts and future directions. Prog Cardiovasc Dis. 2018;60:580–5.
26. Lejay A, Ohana M, Lee JT, Georg Y, Delay C, Lucereau B, Thaveau F, Gaertner S, Chakfé N, Groupe Européen de Recherche sur les Prothèses Appliquées à la Chirurgie Vasculaire (GEPROVAS). Popliteal artery entrapment syndrome. J Cardiovasc Surg. 2014;55:225–37.
27. Li S, King BN, Velasco N, Kumar Y, Gupta N. Cystic adventitial disease-case series and review of literature. Ann Transl Med. 2017;5:327.
28. Fontaine R, Kim M, Kieny R. Surgical treatment of peripheral circulation disorders [in German]. Helv Chir Acta. 1954;21:499–533.
29. Rutherford RB, Flanigan DP, Gupta SK, et al. Suggested standards for reports dealing with lower extremity ischemia. J Vasc Surg. 1986;4:80–94.
30. Rutherford RB, Baker JD, Ernst C, et al. Recommended standards for reports dealing with lower extremity ischemia: revised version. J Vasc Surg. 1997;26:517–38.

Permissions

All chapters in this book were first published in DCBHV, by Springer; hereby published with permission under the Creative Commons Attribution License or equivalent. Every chapter published in this book has been scrutinized by our experts. Their significance has been extensively debated. The topics covered herein carry significant findings which will fuel the growth of the discipline. They may even be implemented as practical applications or may be referred to as a beginning point for another development.

The contributors of this book come from diverse backgrounds, making this book a truly international effort. This book will bring forth new frontiers with its revolutionizing research information and detailed analysis of the nascent developments around the world.

We would like to thank all the contributing authors for lending their expertise to make the book truly unique. They have played a crucial role in the development of this book. Without their invaluable contributions this book wouldn't have been possible. They have made vital efforts to compile up to date information on the varied aspects of this subject to make this book a valuable addition to the collection of many professionals and students.

This book was conceptualized with the vision of imparting up-to-date information and advanced data in this field. To ensure the same, a matchless editorial board was set up. Every individual on the board went through rigorous rounds of assessment to prove their worth. After which they invested a large part of their time researching and compiling the most relevant data for our readers.

The editorial board has been involved in producing this book since its inception. They have spent rigorous hours researching and exploring the diverse topics which have resulted in the successful publishing of this book. They have passed on their knowledge of decades through this book. To expedite this challenging task, the publisher supported the team at every step. A small team of assistant editors was also appointed to further simplify the editing procedure and attain best results for the readers.

Apart from the editorial board, the designing team has also invested a significant amount of their time in understanding the subject and creating the most relevant covers. They scrutinized every image to scout for the most suitable representation of the subject and create an appropriate cover for the book.

The publishing team has been an ardent support to the editorial, designing and production team. Their endless efforts to recruit the best for this project, has resulted in the accomplishment of this book. They are a veteran in the field of academics and their pool of knowledge is as vast as their experience in printing. Their expertise and guidance has proved useful at every step. Their uncompromising quality standards have made this book an exceptional effort. Their encouragement from time to time has been an inspiration for everyone.

The publisher and the editorial board hope that this book will prove to be a valuable piece of knowledge for researchers, students, practitioners and scholars across the globe.

List of Contributors

Jeffrey S. Klein
Department of Radiology, University of Vermont College of Medicine, Burlington, VT, USA

Melissa L. Rosado-de-Christenson
Department of Radiology, Saint Luke's Hospital of Kansas City, Kansas City, MO, USA
Department of Radiology, University of Missouri-Kansas City, Kansas City, MO, USA

Denis Tack
Department of Radiology, Epicura, Ath, Belgium

Nigel Howarth
Institut de Radiologie, Clinique des Grangettes, Genève, Switzerland

Sanjeev Bhalla
Mallinckrodt Institute of Radiology, Washington University, Saint Louis, MO, USA

Edith Marom
Radiology Department, The Chaim Sheba Medical Center, Tel Aviv University, Ramat Gan, Israel

Sujal R. Desai
Royal Brompton Hospital, London, UK

Helmut Prosch
Department of Biomedical Imaging and Image-guided Therapy, Medical University of Vienna, Vienna, Austria

Jeffrey R. Galvin
University of Maryland, Silver Spring, MD, USA

Gerald F. Abbott
Thoracic Imaging FND-202, Massachusetts General Hospital, Boston, MA, USA
St George's Medical School, University of London, London, UK

Ioannis Vlahos
Department of Radiology, St. George's Hospital and NHS Trust, St George's Medical School, University of London, London, UK

Philippe A. Grenier
Department Radiology, Sorbonne Université - Hôpital Pitié-Salpêtrière, Paris, France

Jeffrey P. Kanne
Department of Radiology, University of Wisconsin School of Medicine and Public Health, Madison, WI, USA

Tomás Franquet
Department of Radiology, Hospital de Sant Pau. Universidad Autonoma de Barcelona, Barcelona, Spain

Johnathan H. Chung
Department of Radiology, The University of Chicago Medicine, Chicago, IL, USA

Brett W. Carter and Jeremy J. Erasmus
Department of Diagnostic Radiology, The University of Texas MD Anderson Cancer Center, Houston, TX, USA

Aine M. Kelly
Department of Radiology, University of Michigan, Ann Arbor, MI, USA

Thomas Frauenfelder
Institute of diagnostic and interventional Radiology, University Hospital Zurich, Zurich, Switzerland

Alison Hart and Edward Y. Lee
Department of Radiology, Boston Children's Hospital and Harvard Medical School, Boston, MA, USA

Cornelia Schaefer-Prokop
Department of Radiology, Meander Medical Centre, Amersfoort, Netherlands
Department of Radiology, Radboud University, Nijmegen, Netherlands

Brett M. Elicker
Department of Radiology and Biomedical Imaging, University of California, San Francisco, CA, USA

Loren Ketai
Department of Radiology, University of New Mexico HSC, Albuquerque, NM, USA

Steven L. Primack
Department of Diagnostic Radiology, Oregon Health and Science University, Portland, OR, USA

Fiona J. Gilbert
Department of Radiology, School of Clinical Medicine, University of Cambridge, Cambridge, UK

Katja Pinker-Domenig
Department of Radiology, Breast Imaging Service, Memorial Sloan Kettering Cancer Center, New York, NY, USA

Ulrich Bick
Department of Radiology, Charité - Universitätsmedizin Berlin, Berlin, Germany

Thomas H. Helbich
Department of Biomedical Imaging and Image-guided Therapy, Division of Molecular and Gender Imaging, Medical University of Vienna, Vienna, Austria

Albert de Roos
Department of Radiology, Leiden University Medical Center, Leiden, South Holland, The Netherlands

Konstantin Nikolaou
Department of Diagnostic and Interventional Radiology, University Hospitals Tubingen, Tubingen, Germany

David A. Bluemke
Department of Radiology, University of Wisconsin School of Medicine and Public Health, Madison, WI, USA

Shawn D. Teague
Department of Radiology, National Jewish Health, University of Colorado School of Medicine, Denver, CO, USA

Alexander A. Bankier
Department of Radiology, Beth Israel Deaconess Medical Center, Harvard Medical School, Boston, MA, USA

Carole Dennie
Department of Medical Imaging, The Ottawa Hospital, University of Ottawa, Ottawa, ON, Canada

Thomas M. Grist
Department of Radiology, University of Wisconsin School of Medicine and Public Health, Madison, WI, USA

Geoffrey D. Rubin
Department of Radiology, Duke University School of Medicine, Durham, NC, USA

Thorsten Bley
Institut für Diagnostische und Interventionelle Radiologie, Universitätsklinikum Würzburg, Würzburg, Deutschland

Justus Roos
Radiologie und Nuklearmedizin, Institut für Radiologie und Nuklearmedizin, Luzerner Kantonsspital, Luzern, Switzerland

Tim Leiner
Department of Radiology, Utrecht University Medical Center, Utrecht, The Netherlands

James C. Carr
Department of Radiology, Northwestern Memorial Hospital, Chicago, IL, USA

Index

www.ingramcontent.com/pod-product-compliance
Lightning Source LLC
LaVergne TN
LVHW060529210926
848485LV00005B/1170
* 9 7 8 1 6 3 9 8 7 1 5 9 9 *